S0-CRS-920

NINTH SYMPOSIUM
ON ADVANCED MEDICINE

MEDCOM SYMPOSIUM SERIES

NINTH SYMPOSIUM ON ADVANCED MEDICINE

Proceedings of a Conference
held at the Royal College of Physicians of London
February 19-23, 1973

Edited by Geoffrey Walker, MD, MRCP

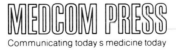

Communicating today s medicine today

© The Royal College of Physicians of London, 1973

Ninth Symposium on Advanced Medicine

First published 1973
by Pitman Medical Publishing Company
© The Royal College of Physicians of London, 1973
Reprinted by permission of Pitman Medical Publishing Company

MEDC⊕M®

World leader in multimedia medical education programs
2 Hammarskjöld Plaza
New York, New York 10017 (212) 832-1400

PRINTED IN THE UNITED STATES OF AMERICA

No part of this publication may be reproduced, stored in a retrieval system
or transmitted, in any form or by any means, electronic, mechanical,
photocopying, recording or otherwise, without the prior written permission
of the publisher.

ISBN 0-8463-0149-0

Editor's Foreword

The Ninth Symposium on Advanced Medicine, held at the Royal College of Physicians in February 1973, proved to be extremely popular and, like its predecessors, incorporated recent advances in various fields while maintaining a strict relevance to the practice of medicine. The participants found the interchange of ideas, both during the formal discussions after individual papers and, in particular, in the panel discussions at the end of each session, to be of great value.

I would like to convey my sincere thanks, on behalf of the College, to the Chairmen and Speakers who responded admirably to the spirit of the Symposium, and provided us with such enjoyable and stimulating material and ideas. We are also indebted to those who participated in the "Talking to the Experts" sessions which were again well received by all who took part.

I am also grateful to Dr Peter Ball, Assistant Registrar of the College, for his help, and to his secretary, Miss Ann Kimber for her invaluable assistance and calm efficiency.

At the end of the book an index to all previous volumes is included and I am indebted to last year's editor, Dr Graham Neale, whose work this largely reflects. I am sure this will prove of use to physicians wishing to refer back to the wide range of subjects covered over the past nine years.

Finally, it is my very great pleasure to thank Mrs Betty Dickens of Pitman Medical for her untiring and skilful efforts and advice which have enabled us to produce these Proceedings so soon after the actual conference that it constitutes an all-time record.

Participants

CHAIRMEN

E G L Bywaters
MD, FRCP

Professor of Rheumatology, Royal Postgraduate Medical School, Hammersmith Hospital, London. Director, MRC Rheumatism Unit, Taplow, Bucks

C A Clarke
CBE, MD, PRCP, FRS

President of the Royal College of Physicians

A Goldberg
DSc, MD, FRCP (Glas., Ed. and Lond), FRSE

Regius Professor of Materia Medica, University of Glasgow, Stobhill General Hospital, Glasgow

D G Grahame-Smith
MB, PhD, FRCP

Rhodes Professor of Clinical Pharmacology, Radcliffe Infirmary, Oxford

M S Losowsky
MD, FRCP

Professor of Medicine, St James's Hospital, Leeds

A Stuart Mason
MD, FRCP

Consultant Endocrinologist, The London Hospital, London

J G Scadding
MD, FRCP

Emeritus Professor of Medicine, University of London

SPEAKERS

Surgeon Commander
D M Ackery,
Royal Navy,
MA, MB, MSc

Honorary Consultant in Nuclear Medicine, Southampton University Hospitals

A W Asscher
MD, BSc, FRCP

Reader in Medicine, KRUF Institute of Renal Disease, Welsh National School of Medicine, Royal Infirmary, Cardiff

A G Bearn
MD, FRCP

Chairman, Department of Medicine, New York Hospital—Cornell Medical Center, 525 East 68th Street, New York, NY 10021, USA

A J Bellingham
MB, MRCP

Senior Lecturer, Department of Clinical Haematology, University College Hospital Medical School, London

A Bennett
PhD

Senior Lecturer in Basic Science, King's College Hospital Medical School, London

S R Bloom,
MA, MB, MRCP

MRC Clinical Research Fellow, The Middlesex Hospital, London

C C Booth,
MD, FRCP

Professor of Medicine, Royal Postgraduate Medical School, Hammersmith Hospital, London

E D R Campbell,
FRCP

Consultant Physician, Department of Rheumatology, Royal Free Hospital, London

R D Catterall
FRCP (Ed.)

Director and Physician, Department of Venereology, James Pringle House, The Middlesex Hospital, London

I Chanarin,
MD, MCPath

Consultant Haematologist, Northwick Park Hospital, Harrow, Middlesex

T J H Clark,
MD, BSc, MRCP

Consultant Physician, Guy's and Brompton Hospitals, London

M E Conolly
MD, MRCP

Lecturer in Clinical Pharmacology, Royal Postgraduate Medical School, Hammersmith Hospital, London

Deborah Doniach
MD, FRCP

Reader in Immunopathology, The Middlesex Hospital Medical School, London

R H Dowling
MD, MRCP

Lecturer in Medicine and Consultant Physician, Royal Postgraduate Medical School, Hammersmith Hospital, London

P T Flute
MD, MCPath

Professor of Haematology, St George's Hospital, London

D L Gardner
MD, FRCP (Ed.)

Professor of Pathology, The Queen's University of Belfast, Belfast, UK

S Godfrey,
MD, PhD, MRCP

Senior Lecturer and Honorary Consultant Paediatrician, Cardiothoracic Institute, Brompton Hospital, London

D G Grahame-Smith
MB, PhD, FRCP

Rhodes Professor of Clinical Pharmacology, Radcliffe Infirmary, Oxford

W R Greig,
MD, PhD, FRCP
(Glas.) MRCP (Ed.)

Senior Lecturer in Medicine and Consultant Physician, University Department of Medicine, Royal Infirmary, Glasgow

R Hall,
BSc, MD, FRCP

Professor of Medicine, University of Newcastle upon Tyne, Newcastle upon Tyne

K W Heaton
MD, MRCP

Consultant Senior Lecturer in Medicine, Department of Medicine, Royal Infirmary, Bristol, 2

G R V Hughes,
MB, MRCP

Senior Registrar and Clinical Tutor in Medicine, Royal Postgraduate Medical School, Hammersmith Hospital, London

J M B Hughes,
MB, MRCP

Lecturer in Medicine and Radiology, Royal Postgraduate Medical School, Hammersmith Hospital, London

P Hugh-Jones
MD, FRCP

Consultant Physician and Director, Chest Unit, King's College Hospital, London

P Isaac
MB, MRCP

Member of the MRC Clinical Pharmacology Unit, Radcliffe Infirmary, Oxford

R J Jarrett
MA, MD, MFCM

Lecturer, Departments of Medicine and Community Medicine, Guy's Hospital, London

M Lader
BSc, PhD, MD

Honorary Senior Lecturer, Institute of Psychiatry, The Maudsley Hospital, London

J Landon,
MD, MRCP

Professor of Chemical Pathology, St Bartholomew's Hospital, London

A G E Pearse,
MA, MD, FRCP,
FRCPath

Professor of Histochemistry, Royal Postgraduate Medical School, Hammersmith Hospital, London

I M Roitt
DSc, MRCPath

Professor of Immunology, The Middlesex Hospital Medical School, London

G A Rose,
DM, FRCP, FFCM

Professor of Epidemiology and Preventive Medicine, St Mary's Hospital Medical School, London

G M Sterling
MD, MRCP

Senior Lecturer in Medicine, Southampton University Hospitals, Southampton

D J Weatherall
MD, FRCP, MRCPath

Professor of Haematology, The University of Liverpool, Liverpool

N J Y Woodhouse
MRCP, MB

Lecturer, Department of Medicine, King's College Hospital, London

Eleanor Zaimis
MD, MRCP

Professor of Pharmacology, Royal Free Hospital Medical School, London

Contents

PART I

THYROID DISEASE
Chairman: Dr A Stuart Mason

Present Status of *In Vitro* Tests of Thyroid Function

J LANDON, G M BESSER, VIVIAN CHAN, D GOLDIE

INTRODUCTION

The problem of assessing thyroid function is of importance to physicians in a wide range of specialities and also to clinical chemists and physicists. This is partly because thyroid abnormalities are among the most common endocrine disorders, and partly because of the need to diagnose and treat thyroid dysfunction early, before it has caused gross clinical manifestations. Thus the clinician requires access to a range of thyroid function tests to enable him to confirm his clinical suspicions in patients presenting with features suggestive of thyroid dysfunction; to screen subjects at risk, such as patients with various types of autoimmune disease or who have had thyroid surgery; to differentiate between primary and secondary hypothyroidism and to assess the effectiveness of therapy. Diagnostic techniques are better developed and more widely available than ever before but the multiplicity of such procedures is in itself confusing. An additional problem is the different range of values quoted by various authors, due to lack of universal standards and the variety of analytical techniques employed.

The purpose of this paper is to present an account of the in vitro tests most commonly employed in the United Kingdom to assess thyroid function. In order to facilitate understanding of these tests, it is first necessary to summarise some facts concerning the physiology and pathophysiology of the hypothalamic-pituitary-thyroid axis.

PHYSIOLOGICAL CONSIDERATIONS

It is now nearly fifty years since Harrington (1926) elucidated the chemical structure of thyroxine (T4). Since then, the complex sequence of reactions involved in the synthesis of T4 within the thyroid gland has been determined. It has also been shown that, following its release, the great majority circulates bound to various proteins including thyroxine-binding globulin (TBG), thyroxine-binding prealbumin (TBPA) and albumin. Indeed, only some 0.05% of the circulating T4 is in what is considered to be the physiologically active,

3

unbound (free) form. More recently, Gross and Pitt-Rivers (1952) identified the more potent thyroid hormone, tri-iodothyronine (T3). This circulates bound to TBG and albumin (but not TBPA) with about 0.5% of its molecules in the free form. There is now extensive evidence that T3 is derived partly from the thyroid and partly from peripheral monodeiodination of T4 (Pitt-Rivers et al, 1955; Sterling et al, 1970).

The reaction between the thyroid hormones and circulating binding proteins is reversible (Robbins & Rall, 1957) and governed by the Law of Mass Action. Many of the problems which arise in the in vitro assessment of thyroid function are due to the fact that most of the T3 and T4 circulates in a bound form, while only the relatively minute free fractions are thought to be involved in feedback control and metabolic activity. Thus, measurements of total T3 and T4 determine predominantly the bound hormones and factors that influence binding (including medication with phenytoin and salicylates) may transiently raise the circulating concentration of the free hormones, without this being apparent. Conversely, total levels of T3 and T4, but not necessarily their free fractions, are markedly influenced by the concentration of the thyroid-binding proteins. For example, a subject may have normal free hormone levels and, therefore, be euthyroid, despite having low total T3 and T4 values (when thyroid-binding protein concentrations are decreased, as in protein deficiency states, severe illness, hepatic dysfunction or following the administration of androgens) or high values (when thyroid-binding protein concentrations are raised, as in pregnancy or during oestrogen administration.

Thyroid function is controlled by the anterior pituitary glycoprotein, thyroid stimulating hormone (TSH), which stimulates virtually all steps of thyroid hormone biosynthesis. Two physiological control systems have been demonstrated:

(a) a negative feedback mechanism, whereby the concentration of free T3 influences the anterior pituitary thyrotroph cells directly, to inhibit the release of TSH, and (b) a neurohormonal mechanism, whereby a hypothalamic hormone, the tripeptide thyrotrophin-releasing hormone (TRH), reaches the anterior pituitary via the hypothalamic-hypophyseal portal circulation, and stimulates the release of TSH.

PATHOPHYSIOLOGY

THYROID OVERACTIVITY

It seems likely that this is often due to the presence of abnormal thyroid stimulators of autoimmune origin, produced by thymic and lymphoid cells. This is the subject of a later paper by Dr Doniach. Occasionally hyperthyroidism may result from the autonomous oversecretion of thyroid hormones by a thyroid tumour. Circulating levels of both total and free T3 and

T4 are usually raised, while TSH levels are low (due to suppression of its release via the negative feedback system). Recently a new form of hyperthyroidism, T3-thyrotoxicosis, has been described (Hollander et al, 1969; Sterling et al, 1970) and is due to the selective hypersecretion of tri-iodothyronine. These patients may have normal or even low levels of total T4 although, of course, their levels of both total and free T3 are markedly elevated.

THYROID UNDERACTIVITY

Hypothyroidism may be primary (as a result of autoimmune disease, thyroidectomy, or impaired thyroid hormone synthesis) or secondary to pituitary or hypothalamic dysfunction. All types are associated with low total and free thyroid hormone levels. However, circulating TSH values are markedly elevated in primary hypothyroidism but low or undetectable in the secondary group.

GENERAL COMMENTS CONCERNING IN VITRO THYROID FUNCTION TESTS

It will be apparent from the above, and from Table I, that no problems would arise in the diagnosis of thyroid function if there were available simple, inexpensive assays of adequate sensitivity to determine basal circulating levels of TRH, TSH, autoimmune thyroid stimulators and free T3 and T4.

Table I. Results of ideal in vitro thyroid function
tests in thyroid disorders

	TSH	Autoimmune Thyroid Stimulators	Free T3	Free T4
Thyroid Overactivity				
Thyrotoxicosis	Low	High	High	High
T3-thyrotoxicosis	Low	High	Very High	Normal or high
Due to a thyroid neoplasm	Low	U.D.*	High	High
Thyroid Underactivity				
Primary	Very high	U.D.	Low	Low
Secondary to pituitary or hypothalamic dysfunction	Low	U.D.	Low	Low
* U.D. = undetectable				

Unfortunately, available assays for free T3 and T4 involve dialysis or ultracentrifugation, and are too complex for routine application; circulating levels of the autoimmune thyroid stimulators can be determined only by difficult and time-consuming bioassays; and there is no assay for TRH (to help differentiate between the hypothalamic and pituitary causes of hypothyroidism) which is sufficiently sensitive to cope with the marked dilution that follows drainage of blood from the hypothalamic-hypophyseal portal circulation into the systemic circulation. Satisfactory radioimmunoassays have, however, been developed for TSH although, at present, they are available in only a few centres.

Table II. In vitro tests of pituitary-thyroid function

Name of Test	Abbreviation	Normal Range*
A. To assess hypothalamic-pituitary function		
Radioimmunoassay of circulating TSH	TSH (RIA)	< 0.4 - 3.0 μU/ml +
B. To determine total circulating levels of thyroid hormones		
(a) Chemical - Protein bound iodine	PBI	4 - 8 μg/100 ml
(b) Isotopic - Thyroxine by competitive protein binding	T4 (CPBA)	4.5 - 13.5 μg/100 ml
- Tri-iodothyronine by radioimmunoassay	T3 (RIA)	90 - 180 ng/100 ml
C. To assess the degree of saturation of the thyroid-hormone binding proteins		
Thyroid hormone binding test (Thyopac 3)	THBT	95 - 120%
D. To assess, indirectly, circulating levels of free T3 and T4		
Free thyroxine index	FT4I	4 - 8
Effective thyroxine ratio	ETR	**
Urinary thyroxine excretion	Urinary T4 (CPBA)	4.5 - 13.5 μg/24 hr
Urinary tri-iodothyronine excretion	Urinary T3 (RIA)	2 - 4.5 μg/24 hr +

* The normal range will vary depending on the analytical procedures and standards used – thus, it should be determined by each laboratory providing a thyroid service.

** Not yet performed in our laboratory.

\+ Results vary greatly depending on the antiserum used.

The assays most commonly employed in this country, to assess hypo-thalamic-pituitary-thyroid function, are listed in Table II. In addition to radioimmunoassays for TSH, they comprise procedures designed to determine circulating levels of total T3 and T4, either by chemical or isotopic means; techniques to assess the degree of saturation of the thyroid-hormone binding proteins; and several procedures to determine, indirectly, circulating levels of the free thyroid hormones. Confusion often arises because of the different names and abbreviations used for these tests. In 1971, the American Thyroid Association proposed a new nomenclature (Solomon et al, 1972), in which the chemical species being measured and the method employed are both clearly stated. Thus, for radioimmunoassays of tri-iodothyronine, the chemical form is stated first, followed by the method in parenthesis; T3 (RIA). In many people's view, their nomenclature requires slight modification. For example, use of the term T3 uptake for procedures designed to assess the degree of saturation of the binding-proteins, may be mistaken as the neck-uptake of ^{131}I-T3 or it may lead the inexperienced clinician into thinking that the results indicate the circulating levels of T3. For these reasons, we prefer the simpler and more informative name, 'thyroid hormone binding test'; THBT (Table II).

6

Another problem is the different range of values obtained by different laboratories, due to such factors as the variety of assay procedures available for many of these determinations; a lack of International Reference Standards; and, at present, the absence of a National Quality Control Service of the type that has proved so valuable for more routine clinical assays. It is essential, therefore, for all laboratories providing an in vitro thyroid service to establish their own normal ranges and system of quality control. There are also advantages in attempting to organise such services on an Area and Regional basis and to limit the analytical procedures employed in this country, in order to facilitate the interpretation of data from different hospitals.

INDIVIDUAL IN VITRO THYROID FUNCTION TESTS

Every determination must be looked at with regard to its specificity, sensitivity, precision and accuracy; its practicality (cost, simplicity and the number of assays that can be performed in a working week) and the factors, other than thyroid dysfunction, that can influence the results obtained.

(A) TESTS DESIGNED TO ASSESS HYPOTHALAMIC-PITUITARY FUNCTION

Thyroid-stimulating hormone by radioimmunoassay - TSH (RIA)

Radioimmunoassays for TSH were introduced by Odell and his colleagues (1965) and by Utiger (1965). They have proved the single most valuable recent addition to the range of in vitro function tests, partly because TSH levels are not significantly influenced by factors outside the hypothalamic-pituitary-thyroid axis and partly because they rapidly reflect changes in the function of the axis (since the plasma clearance half-time for TSH is only 10 to 20 min as compared with several days for T4). The assay technique depends upon competition between endogenous hormone (or standards) and a fixed amount of ^{125}I-or ^{131}I-labelled TSH for a constant, limited number of binding sites on the antibodies contained in the serum of an animal (usually a rabbit) previously immunised with TSH. Our normal range, employing our own reagents, is less than 0.4 to 3.0 $\mu U/ml$. Patients with all forms of thyrotoxicosis or with secondary hypothyroidism have low levels (less than 0.4 $\mu U/ml$) whereas those with primary hypothyroidism have markedly elevated values.

The clinical value of basal TSH determinations and of their response to exogenous TRH, is considered in detail in the next paper, by Professor Hall. Nonetheless it seems worthwhile making two points concerning the assay of TSH in this general review. First, it is particularly important for a laboratory to establish its own normal range - results can vary considerably, depending on the antiserum used, because TSH shares a common α-subunit with luteinising hormone, follicle-stimulating hormone and human chorionic gonadotrophin, and antisera may or may not bind these other glycoproteins. Second, supplies of purified TSH and suitable antisera are in short supply and it is probably better, therefore, for many laboratories to send their samples for TSH assays to a few centres – at least, until good diagnostic kits become available.

(B) TESTS DESIGNED TO DETERMINE TOTAL CIRCULATING LEVELS OF THE THYROID HORMONES

Protein bound iodine (PBI)

Iodine comprises 65.3% of the T4 molecule and its measurement, by chemical means, provides an indirect assessment of the serum thyroid hormone concentration. Serum is pretreated, usually with an anion exchange resin, to remove inorganic iodide; the serum proteins are digested to release bound iodine; and the liberated iodine is then measured by its catalytic effect on the reduction of yellow ceric to colourless cerous ions by arsenious acid (Sandell & Kolthoff, 1937). The normal range varies slightly in different hospitals and, in our own, is 4 to 8 μg/100 ml.

There is no place for manual PBI methods now that more precise automated procedures are available, which enable several hundred determinations in a working week at low cost (25 p per assay) and with high precision ('between-assay' coefficient of variation approx. 3%). Results are influenced by many factors other than the thyroid status of the patient (Table III) and, in particular, by changes in circulating levels of the thyroid hormone binding proteins and by the presence of high concentrations of inorganic iodides due to the prior administration of drugs (such as enterovioform and various cough mixtures) or of contrast media. The assay of butanol extractable iodine (BEI) is more specific, because inorganic iodine and some other contaminating fractions are removed prior to assay. It is, however, more time-consuming and less precise than PBI determination, and is no longer employed in this country.

Total thyroxine by competitive protein binding-T4 (CPBA) - Thyopac 4

The direct measurement of circulating levels of total T4 was pioneered by Ekins (1960). The endogenous thyroid hormones are extracted from plasma or serum and assayed by competitive protein binding. This technique is similar to radioimmunoassay with the exception that thyroxine-binding globulins, rather than an antibody, are employed as the binding ligand. Our normal range, employing the Thyopac 4 kit marketed by the Radiochemical Centre, is 4.5 to 13.5 μg/100 ml.

As with the PBI, decreased values are found in patients with primary or secondary hypothyroidism and elevated values in patients with

8

Table III. Summary of some factors, other than thyroid status, that influence various in-vitro thyroid function tests

Test	Organic and inorganic iodides (and other halogens)	Heavy metals (gold, mercury in diuretics etc)	Drugs which compete for TBG binding sites	Drugs or situations that: Increase TBG (Oestrogen, Pregnancy, Genetic)	Decrease TBG (Androgens, Corticosteroids, Starvation, Genetic)	Severe Proteinuria
TSH (RIA)	Normal	Normal	Transient decrease then normal	Normal	Normal	Normal
PBI	High	Low	Low	High	Low	Low
T4 (CPBA)	Normal	Normal	Low	High	Low	Low
T3 (RIA)	Normal	Normal	Low	High	Low	Low
THBT (Thyopac 3)	Normal	Normal	High	High	Low	Low
FT4I	High if based on PBI	Low values if based on PBI	Normal	Normal	Normal	Normal
ETR	Normal	Normal	Normal	Normal	Normal	Normal
Urinary T4 (CPBA)	Normal	Normal	High	Normal	Normal	High
Urinary T3 (RIA)	Normal	Normal	High	Normal	Normal	High

thyrotoxicosis – except when this is due predominantly to T3. The test is also influenced by changes in the circulating levels of the thyroid-hormone binding proteins. However, it has the great advantage over the chemical assay that results are not affected by the presence in the sample of inorganic iodides or heavy metals.

Total tri-iodothyronine by radioimmunoassay - T3 (RIA)

Very recently antisera have been prepared against T3 by immunising animals with a T3-protein or synthetic poly-amino acid conjugate. This has enabled radioimmunoassays to be established for the hormone, suitable for use with unextracted samples. A compound such as 8-anilino-1-naph-thalene sulphonic acid must be added to the reaction system to displace T3 from its binding proteins and to stop the latter interfering with the assay (Chopra et al, 1972). The assay is subject to a variety of artefacts and suitable antisera are difficult to obtain. Consequently, the technique is available only in a few centres.

(C) TESTS DESIGNED TO ASSESS THE DEGREE OF SATURATION OF THE THYROID-HORMONE BINDING PROTEINS

Thyroid hormone binding test (THBT): Thyopac 3

In all tests of this type exogenous labelled hormone is incubated with a sample of the patient's plasma or serum, when it partitions between the bound and free fractions according to the number of unoccupied binding sites. This is then assessed by adsorbing the free fraction onto a secondary binding material such as the patient's red blood cells, an ion exchange resin or Sephadex.

In this country the Thyopac 3 kit, marketed by the Radiochemical Centre at Amersham, is most widely used and has the considerable advantages over other procedures that it is simple, quick and the results are not temperature or time dependent (Chan et al, 1972a). Its name, Thyopac 3, has the disadvantage that (by analogy with the Thyopac 4 kit) the inexperienced clinician may believe that it provides him with an index of circulating T3 levels. It should also be noted that, in contrast with other tests of this type, the fraction of ^{125}I-T3 bound to the thyroid hormone binding proteins is measured, rather than the free fraction adsorbed by the secondary binder, ie. the results are directly proportional to the concentration of unoccupied binding sites. Results are expressed as a ratio in terms of a reference serum and, in normal subjects, range from 95 to 120%. When there is an excess of endogenous thyroid hormones, as in thyrotoxicosis, the protein binding sites are relatively saturated and less of the added, labelled hormone is bound. Consequently fewer counts are obtained than normal and results are less than 95%. The reverse is found in hypothyroidism. This test is also affected by changes in concentration of the thyroid-hormone binding proteins. Thus an increase, as occurs in pregnancy or during administration of oestrogens, results in a rise in the number of available unoccupied binding sites and an increase in the radioactive counts obtained, with values in excess of 120%. Obviously a decrease in binding protein levels has the reverse effect, as do drugs (such as salicylates, phenytoin and phenylbutazone) which themselves occupy some of the binding sites.

(D) TESTS DESIGNED TO ASSESS, INDIRECTLY, CIRCULATING
     LEVELS OF FREE T3 AND T4

It has been stressed previously in this paper that only the free thyroid hormones in the circulation are thought to be physiologically active, and thus determine the thyroid status of the subject. The difficulty of assessing free hormone levels directly has led to a number of indirect approaches to the problem.

The free thyroxine index - FT4I

The results of PBI and THBT were used by Clark and Horn (1965) to compute the FT4I, which was subsequently shown to correlate well with direct determinations of free T4 (Wellby & O'Halloran, 1966). It can be used in conjunction with T4 (CPBA) as well as with PBI results and, when the Thyopac 3 is employed as the thyroid hormone binding test:

$$\text{FT4I} = \frac{\text{PBI or T4 (Thyopac 4)}}{\text{THBT (Thyopac 3)}} \times \text{Mean Normal THBT}$$

It is a most useful concept since it helps eliminate the misleading results found both with PBI and THBT due to changes in the concentration of circulating thyroid hormone binding proteins. For example, although an increase in TBG raises the PBI (and total T4 concentration) it also increases the results of the thyroid hormone binding test and, when the first is divided by the second, the same index is found as in normal subjects. In thyrotoxicosis, however, while the PBI (and total T4 concentration) is raised, the result of the THBT is lowered and the FT4I helps to further separate this group from the normal. The index is also of value in differentiating between those subjects with low PBI (or T4 levels) due to hypothyroidism from those due to decreased levels of circulating binding proteins.

THE EFFECTIVE THYROXINE RATIO - ETR

Recently, Mallinckrodt has introduced a new parameter of thyroid function, known as the effective thyroxine ratio (ETR). In this, the patient's serum T4 is estimated by competitive protein binding in the presence of a very small volume of the patient's unextracted serum. The presence of the unextracted serum disturbs the concentration of binding protein in the system to an extent determined by the concentration of the patient's unoccupied TBG binding sites and hence 'corrects' the T4 level in proportion to the available TBG binding sites. The results are expressed in terms of a ratio between the patient's serum and a pool sample which is given an arbitrary value of one. In effect, this test is a means of combining a serum T4 and THBT in a single tube. The ratio provides an accurate definition of thyroid status, irrespective of changes in the thyroid hormone binding proteins (Thorson et al, 1972). Its advantage is that it involves only one assay, whereas two are required to determine the FT4I. Its disadvantage is that it does not provide separate measurements of circulating total T4 and of free binding site concentration. The place of the ETR in routine clinical practice is yet to be established.

URINARY T4 (CPBA) AND URINARY T3 (RIA)

Finally, it is possible that the assay of urinary T4 (Chan & Landon, 1972) and urinary T3 (Chan et al, 1972b) offers another indirect means of estimating circulating levels of free T3 and T4. This approach is based on the assumption that only the free hormone fractions are filtered by the renal glomeruli and excreted in the urine. Initial results have proved encouraging. However, 24 hr urine collections are required and the place of urinary T3 and T4 assays in routine clinical practice is yet to be established.

CHOICE AND INTERPRETATION OF IN VITRO THYROID FUNCTION TESTS IN CLINICAL PRACTICE

The choice of in vitro thyroid function tests employed in a given clinical situation varies considerably, and depends both on the facilities of the laboratory providing the service and the wishes of individual clinicians. Our own approach, set out below, is based on the relatively high incidence of thyroid dysfunction, close collaboration between clinical and laboratory staff and the wish to minimise any inconvenience to patients by restricting the tests performed to a minimum compatible with establishing the diagnosis.

SCREENING

In addition to assessing thyroid function in all patients with clinical evidence suggestive of hypo- or hyperthyroidism, it is our policy to encourage clinicians to screen the majority of their in-patients and out-patients, especially the elderly and those with evidence of autoimmune diseases or a previous history of thyroid trouble. A PBI and THBT (Thyopac 3) is performed on all samples sent for screening, and should be followed by a competitive protein binding assay for T4 (Thyopac 4) for all samples in which the PBI cannot be determined (because of contamination), and for all samples in which a slightly elevated PBI level is found – to ensure that this is not due to minor degrees of contamination with inorganic iodide, etc. The FT4I is then calculated from these results. All these assays are under the direction of a single individual and are performed in one department, to avoid the chaos that may follow samples being sent to different parts of a hospital. This approach has the merit of administrative simplicity, and of excluding abnormalities in individual tests due either to contamination or to changes in circulating levels of thyroid-hormone binding proteins.

FURTHER IN VITRO TESTING

Patients can be divided into seven groups on the basis of the clinical assessment and the results of the screening tests outlined above (Table IV). Of these, three are clear-cut, with by far the largest group being subjects who are euthyroid both on clinical and biochemical grounds and for whom no further investigations are required. Patients with clinical evidence of hypothyroidism in which the diagnosis is confirmed by the screening tests, require basal plasma TSH determinations to differentiate between the primary and secondary forms of the disorder. Appropriate immunological studies for evidence of autoimmunity should be performed on those with primary hypothyroidism, while procedures designed to assess other aspects of hypothalamic-pituitary function are mandatory in the secondary group. It must be remembered that administration of thyroxine alone to a patient with severe pituitary hypofunction can precipitate an acute adrenal crisis. The third clear-cut group comprises patients with clinical and biochemical evidence of hyperthyroidism. Prior to instituting therapy, in borderline cases, it is wise to prove the diagnosis more completely, for example by

Table IV. Choice of available in vitro thyroid function tests and results in various groups

Clinical Assessment	Biochemical Assessment					
	Screening Tests					Further Tests Required
	PBI	T4	THBT	FT4I	Summary	
Hyperthyroid	High	High	Low	High	Hyperthyroid	TSH response to TRH
Hyperthyroid	Normal	-	Normal	Normal	Euthyroid	TSH response to TRH ? T3 thyrotoxicosis Plasma (and possibly urine) T3
Euthyroid	High	High	Low	High	Hyperthyroid	Repeat screening tests Follow-up
Euthyroid	Normal	-	Normal	Normal	Euthyroid	None
Euthyroid	Low	-	High	Low	Hypothyroid	Basal TSH ? subclinical hypothyroidism Follow-up
Hypothyroid	Normal	-	Normal	Normal	Euthyroid	Repeat screening tests Consider other causes for the signs and symptoms
Hypothyroid	Low	-	High	Low	Hypothyroid	Basal TSH If primary do autoantibody studies; if secondary perform other tests of hypothalamic-pituitary function

determining the TSH response to TRH. If basal levels are low and fail to rise significantly during the test, then there is no need to investigate the patient further, unless the possibility of a thyroid tumour exists.

The remaining four groups pose more problems in that they comprise subjects with a disparity between their clinical and biochemical assessment. Clinical evidence of hyperthyroidism in association with normal or border-line PBI, T4, THBT and FT4I values, raises the possibility of T3-thyro-toxicosis, and it must be remembered that, in this condition, the neck up-take of radioactive iodine may be normal. This diagnosis should be con-firmed by demonstrating low basal TSH levels, an absent TSH response to TRH and elevated plasma (and possibly urine) T3 values. Subjects without symptoms, but with screening tests indicative of hypothyroidism may belong to the subclinical group discussed by Professor Hall in the next paper, and require basal TSH determinations and careful follow-up. Conversely, another diagnosis must be considered for those with signs and symptoms suggestive of hypothyroidism but with normal test results. Tests should be repeated in the final group (clinically euthyroid with tests suggestive of hyperthyroidism) but, if still abnormal, warrant follow-up rather than therapy.

SUMMARY

The large number of in vitro thyroid function tests currently available reflects the absence of simple and precise assays for the free fractions of circulating tri-iodothyronine and thyroxine. Problems in the interpretation of the tests may arise due to prior administration of drugs that contain inorganic iodide, or influence the binding of the thyroid hormones, and by drugs or physiological situations which cause alterations in the circulating concentrations of the thyroid-hormone binding proteins.

Despite the inadequacies of individual tests, it is usually possible to accurately evaluate thyroid status by employing several. In our experience a combination of a protein bound iodine determination, a thyroid hormone binding test, the assay of the circulating total thyroxine (in certain circumstances) and calculation of the free thyroxine index, enable those patients that require more sophisticated test procedures to be singled out. Other tests that may be indicated include determination of basal thyroid stimulating hormone levels and their response to thyrotrophin-releasing hormone, and radioimmunoassay for plasma and, possibly, urinary tri-iodothyronine.

ACKNOWLEDGEMENTS

We gratefully acknowledge the skilled technical assistance of Malcolm Self and other members of the Analytical Section of the Department of Chemical Pathology and generous financial support from the Medical Research Council and the Board of Governors of St Bartholomew's Hospital.

REFERENCES

Chan, V., McAlister, J. and Landon, J. (1972a) Journal of Clinical Pathology, **25**, 30

Chan, V. and Landon, J. (1972) Lancet, **i**, 4

Chan, V., Besser, G. M., Landon, J. and Ekins, R. P. (1972b) Lancet, **ii**, 253

Chopra, I. J., Ho, R. S. and Lam, R. (1972) Journal of Laboratory and Clinical Medicine, **80**, 729

Clark, F. and Horn, D. B. (1965) Journal of Clinical Endocrinology and Metabolism, **25**, 39

Ekins, R. P. (1960) Clinica Chimica Acta, **5**, 453

Gross, J. and Pitt-Rivers, R. (1952) Lancet, **i**, 439

Harrington, C. R. (1926) Biochemical Journal, **20**, 293

Hollander, C. S., Nihei, N. and Burday, S. Z. (1969) Clinical Research, **17**, 286

Odell, W. D., Wilber, J. F. and Paul, W. E. (1965) Journal of Clinical Endocrinology and Metabolism, **25**, 1179

Pitt-Rivers, R., Stanbury, J. B. and Rapp, B. (1955) Journal of Clinical Endocrinology and Metabolism, **15**, 616

Robbins, J. and Rall, J. E. (1957) Recent Progress in Hormone Research, **13**, 161

Sandell, E. B. and Kolthoff, I. M. (1937) Microchim Acta, **1**, 9

Solomon, D. H., Benotti, J., Detroot, L. J., Greer, M. A., Pileggi, V. J., Pittman, J. A., Robbins, J., Selenkow, H. A., Sterling, K. and Volpe, R. (1972) Journal of Clinical Endocrinology and Metabolism, **34**, 844

Sterling, K., Brenner, M. A. and Newman, E. S. (1970) Science, **169**, 1099

Sterling, K., Refetoff, S. and Selenkow, H. A. (1970) Journal of the American Medical Association, **213**, 571

Thorson, S. C., Mincey, E. K., McIntosh, H. W. and Morrison, R. T. (1972) British Medical Journal, **2**, 67

Utiger, R. D. (1965) Journal of Clinical Investigation, **44**, 1277

Wellby, M. and O'Halloran, M. W. (1966) British Medical Journal, **2**, 668

The Role of TSH and TRH in Thyroid Disease

REGINALD HALL, D C EVERED, W M G TUNBRIDGE

THYROID-STIMULATING HORMONE

Thyroid-stimulating hormone (TSH) levels in the circulation can now be measured by a sensitive, specific radioimmunoassay. The requirements for a TSH immunoassay are:

1) **TSH for iodination** — a highly purified TSH preparation suitable for labelling can be obtained from the National Pituitary Agency, USA.

2) **Anti-TSH antisera** are available from the Medical Research Council (MRC) and the NPA. These are rabbit anti-human TSH antisera.

3) **Standard TSH** is available from the MRC. Standard 68/38 is suitable, a human TSH standard should always be used.

4) **Precipitating antibodies** are available from commercial laboratories but must always be tested before use under assay conditions.

5) **Radioiodine for labelling** by the standard Hunter and Greenwood technique is available from the Radiochemical Centre at Amersham. Most workers now prefer to use ^{125}I for labelling; fresh, carrier-free iodine should always be used. An outline of the assay techniques and problems has been given by Hall (1972).

Problems of the TSH immunoassay

Current TSH assays are suitable for routine clinical use but they have a number of limitations which must be clearly recognised.

1) **Specificity.** Most anti-TSH antisera show cross-reaction with the other glycoprotein hormones (LH, FSH and HCG). To correct for this, HCG is added in the first incubation although this procedure sometimes leads to reduced assay sensitivity.

2) **Sensitivity.** The major drawback of current TSH assays is their lack of

15

sensitivity, many are unable to detect TSH in normal sera or grossly overestimate the level and probably all assays are subject to non-specific interference and overestimate normal TSH levels. Because of this lack of sensitivity, measurements of TSH are not helpful in separating low TSH levels from those within the normal range.

3) **Time of incubation.** Few TSH assays can be completed within less than one week of receipt of the specimen which diminishes the value of this measurement in routine clinical practice.

4) **Stability of labelled TSH.** Labelled TSH deteriorates and few labelled TSH preparations can be used for more than two weeks despite the 60 day half-life of ^{125}I.

5) **Variability of results.** Although intra-assay variation is small, results of consecutive TSH assays in the same laboratory often show disturbing variability, particularly in measurements of levels in or near to the normal range. Between-laboratory comparisons are rarely published but show even wider variations as a result of different assay techniques and different materials used, particularly the anti-TSH antisera.

Measurement of TSH

1) **Euthyroid subjects.** Normal TSH values are probably $< 1\mu U$ per ml, a level below the limit of sensitivity of most current TSH assays. It is now recognised that lower values for TSH are obtained in assays in which the standard curve is set up in serum obtained from controls treated with triiodothyronine which is 'free' of TSH. In the authors' laboratory, normal TSH levels range from undetectable to about $4\mu U$ per ml (of MRC 68/38) with a mean of $1.6\mu U$ per ml.

There do not appear to be any significant differences in TSH levels between men, women and children over the age of one year. Preliminary studies suggest that TSH levels are higher in the elderly. Shortly after birth there is a rapid but transient rise in serum TSH, due at least in part to the stimulus of cold. It is now clear that serum TSH levels, like those of growth hormone, show a circadian rhythm, peak levels occurring between 2 and 4 am and minimum levels between 6 and 8 pm. The rise follows about two hours after the onset of sleep and additional peaks can be observed in subjects who sleep during the day (Patel et al, 1972).

2) **Non-toxic goitre.** The majority of patients with non-toxic goitres have normal TSH levels and the role of TSH in the production of such goitres is unknown. Patients with goitre who do show a raised TSH level are usually found to be suffering from auto-immune thyroid disease (or endemic goitre in iodine deficient areas) or more rarely have been exposed to some goitrogen or have an intrathyroidal enzyme defect.

3) **Hypothyroidism.** The major value of serum TSH measurements lies in the exclusion of primary thyroid failure. All patients with thyroid failure due to thyroid disease have a raised serum TSH level, so the finding of a normal TSH level in a patient suspected of thyroid failure excludes this diagnosis. Obviously hypothyroidism on the basis of pituitary or hypothalamic disease is associated with low or normal TSH levels. However, it must be stressed that a raised TSH level, although implying some departure from optimum circulating thyroid hormone levels which may or may not have been compensated for, does not in itself indicate the presence of clinical hypothyroidism and is therefore not necessarily an indication for treatment. Evered and Hall (1972) have classified thyroid failure into three grades:

1) **Overt hypothyroidism** (or myxoedema) when the classical features of thyroid failure are present, routine thyroid function tests are abnormal and the serum TSH level is high. This represents a major degree of thyroid failure but is rarer than the lesser grades of hypothyroidism.

2) **Mild hypothyroidism** where the clinical features are non-specific and a firm clinical diagnosis cannot be made. Routine thyroid function tests are often normal or in the equivocal range, but the serum TSH level is always elevated. About half of these patients have a 'normal' thyroid reserve as measured by the TSH stimulation test, so this is not very helpful in diagnosis. Patients in this category obtain symptomatic benefit from thyroid hormone treatment.

3) **Subclinical hypothyroidism** is defined as an asymptomatic state where routine thyroid function tests are normal but the serum TSH level is raised. It has been suggested on the basis of hospital studies, that patients in this category are at risk for ischaemic heart disease, but this conclusion cannot be accepted until it has been validated from studies in the general population, which the authors and their colleagues are carrying out at present. This category may mimic mild hypothyroidism if, for example, a patient with subclinical hypothyroidism becomes depressed or develops other non-specific symptoms compatible with hypothyroidism. In this situation the only method of differentiating the groups is by a carefully controlled trial of l-thyroxine. If the patient's symptoms respond to l-thyroxine it is likely that he falls into the category of mild hypothyroidism, although the possibility of a placebo effect must not be overlooked. It would be too cumbersome to use a double blind trial of l-thyroxine against placebo in all of these patients and at present it seems reasonable to accept that a patient with non-specific symptoms who has a raised TSH and responds to l-thyroxine should have long-term treatment with thyroid hormone. What is needed is some peripheral tissue response test which correlates closely with the patient's symptoms but none is available at present.

Patients with autoimmune thyroid disease and those who have received destructive therapy to the thyroid but who have normal TSH levels, must be considered to be at risk for the development of thyroid failure. This progression is probably uncommon in those with autoimmune thyroid disease but quite frequent in those who have received destructive therapy. The time-course of the progression is unknown in autoimmune thyroid disease but is generally well established in patients treated by radioiodine or partial thyroidectomy.

4) Hyperthyroidism is only very rarely due to overproduction of TSH. A few patients with pituitary tumours or hypothalamic dysfunction have been described where hyperthyroidism has been associated with raised circulating levels of TSH. The vast majority of patients with hyperthyroidism have low (or normal) TSH levels, but as mentioned earlier, because of the limitation of assay sensitivity, low TSH levels cannot be separated from normal and hence isolated TSH estimations have no place at present in the diagnosis of hyperthyroidism. The use of TSH measurements after TRH in the recognition of hyperthyroidism will be considered later.

Other Thyroid Stimulators

TSH is by no means the only thyroid-stimulating agent; other stimulators of the thyroid have also been described, including:

1) **Long-acting thyroid stimulator (LATS)**, an IgG molecule present in the circulation in some patients with Graves' disease and occasionally in their apparently healthy relatives. It is known to stimulate the thyroid in animals and in man. At present its role in the pathogenesis of the hyperthyroidism of Graves' disease is uncertain, but it would seem improbable that a thyroid-stimulating immunoglobulin was present as an epiphenomenon.

2) **Human molar thyrotrophin (HMT)** is a larger-molecular weight compound present in some hydatidiform moles. It can be detected in the serum of patients with hyperthyroidism associated with moles and also in the urine of normal pregnant women.

3) **Human chorionic thyrotrophin (HCT)** has a molecular weight similar to that of pituitary TSH and shows some similarities in structure as tested by immunoassay. It may be derived from HMT although this is still not proven.

The role of these two trophoblast-derived thyroid stimulators in normal pregnancy is uncertain at the present time.

Structure of TSH

It has now been shown that TSH, like the other glycoprotein hormones, is made up of two subunits, designated α and β. The α-subunit is common to HCG, LH and FSH, whereas the β-subunit, which confers biological activity differs in the various hormones. In theory it might be expected that a more specific radio-immunoassay could be developed by using β-subunit specific antibodies, but so far this has not proved possible.

Control of TSH Secretion

TSH secretion is normally controlled by a feedback mechanism by thyroid hormones acting on the anterior pituitary, modulating its responsiveness to thyrotrophin-releasing hormone (Figure 1). In primary thyroid failure where circulating thyroid hormone levels are lowered there is an increased circulating level of TSH and an increase in pituitary TSH stores, and TRH injection causes an exaggerated and prolonged rise in serum TSH. In primary pituitary failure low levels of circulating thyroid hormone are accompanied by low serum TSH but it is uncertain whether there is an increased compensatory TRH drive. In hyperthyroidism the high levels of thyroid hormones inhibit the effect of TRH on TSH release and the serum TSH level is low. Recently a direct in vitro stimulatory effect of thyroxine on hypothalamic TRH secretion has been described; the clinical significance of this is at present unknown. TRH probably affects both TSH synthesis and TSH release, the latter certainly, by some mechanism mediated by cyclic AMP. The effects of thyroid hormones in blocking TRH-mediated TSH release is dose-dependent and can be overcome by inhibitors of protein synthesis suggesting that a protein intermediate is responsible for the inhibition.

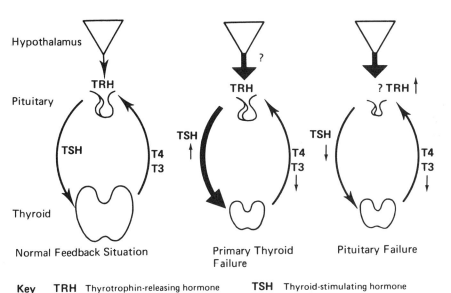

Key	TRH	Thyrotrophin-releasing hormone	TSH	Thyroid-stimulating hormone
	T4	Thyroxine	T3	Triiodothyronine

Figure 1. Hypothalamic-pituitary-thyroid relationships in health and disease

19

THYROTROPHIN-RELEASING HORMONE (TRH)

TRH is a tripeptide, pyroglutamyl-histidyl-prolinamide which has been isolated from the median eminence of many species. Its structure appears to be identical in different species and it is easily synthesised. TRH is produced in the neurones of a wide area of the hypothalamus and transported from there to the median eminence where it is stored. Under appropriate stimuli TRH is released into the portal circulation and carried to the thyrotroph cells of the anterior lobe where it exerts its action on TSH synthesis and release. It has structural similarities to the decapeptide LH/FSH-RH which also has a pyroglutamyl structure at one end of the molecule and an amide group, as part of glycinamide, at the other end.

Specificity of TRH

TRH is not entirely specific for TSH. It constantly releases prolactin (PRO) with a time course similar to that of TSH release. Occasionally LH is released in women, a finding which may be explained by the similarity in structure of TRH and LH/FSH-RH. It has no consistent effect on Growth Hormone (GH) release in normal subjects other than those which might be ascribed to random fluctuations in GH levels or stress-induced release. However in patients with acromegaly TRH often induces a marked rise in serum GH levels. TRH has no effect on the release of neurophysin or ACTH and during pregnancy has no effect on HCT.

Side-effects of TRH

No major side-effects have resulted from the intravenous or oral administration of TRH. It causes minor transient side-effects in the majority of subjects when it is administered by rapid intravenous injection. These include nausea, facial flushing and a desire to pass urine. They may be ascribed to a direct action of the bolus of TRH on plain muscle of the gastrointestinal and genito-urinary tracts since this has been demonstrated in vitro. It is obviously wise to avoid administration of TRH during pregnancy although it has been administered to a number of pregnant women without adverse effect on the foetus.

Clinical Applications of TRH

These can be divided into diagnostic and therapeutic categories. TRH is helpful in the diagnosis of thyroid disease (Ormston et al, 1971) and as a test of pituitary-hypothalamic function (Hall et al, 1972). The response to TRH can be monitored by measurements of serum TSH levels after intravenous or oral TRH or by measurement of TSH-induced changes of thyroxine or tri-iodothyronine (Lawton et al, 1973). Preliminary studies suggest that TRH might be of value in the treatment of depression. It is convenient to consider the diagnostic applications of TRH under the following headings (its use in pituitary-hypothalamic disease will only be briefly considered):

(a) Normal subjects
(b) Patients with thyroid disease
  Hypothyroidism
  Hyperthyroidism
  Causes of an absent or impaired response in subjects who are clinically
    euthyroid.

(a) Normal Subjects

It is necessary for each laboratory measuring TSH to establish its own
normal range of responses to TRH.

Pattern of response to TRH. After intravenous injection of TRH there is a
rapid rise of serum TSH levels in normal subjects, detectable at five minutes
and peaking at about 20 minutes, returning to baseline values by two to four
hours. It is for this reason that in the widely-used intravenous TRH test,
specimens are taken for TSH measurements before TRH, at 20 minutes (peak
response) and at 60 minutes (to detect delayed responses). After oral TRH,
the TSH rise occurs later and is more prolonged. Intervals of at least one
week should be allowed between repeat tests.

Pattern of response of thyroid hormones to TRH. TRH administration releases
TSH, which in turn leads to release of T4 and T3 from the thyroid. Lawton
et al (1973) have shown that the serum T3 level consistently peaks between
two and four hours after $200\mu g$ of intravenous TRH. Thus a simple intravenous
TRH test using a rapid injection of $200\mu g$ of TRH with samples at 20 minutes
for TSH and at three hours for T3 provides a test of the integrity of the pituitary thyroid axis. The increase in serum T4 concentration after intravenous
TRH is a less reliable index of thyroid response. Measurements of serum
T4 six or twenty-four hours after 40mg of oral TRH can be used as an alternative test.

Pattern of thyroid radioiodine uptake response to TRH. After administration
of a series of large doses of oral TRH a rise in thyroidal radioiodine uptake
can be demonstrated but this procedure is too cumbersome for routine use.

Response to TRH in males and females. Women show a greater rise in TSH
than men at time intervals of 20 and 60 minutes after intravenous TRH. This
effect is due to the higher oestrogen levels in women and the response in men
can be enhanced by oestrogen administration.

Effects of age on TRH response. There is no good evidence that the peak
level of TSH in response to TRH is different in the elderly but because of
higher basal levels in older patients the TSH increment is less. Children
appear to respond similarly to adults.

Effects of circadian rhythm. It has been shown that the TSH response to
TRH, expressed as a percentage of the basal value is greater during the

night than during the day (Jensen & Weeke, 1972). It is best to carry out routine TRH tests at a similar time of the day.

Effects of height, weight and surface area on TRH response. There do not appear to be changes in the TSH response to TRH dependent on these parameters, hence it is satisfactory to use the same dose in all situations.

Effect of dose of TRH on TSH response. The TSH response increases with increasing doses of intravenous TRH to plateau at about 400μg of TRH. Consistent responses to TRH are not found at doses of less than 50μg. With oral TRH a 40mg dose produces a consistent rise of both TSH and T4.

Effect of drugs on TRH response. The TSH response to TRH is enhanced by intravenous theophylline, by oestrogens in men and by overtreatment with antithyroid drugs. It is reduced by pharmacological doses of corticosteroids, by thyroid hormones and by long-term L-DOPA. It is necessary to withdraw T4 for three weeks and T3 for ten days before performing a TRH test.

Effects of basal T4 and TSH levels on response to TRH. The peak TSH response is directly related to the basal TSH level and inversely related to the basal T4 level. This relationship has been shown in normal subjects after oral TRH and in patients with endemic goitre after intravenous TRH.

(b) Patients with Thyroid Disease

Hypothyroidism. Patients with primary hypothyroidism show an exaggerated and prolonged TSH response to TRH. However, the elevated basal TSH level provides sufficient information to help in the diagnosis of symptomatic hypothyroidism.

Hyperthyroidism. Because of the increased circulating levels of T4 and T3, patients with hyperthyroidism fail to respond to a small (200μg) dose of TRH. The inhibition of response is dose-dependent and occasional patients with mild hyperthyroidism have responded to large doses of intravenous or oral TRH. The rapid intravenous TRH test is of particular value in excluding a diagnosis of hyperthyroidism. A normal response excludes hyperthyroidism but it must be stressed that an absent or impaired response, while commonly due to hyperthyroidism, may have other explanations. In patients with the syndrome of T3 toxicosis who have a normal serum PBI, T4 and thyroxine-binding globulin, but raised T3 levels, an absent response to TRH can provide confirmation of a clinical diagnosis of hyperthyroidism if a serum T3 measurement is not available. It has been shown that the results of the TRH test correlate well with those of the T3 suppression test. A normal TRH test is correlated with normal suppressibility, and an absent or impaired TSH response to TRH correlates with impaired or absent suppression by T3. In view of this correlation the TRH test is to be preferred to the T3 suppression test since it is safer and more rapid and convenient to the patient.

Causes of an absent or impaired response in patients who are clinically

euthyroid. As stated above, an absent or impaired TSH response to TRH does not necessarily indicate that the patient is hyperthyroid. Absent or impaired responses without hyperthyroidism are sometimes found in the following clinical situations: Ophthalmic Graves' disease; Graves' disease, euthyroid after therapy; Autonomous thyroid adenoma; Multinodular goitre; Hypothyroid patients receiving more than the optimal replacement dose of l-thyroxine.

In the majority of these situations, measurements of serum T4 and T3 indicate that the level of one or other of the thyroid hormones is higher than the normal population mean. Like the T3 suppression test, the TRH test is also of value in the diagnosis of unilateral exophthalmos — a common presentation of ophthalmic Graves' disease.

Response to TRH in Secondary Hypothyroidism

TRH can be used as a test of pituitary TSH reserve. In patients with hypothyroidism due to pituitary disease there is no response to TRH. However, failure of response to TRH should not be equated with clinical hypothyroidism; it indicates patients who are at risk for the development of hypothyroidism. A normal response to TRH excludes pituitary hypothyroidism. Patients with hypothalamic disease in whom the pituitary is intact may have a normal TSH response to TRH. Patients with acromegaly, especially those who have received some form of destructive therapy, often fail to respond to TRH, yet only a small minority develop clinical hypothyroidism.

Spectrum of Thyroid Disease

Studies of serum TSH and its response to TRH coupled with measurements of circulating T3 and T4 have made it apparent that there is a spectrum of thyroid function between normality and overt thyroid disease (Figure 2). It has long been accepted that hypothyroidism is a graded phenomenon, but only recently has evidence accumulated indicating that hyperthyroidism is also graded in this way.

The pattern of TSH response to TRH is dependent on the circulating levels of thyroid hormones. An increase in thyroid hormone levels depresses the basal TSH and reduces or abolishes the response to TRH whereas a decrease in thyroid hormones is associated with an increased basal TSH and an exaggerated response to TRH. What then constitutes an increase or a decrease in circulating thyroid hormone levels? It was shown by Snyder and Utiger (1972) that treatment of normal subjects with small doses of T3 and T4 (15μg of T3 and 60μg of T4 daily) caused a marked decrease in their response to TRH. The serum T3 levels of these subjects were elevated above their pretreatment values but were still within the normal range and their serum T4 levels were unchanged. Similarly Ormston et al (1972) have shown that some patients with ophthalmic Graves' disease who are euthyroid have

23

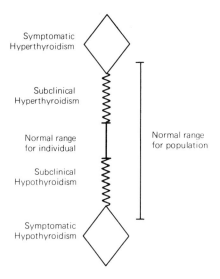

Figure 2. Spectrum of thyroid disease

minimal elevation of the serum T3 level and an impaired or absent response to TRH. It is apparent, therefore, that the range of serum T3 and T4 concentrations in which the TSH response to TRH is normal is very small. This range will vary from individual to individual and will be much narrower than the normal range for the general population (Figure 3), being finely regulated

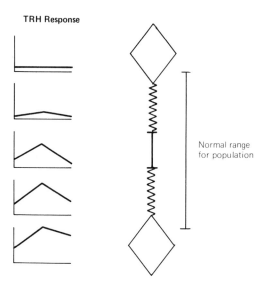

Figure 3. TRH response in spectrum of thyroid disease

by the TSH-mediated feedback mechanism. It probably remains unchanged for long periods of time although the setting may change in old age or show a seasonal variation.

Minor deviations from the individual range are associated with small changes in TSH levels and a more obvious alteration in the TSH response to TRH. Small upward deviations of thyroid hormones lead to a state of 'subclinical hyperthyroidism', defined as an asymptomatic condition associated with an absent or impaired response to TRH and supraoptimal levels of T3 and/or T4 for the individual. A further increase of T3 and T4 is required before clinical hyperthyroidism is produced. Subclinical hyperthyroidism may be recognised in some of the following situations:

Preceding symptomatic hyperthyroidism
Ophthalmic Graves' disease
Autonomous thyroid adenoma (subclinical toxic adenoma)
Multinodular goitre
During poorly controlled antithyroid treatment
After destructive therapy to the thyroid
During replacement therapy with l-thyroxine
0.2 - 0.4mg daily for hypothyroidism

The clinical significance of subclinical hyperthyroidism is unknown. Some patients are at risk for the development of overt hyperthyroidism, but in others, particularly some with ophthalmic Graves' disease, this condition may persist for many years. It appears to be a feature of thyroid function in any gland not regulated by the normal finely-balanced feedback process. The level of circulating thyroid hormones will then depend on other factors such as the size (mass) of the thyroid adenoma, the iodine supply in the diet, and possibly on other thyroid-stimulating agents such as the long-acting thyroid stimulator.

There is no doubt that slight increases of thyroid hormone levels may have deleterious effects in some patients with ischaemic heart disease or a tendency to supraventricular tachycardia, but it remains uncertain whether they confer any biological disadvantage in the majority of subjects. Again long-standing hyperthyroidism occasionally leads to osteoporosis but this is uncommon. It remains to be seen whether a prolonged state of subclinical hyperthyroidism will affect the skeleton. Further long-term studies are required to elucidate the sequelae, if any, of a prolonged state of subclinical hyperthyroidism.

A similar situation exists so far as hypothyroidism is concerned (see before). Lowered levels of circulating thyroid hormones may be associated with raised TSH levels in asymptomatic subjects — subclinical hypothyroidism. In others the level of circulating thyroid hormone is apparently normal yet the TSH level is raised. Does this represent full compensation or is the

25

thyroid hormone level still suboptimal for a given individual? These possibilities require to be resolved. Again we know relatively little of the role of T4 compared with T3 in regulating the feedback mechanism. In some situations, T3 appears pre-eminent. For example in rats, blockage of peripheral deiodination of T4 to T3 by propylthiouracil prevents inhibition of the TRH response by T4. However in some patients with early thyroid failure and large goitres, the serum TSH level is elevated in association with an elevated serum T3, a situation which is difficult to explain at present.

If the spectrum of thyroid function and disease is accepted, it becomes obvious that it is often difficult to define the precise thyroid status of an individual with such crude tools as clinical diagnostic indices or routine thyroid function tests. In the past minor degrees of thyroid dysfunction have often been overlooked, and this is perhaps just as well because the need to treat them is as yet unproven.

CONCLUSIONS

The measurements of serum TSH levels and their response to TRH provide valuable information in the diagnosis of thyroid disease and give new insight into the mechanisms controlling the secretion of TSH and the action of this hormone on the thyroid.

REFERENCES

Evered, D. and Hall, R. (1972) British Medical Journal, 1, 290
Hall, R. (1972) Clinical Endocrinology, 1, 115
Hall, R., Ormston, B. J., Besser, G. M., Cryer, R. J. and McKendrick,
    M. (1972) Lancet, 1, 759
Jensen, S. E. and Weeke, J. (1972) Israel Journal of Medical Sciences,
    8, 48
Lawton, N. F., Ellis, S. M. and Sufi, S. (1973) Clinical Endocrinology,
    2, 57
Ormston, B. J., Garry, R., Cryer, R. J., Besser, G. M. and Hall, R.
    (1971) Lancet, 11, 10
Ormston, B. J., Alexander, L., Evered, D. C., Clark, F., Bird, T.,
    Fernandez, M. and Hall, R. (1972) Israel Journal of Medical Sciences,
    8, 49
Patel, Y. C., Alford, F. P. and Burger, H. G. (1972) Clinical Science,
    43, 71
Snyder, P. J. and Utiger, R. D. (1972) Journal of Clinical Investigation,
    51, 2077

Progress Report on Thyroid Autoimmune Disease

DEBORAH DONIACH

Thyroid autoimmunity has been reviewed so extensively (Doniach & Roitt, 1969; Shulman, 1971; Beall & Solomon, 1971) that this short survey will cover only advances made in the past few years. These will be discussed first in relation to lymphoid thyroiditis, which includes all the variants of goitrous or Hashimoto's thyroiditis and myxoedema with thyroid atrophy and, secondly, in connection with Graves' disease where recent findings show particular promise.

AUTOIMMUNE THYROIDITIS

THYROID SPECIFIC ANTIGENS AND DIAGNOSTIC ANTIBODY TESTS

In addition to the three old-established autoantigens, ie thyroglobulin, microsomal (cytoplasmic) and 2nd colloid (CA2), separate antibodies have been found in the serum of thyroiditis patients which react with a thyroid specific cell surface antigen (Fagraeus & Jonsson, 1970). These antibodies have to be detected on live suspensions of human thyroid cells, by immunofluorescence, where they produce an interrupted line of staining around each cell. They can also be detected by a complicated, mixed haemadsorption test using monolayer cell-cultures. The special interest of this system is theoretical. Any immunological attack taking place in vivo must involve antigen accessible on the outer membrane as live cells are impermeable to antibodies. If cell-mediated cytotoxicity is envisaged, killing by sensitised lymphocytes is also via surface antigen. Another point worthy of mention is that no connection could be demonstrated between the surface antibodies and long-acting thyroid stimulator (LATS) which apparently reacts with a different receptor (Fagraeus et al, 1970) and cannot be seen by fluorescence.

Until recently, antibodies to thyroglobulin and the microsomal antigen were best detected by tanned red cell agglutination (TRC) and immunofluorescence respectively, while the complement fixation test was used for semi-quantitative titration of the microsomal antibodies. Less than 1% of Hashimoto patients were missed when these screening tests were employed for the differentiation from other non-toxic goitres, and in the majority of cases also from cancer. The older Ouchterlony precipitin method and the equally insensitive Latex-thyroglobulin-antibody test cannot be used by themselves as nearly half the thyroiditis patients have only traces of or no thyroglobulin antibodies in their serum, though they practically all show positive fluorescence on thyroid cytoplasm and colloid (CA2 antigen). The differential diagnosis of primary myxoedema from obesity, depressive states, pituitary failure, etc requires sensitive methods as many patients have very low antibody titres, although extremely high antibody levels are occasionally seen even in myxoedema coma.

At least 25% of cases with long-standing thyroid atrophy give negative results by the tests mentioned above, especially if the patients have been treated with thyroxine (Papapetrou et al, 1972). For this reason the radioimmunoassays developed by Mori and co-workers (1970, 1971) for the determination of thyroglobulin and microsomal antibodies will probably supercede all other methods, especially when the reagents become available in the form of commercial kits. These new tests give 100% positive results in Hashimoto's goitre, myxoedema and thyrotoxicosis and in about 25% of mixed hospital patients. Diffuse thyroiditis is generally associated with higher titres than subclinical focal lesions, and if the positive sera are assayed for TSH in addition to the antibodies, it will prove possible to diagnose all cases requiring thyroxine replacement on a single sample of 5ml of blood. In the selected population of hospital patients with symptoms, approximately half of those found to have thyroid antibodies have slightly or moderately elevated serum TSH values, even when hypothyroidism is not suspected clinically (Lawton et al, 1973). The TRH test is rarely abnormal in patients with serum TSH levels below $5-10\mu U/ml$ and a proportion of cases with a low thyroid reserve are well-compensated and may not require thyroxine for some years (Gordin et al, 1972). This is particularly striking in post-^{131}I hypothyroidism.

Sensitive thyroid antibody tests are helpful in distinguishing anxiety states from thyrotoxicosis and local orbital lesions from unilateral endocrine exophthalmos. Here again, sera with positive antibody tests could be tested for TSH since a Graves' diathesis is usually shown up by a TSH level below $5\mu U/ml$ and low responsiveness to TRH.

CELL MEDIATED HYPERSENSITIVITY (CMH) IN THYROIDITIS

Two methods for the study of CMH are applicable to human patients: the lymphocyte transformation test (LTT) and the leucocyte migration inhibition test (LMT). Several authors have reported lymphocyte transformation in thyroid patients with thyroid extracts and thyroglobulin (Ehrenfeld et al, 1971).

There is still some doubt as to whether the antigen causes direct blast trans-formation of the T lymphocytes or whether sensitised B cells are triggered.

The leucocyte migration inhibition test of Bendixen and Søborg (1969) is thought to reflect cell-mediated immunity in the human and the ability of the patient's T-lymphocytes to secrete a migration inhibition factor (MIF). A correlation has been demonstrated between a positive LMT and cutaneous delayed hypersensitivity reactions to Brucella and to tuberculin protein. The test has also been applied to the investigation of autoimmune disorders where cellular immune mechanisms directed against tissue components may have an important pathogenic role. There is evidence of migration inhibition with the appropriate tissues in Addison's disease, Sjögren's syndrome, glomeru-lonephritis, pernicious anaemia, primary biliary cirrhosis, active chronic hepatitis, ulcerative colitis, diabetes mellitus, and several studies have appeared using this test in thyroiditis (Calder et al,1972; Wartenberg et al, 1973a). In our hands the test gave good results with thyroid microsomes while thyroglobulin was ineffective. All Hashimoto, primary myxoedema and thyrotoxic patients showed some migration inhibition with thyroid micro-somes. This was organ-specific in the sense that liver microsomes had no effect. Lymphocytes from normal subjects did not react with thyroid or liver subcellular fractions. The LMT is not an easy method and to get quantitative results it is necessary to set up tissue culture chambers with at least three doses of antigen in quadruplicate for each patient. Doing the test in this care-ful way made it possible to obtain some interesting clinical correlations with different variants of Hashimoto's thyroiditis and to throw some light on the varying responsiveness of these goitres to thyroxine replacement therapy.

It has been known for some years that Hashimoto's disease can be broadly classified into a milder 'hypercellular' or 'oxyphil' variant, and a more severe form termed 'fibrous'. This is obviously an oversimplified view and in reality the disease forms a spectrum with many intermediate cases. Typical examples of each variant differ from each other clinically, histologically and in their serum autoantibody pattern as shown in Table I. Studies with the leucocyte migration inhibition test have suggested that patients with the milder form of the disease tend to have more pronounced CMH to thyroid microsomes and, furthermore, the few patients in whom the goitre failed to become smaller after prolonged thyroxine in full replace-ment doses, showed the most intense migration inhibition (Figure 1).

An interesting but unexplained phenomenon is the positive LMT obtained in thyroiditis and thyrotoxicosis with liver mitochondria (Calder et al,1972; Wartenberg et al,1973b). This appears to correspond quantitatively with the organ specific CMH to thyroid microsomes, so that the most intense migration inhibition was again found in patients with low or absent thyroglo-bulin antibodies, particularly in the few cases with T4 resistant goitres.

Table I. Comparison of two variants of Hashimoto's thyroiditis

	Hypercellular or oxyphil	Fibrous
Sex Ratio	20F /1M	5-7F /1M
Incidence	Fairly common	Rare
GOITRE		
Size	Usually moderate or small	Some very large
Consistency	Moderately firm	Very firm with irregular surface
Pain /tenderness	Occasionally	None
THYROID FUNCTION	Euthyroid	Often hypothyroid
Response to Thyroxine		
Majority	Slow reduction goitre size	Often rapid
Minority	No change	Resistant to Thyroxine
HISTOLOGY		
Cellular infiltrate	Mainly lymphocytes with germinal centres	Mainly plasma cells
Oxyphil change	Prominent	Usually present
Fibrosis	Minimal	Marked
IMMUNOLOGY		
Thyroglobulin antibodies	Trace or absent	Precipitin test positive in over 90% High TRC titres
Microsomal antibodies	Moderate titres	Moderate or high
Leucocyte migration with thyroid microsomes	Strong inhibition	Weak response

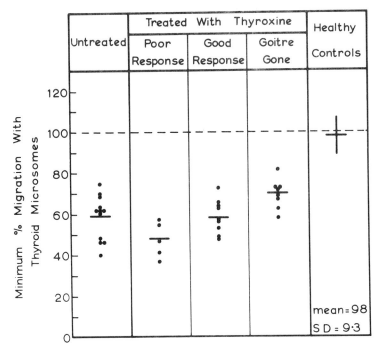

Figure 1. Correlation of leucocyte migration inhibition (LMT) in response to thyroid microsomes, with the regression of the goitre on prolonged thyroxine therapy in 34 cases of autoimmune thyroiditis and 47 normal controls. Cases with positive CFT but low or absent thyroglobulin antibodies gave the best migration inhibition. (Reproduced by kind permission of the Editor, International Archives of Allergy and Immunology. Wartenberg et al, 1973a)

PATHOGENESIS OF THYROIDITIS

The pathogenetic mechanisms operating in autoimmune thyroiditis are far from clear in the human subject. In the spontaneous thyroiditis of obese chickens which has proved to be such a good experimental model for the human disease (Rose et al, 1971), there is a strict bursal dependence implying a more important role for the B or antibody making lymphocytes. However, in the experimental organ-specific auto-allergies in rodents, the effects of neonatal thymectomy indicate a greater role for CMH and the T-cell system. In the human disease the poor correlation between the intensity of thyroiditis and the titres of circulating antibodies has often been quoted as an argument in favour of a dominant role for cellular immunity, although there is little direct evidence implicating CMH in the killing of thyroid cells. The LMT results outlined above suggest that CMH may play a role in the cases of Hashimoto goitre with low thyroglobulin antibodies whereas the fibrous variant characterised by large amounts of circulating thyroglobulin precipitins may well represent an immune-complex mediated lesion. This becomes more

31

likely when one considers that deposits of immune complexes of granular nature, resembling those seen in nephritis, are observed around the acinar basement membrane in the focal thyroiditis of Graves' disease (Doniach, 1967; Werner et al, 1972). It is possible that cell-mediated hypersensitivity is only one of the pathogenetic factors in a complicated interplay between cellular and humoral components of the autoimmune attack.

GENETIC ASPECTS OF THYROID AUTOIMMUNITY

Chromosome anomalies

Partial defects of CMH, dysgammaglobulinaemia and autoimmune phenomena are not uncommon in patients with chromosome anomalies (Fialkow, 1969). Clinical observations showed an increased prevalence of thyroiditis in ovarian dysgenesis, especially in cases with X isochromosome defects (Guinet et al, 1969). Similarly, mosaics with structurally abnormal sex chromosomes have by far the highest incidence of thyroid antibodies (60%) although positive results are also found in Turner's syndrome with XO karyotype (Doniach et al, 1968). Thyroid function tests reveal an impaired thyroid reserve in a proportion of these cases (McHardy-Young et al, 1970), as they do in normal women with circulating antibodies. In Kleinfelter's syndrome with karyotype XXY no increase in thyroid antibodies has been noted. A high incidence of thyroid antibodies has been reported in Down's syndrome and also in the mothers of these children (Fialkow et al, 1971) suggesting that an abnormal maternal tendency to autoimmunity might be the cause of the chromosome translocation in this type of mental deficiency. A search for minor chromosome defects in Hashimoto patients and for cases of Downs' syndrome in their offspring gave completely negative results in our hands.

Familial aspects of thyroid autoimmune disease

The aggregation of Hashimoto goitre, primary myxoedema and Graves' disease in the same families supports the autoimmune hypothesis. This is now backed up by the genetically determined chicken thyroiditis, where only 8 generations of inbreeding resulted in the regular occurrence of the disease at 3 weeks of age, with obesity and frequent myxoedema (Rose et al, 1971), although Graves' disease has not been observed in animals as yet. Hall was the first to look for antibodies in human families (Hall & Stanbury, 1967; Hall et al, 1972) and the genetic predisposition to thyroid autoimmunity has since been confirmed by many other studies (Doniach et al, 1965a and b). Thyroiditis can be inherited through the mother or father and in affected children the autoimmunity trait is often present on both sides of the family. Evidence also comes from studies in identical twins: for instance the concordance rate for Graves' disease is nearly 60% in monozygotic and only 9% in dizygotic twins of the same sex.

Table II. Evidence for regarding Graves' thyrotoxicosis as a primary autoimmune disease

Circumstantial evidence	Direct evidence
1. Familial incidence, same families as Hashimoto and myxoedema.	Long-acting thyroid stimulator (LATS) detected in serum of up to 80% of primary thyrotoxics after immunoglobulin concentration.
2. Female sex preponderance.	Pathogenic effect of LATS. Placental transmission causes temporary Graves' disease in neonates. Infused LATS
3. Exacerbations and remissions.	stimulates normal human and animal thyroid gland with release of PB131I.
4. Strong association with focal lymphoid thyroiditis and occasional transition to Hashimoto's struma or primary myxoedema.	Extrapituitary origin of thyrotoxicosis. Disease can occur in hypophysectomised subjects. Pituitary gland shows resting thyrotrophs in Graves' disease.
5. Association with other autoimmune disorders: Pernicious anaemia and atrophic gastritis, adrenal atrophy, myasthenia gravis, SLE, rheumatoid arthritis, Sjögren's dermatomyositis, haemolytic anaemia, thrombocytopenic purpura, "lupoid hepatitis".	Distinction of LATS from TSH. Half-life of injected LATS 7 hours, that of TSH about 5 minutes in animals. LATS cannot be extracted from pituitary or other human organs (except lymphoid cells). LATS recovered in 7S peak and TSH in 4S peak on gel filtration. Anti-TSH serum inactivates TSH and leaves LATS intact.
6. Associated stigmata, eg vitiligo, as in Hashimoto and myxoedema families.	Antibody nature of LATS. Biologic activity is in IgG of patient's serum. It is inactivated by anti-IgG serum, which
7. Antibodies of thyroiditis also found in low titres in virtually all thyrotoxics. Higher titres in severe persistent cases.	does not affect TSH. Thyroid stimulating activity present in Fab fragment obtained by papain digestion of thyrotoxic IgG. After absorption on thyroid microsomes, activity can be
8. Normal men and children have lower incidence of thyroid antibodies than women, while in thyrotoxic men and children these tend to be higher than in the average female case.	eluted at pH 3.5. Treatment with steroids leads to disappearance of LATS, with return to pretreatment levels on stopping drug, as for other autoantibodies.
9. Incidence of gastric parietal cell antibodies (33%) identical with that in lymphoid thyroiditis, independent of treatment or sex and age.	LATS-Protector. Thyrotoxic IgG lacking LATS activity, able to stimulate colloid droplet formation in human but not animal thyroid slices.
10. Familial aggregation of autoantibodies same as in Hashimoto families.	Thyroid specificity of LATS. Activity absorbed out completely with thyroid tissue although LATS-Protector blocks this
11. Myositis of extraocular muscles in progressive exophthalmos, histologic similarity with lupus myositis and dermatomyositis.	reaction. Up to 30% inactivated with excess other organ extracts by non-immunologic mechanisms.
12. Enlargement of thymus with hyperplasia and germinal centres.	

33

In view of the growing importance of transplantation antigens in determining the sensitivity to infection in inbred animals and the finding of an
increase in HLA-1 and HLA-8 tissue types in lupus erythematosus and
lupoid hepatitis, 69 Hashimoto patients were tissue typed (Van Rood & Doniach,
unpublished): no difference could be demonstrated between the patients and
the general population in any of the antigens tested.

AUTOIMMUNE PATHOGENESIS OF GRAVES' DISEASE

The arguments for regarding thyrotoxicosis as a primary autoimmune disorder are summarised in Table II. The real impetus for this hypothesis was
the discovery and elucidation of thyroid stimulating globulins by Adams and
Purves (cf Adams, 1965; Adams & Kennedy, 1971) and many workers who
followed them.

LONG-ACTING THYROID STIMULATOR (LATS)

This non-species specific, stimulating IgG is detected by the McKenzie mouse
bioassay (cf McKenzie, 1972) in which blood ^{131}I-counts are measured before
and after injection of thyrotoxic serum or preferably immunoglobulins. LATS
is detectable in about 20-40% of thyrotoxic sera and the highest values (over
2,000% of preinjection counts) are seen in ^{131}I-refractory patients with pre-
tibial myxoedema. Concentration of IgG can increase the detectability of this
stimulator but leaves a substantial proportion of thyrotoxic patients in whom
it cannot be responsible for the hyperactivity of the gland. On the other hand
pituitary TSH or hypothalmic stimulation through TRH cannot account for
more than a minute proportion of thyrotoxics if any (Emerson & Utiger, 1972).
In the majority, TRH stimulation tests show an unresponsive pituitary and a
^{131}I-uptake not suppressible by T3, suggesting that the thyroid is being
stimulated autonomously, and in recent years numerous reports have appeared
of thyrotoxicosis developing in patients after hypophysectomy for unrelated
conditions. Perhaps the best evidence that LATS is capable of stimulating
the human thyroid is neonatal thyrotoxicosis where the LATS is transmitted
to the baby via the placenta and the disease subsides parallel with the half-
life of the active IgG. There is little doubt that LATS is an autoantibody
made in lymphoid cells (Wall et al, 1973) and it is likely that it combines
with the thyroid at a TSH-sensitive site (Beall & Solomon, 1971; Smith, 1972;
Benhamou-Glynn et al, 1969; Beall et al, 1969) and activates the adenylcyclase
cyclic AMP system at the cell surface (McKenzie, 1972). The objections to
considering LATS as the direct pathogenetic agent in thyrotoxicosis are that
it cannot be detected in all cases, and more serious perhaps, that LATS has
been present in a few euthyroid exophthalmos cases with suppressible iodine
uptake (Chopra & Solomon, 1970; Wong & Doe, 1972) and in occasional relatives of thyrotoxic patients without apparent overstimulation of their thyroid
glands (Wall et al, 1969).

LATS-protector

Adams found that IgG from thyrotoxic sera, themselves inactive in the LATS assay, could nevertheless block the absorption of LATS by thyroid microsomes in vitro and for this reason he called the new antibody LATS-protector. His finding has now been confirmed by Shishiba et al (1973). It was postulated that this blocking antibody might be human-specific and non-reactive in the mouse, just as LATS failed to cross-react with the chicken when this animal was used for TSH assays.

Human-specific thyroid stimulator (HTS)

Two teams of Japanese workers (Shishiba et al, 1973; Onaya et al, 1972) developed a new in vitro assay for TSH and LATS, which consists of culturing thin slices of human thyroid removed at operation in organ culture and then counting the colloid droplets formed on addition of TSH or other stimulators. They have found that all thyrotoxic sera, tested so far, greatly increased the density of colloid droplets in thyroid cells. IgG from thyrotoxic patients stimulates droplet formation whereas normal immunoglobulins have no effect. What is even more interesting is that no stimulation could be demonstrated in guinea-pig or mouse thyroid slices when LATS-negative thyrotoxic sera were added, while these animal thyroids were fully sensitive to LATS and TSH confirming the human specific nature of LATS-protector. In view of these recent findings there is perhaps no need to postulate that sensitised lymphocytes trigger the thyroid cells directly to produce excess thyroid hormone (Volpe et al, 1972; Solomon & Chopra, 1972).

OTHER STIMULATORS RELATED TO LATS AND HTS GLOBULINS

Although it is the thyroid gland which is primarily affected in Graves' disease, LATS has also been shown to influence a number of other tissues. In the human, the presence of LATS in cases with pre-tibial dermopathy and the improvement of the subcutaneous mucopolysaccharide accumulation with steroid applications suggests a connection. In animals, LATS globulin stimulates the metabolism of retro-orbital and epididymal fat (Hart & McKenzie, 1971). El Kabir and Hockaday (1969) showed that, in mice, repeated injections of LATS IgG caused stimulation of the adrenal cortex independently of the pituitary (El Kabir et al, 1971) and studies in thyrotoxic patients suggest an increased rate of cortisol secretion (Gallagher et al, 1972). The possibility that these side effects indicate a more generalised influence on cell-membranes is suggested by the work of Mehdi et al (1971) who showed a direct increase in membrane permeability of E. Coli by LATS IgG. Endocrine exophthalmos now appears to be causally related to the presence of an IgG distinct from LATS, assayed by its stimulatory effects on the Harderian gland of the guinea-pig (Dandona & El Kabir, 1970; Kohn & Winand, 1972), and by its ability to enhance the binding to retro-orbital tissue of TSH fragments with exophthalmogenic properties (Winand & Kohn, 1972). All these stimulating antibodies form a family of closely related IgGs with a capacity to react with different tissues, many of which are also responsive to pituitary TSH.

CONCLUSIONS

It is thought that thyroid autoimmune disorders are caused by a familial defect in immunological tolerance (Irvine, 1964; Weigle, 1971; Roitt, 1972; Bankhurst et al, 1973) which depends on a number of unknown inherited and acquired factors. Possibly there is a central defect of T-cell function and various other deficiencies at a more peripheral level which direct the attack to particular organs. The role of oncogenic or other incomplete viruses (icrons) in triggering the autoimmune attack is as yet unknown in the human, but is being studied in several spontaneous and experimental autoimmune disorders in inbred animals.

REFERENCES

Adams, D. D . (1965) British Medical Journal, 1, 1015
Adams, D. D. and Kennedy, T. H . (1971) Journal of Clinical Endocrinology, 33, 47
Bankhurst, A. D. , Torrigiani, G. and Allison, A. C. (1973) Lancet, i, 226
Beall, G. N. and Solomon, D. H (1971) in 'Immunological Diseases'. (Ed) Samter et al. Little Brown & Co.
Beall, G. N. , Doniach, D. , Roitt, I. M. and El Kabir, D. J. (1969) Journal of Laboratory and Clinical Medicine, 73, 988
Bendixen, G. and Søborg, M. (1969) Danish Medical Bulletin, 16, 1
Benhamou-Glynn, N. , El Kabir, D. J. , Roitt, I. M. and Doniach, D. (1969) Immunology, 16, 187
Calder, E. A. , McLeman, D. , Barnes, E. W. and Irvine, J. W. (1972) Clinical and Experimental Immunology, 12, 429
Chopra, J. I. and Solomon, D. H . (1970) Annals of Internal Medicine, 73, 985
Dandona, P. and El Kabir, D . J. (1970) Clinical Science, 38, 2P
Doniach, D . (1967) Supplement Journal Clinical Pathology, 20, 385
Doniach, D. and Roitt, I. M. (1969) 'Textbook of Immunopathology'. (Ed) P. A. Miescher and H. Muller Eberhardt. Grune & Stratton, New York
Doniach, D. , Roitt, I. M. and Taylor, K. B. (1965a) Annals of the New York Academy of Science, 124, 605
Doniach, D. , Nilsson, L. R. and Roitt, I. M. (1965b) Acta Paediatrica (Stockholm), 54, 260
Doniach, D. , Roitt, I. M. and Polani, P. E. (1968) Proceedings of the Royal Society of Medicine, 61, 278
Ehrenfeld, E. N. , Klein, E. and Benezra, D. (1971) Journal of Clinical Endocrinology, 32, 115
El Kabir, D. J. and Hockaday, T. D . R . (1969) Nature, 224, 5219
El Kabir, D. J. , Hockaday, T. D. R. , Richards, M. R. , Dandona, P. and Naftolin, F. (1971) Proceedings of the Royal Society of Medicine, 64, 2
Emerson, C. H. and Utiger, R. D . (1972) New England Journal of Medicine, 287, 328
Fagraeus, A. and Jonsson, J. (1970) Immunology, 18, 413
Fagraeus, A. , Jonsson, J. and El Kabir, D. J. (1970) Journal of Clinical Endocrinology, 31, 445

Fialkow, P. J. (1969) American Journal of Human Genetics, **18**, 93
Fialkow, P. J. , Thulin, H. C. , Hecht, F. and Cryant, J. (1971) American
 Journal of Human Genetics, **23**, 67
Gallagher, T. F. , Hellman, L. , Finkelstein, J. , Yoshida, K. , Writzman,
 E. D. , Roffwarg, H. D. and Fukushima, D. K. (1972) Journal of Clinical
 Endocrinology, **34**, 919
Gordin, A. , Heinonen, O. P. , Saarinen, P. and Lamberg, B. A. (1972)
 Lancet, i, 551
Guinet, P. , Tourniaire, J. , Robert, M. and Pousset, G. (1969) La Revue
 Lyonnaise De Medecine, **18**, 437
Hall, R. and Stanbury, J. B. (1967) Clinical and Experimental Immunology,
 2, 719
Hall, R. , Dingle, P. R. and Roberts, D. F. (1972) Clinical Genetics,
 3, 319
Hart, I. R. and McKenzie, J. M. (1971) Endocrinology, **88**, 26
Irvine, W. J. (1964) Quarterly Journal of Experimental Physiology, **49**, 324
Kohn, L. D. and Winand, R. J. (1972) IV International Congress of
 Endocrinology, Excerpta Medica I.C. Series No. 256
Lawton, N. F. , Hall, R. and Doniach, D. (1973) in preparation
McHardy-Young, S. , Doniach, D. and Polani, P. E. (1970) Lancet, ii, 1161
McKenzie, J. M. (1972) Metabolism, **21**, 883
Mehdi, Q. , Hockaday, T. D. R. , Newlands, E. and El Kabir, D. J. (1971)
 Proceedings of the Royal Society of Medicine, **64**, 1268
Mori, T. , Fisher, J. and Kriss, J. P. (1970) Journal of Clinical
 Endocrinology, **31**, 119
Mori, T. and Kriss, J. P. (1971) Journal of Clinical Endocrinology, **33**, 688
Onaya, T. , Kotani, M. ,and Yamada, T. (1972) IV International Congress
 Endocrinology, Excerpta Medica I.C. Series No. 256
Papapetrou, P. D. , Lazarus, J. H. , MacSween, R. N. M. and Marden,
 McG. R . (1972) Lancet, ii, 1045
Roitt, I. M. (1972) 'Essential Immunology'. Blackwell, Oxford
Rose, N. R. , Kite, J. A. , Flanagan, T. D. and Witebsky, E. (1971) in
 'Cellular Interactions in Immune Response'. (Ed) Cohen et al.
 Karger, Basel
Shishiba, Y. , Shimizu, T. , Yoshimura, S. and Shizume, K. (1973) Journal
 of Clinical Endocrinology, **35**, March (in press)
Shulman, S. (1971) Advances in Immunology, **14**, 85
Smith, B. R. (1972) Journal of Endocrinology, **52**, 220
Solomon, D. H. and Chopra, I. J. (1972) Mayo Clinic Proceedings, **47**, 803
Volpe, R. , Edmonds, M. , Lamki, L. , Clarke, P. V. and Row, V. V.
 (1972) Mayo Clinic Proceedings, **47**, 824
Wall, J. R. , Good, B. F . and Hetzel, B. S. (1969) Lancet, ii, 1024
Wall, J. R. , Good, B. F. , Forbes, I. J. and Hetzel, B. S . (1973)
 Clinical and Experimental Immunology, **13** (in press)
Wartenberg, J. , Doniach, D. , Brostoff, J. and Roitt, I. M. (1973a)
 International Archives of Allergy and Immunology (in press)
Wartenberg, J. , Doniach, D. , Brostoff, J. and Roitt, I. M. (1973b)
 Clinical and Experimental Immunology, **13** (in press)
Weigle, W. O. (1971) Clinical and Experimental Immunology, **9**, 437
Werner, S. C. , Wegelius, O. , Fierer, J. A. and Hsu, K. C. (1972)
 New England Journal of Medicine, **287**, 421
Winand, R. J. and Kohn, L. D . (1972) Proceedings of the National Academy
 of Science, **69**, 1711
Wong, E . T. and Doe, R. P. (1972) Annals of Internal Medicine, **76**, 77

Radioactive Iodine Treatment of Thyrotoxicosis: The Current Position

W R GREIG

INTRODUCTION

The clinical syndromes of goitre, hyperthyroidism and exophthalmos were described in the mid-nineteenth century while confirmation that there are remarkable amounts of iodine within the thyroid is due to Baumann (1895-96). Within four years ionising irradiations, in the form of artificially produced X-rays, were described by Roentgen while natural radium radioactivity was described by Curie and Bemont. As might be expected, external X-irradiation was subsequently tried in the treatment of thyrotoxicosis (Pittman, 1934), and George R Murray (1913) in his address to the British Medical Association said "The application of suitable doses of X-rays to the enlarged thyroid gland has in some of my cases proved to be of great value. The gland gradually diminishes in size and symptoms disappear. Atrophic changes in the secretory epithelium and both interstitial and extracapsular fibrosis appear ..... these changes are slow in development so that the full effect of the treatment is not obtained until some months have elapsed ..... in some patients there is great improvement or practical recovery but in others only slight improvement has followed a similar course of treatment. We have still much to learn as to the most appropriate dosage and mode of application of this valuable mode of treatment."

Plummer (1923) showed that when sufficient doses of stable iodide (as Lugol's iodine or currently as potassium iodide tablets) were given for several weeks a temporary remission of thyrotoxicosis could be achieved to allow partial thyroidectomy to be performed. This, together with the growing anxiety about the carcinogenic effects of ionising irradiations, made clinicians reluctant to employ X-ray therapy for a non-malignant disease. They were rather inclined to manage thyrotoxic patients either conservatively with symptomatic treatment only or in cases not settling they advised surgery after a short course of stable iodide (Crile & Crile, 1935). When thyrotoxic patients for some reason could not have surgery they might be referred for

38

radiotherapy but in general this was not encouraged (British Medical Journal, 1931). Effective antithyroid drugs of the thiouracil series (Astwood, 1943) and radioactive iodine (Fermi, 1934; Hertz & Roberts, 1942; Chapman & Evans, 1946) were subsequently introduced.

RADIOACTIVE IODINE TREATMENT OF THYROTOXICOSIS (1950-1970)
VARIETIES OF THYROTOXICOSIS

Much effort has been devoted to the classification of thyrotoxicosis, by cause, but the best that can be achieved is a categorisation under the general heading varieties (McDougall & Greig, 1971; McGirr, 1972). Goitre, diffuse or multi-nodular, with thyrotoxicosis and exophthalmos and sometimes pretibial myxoedema and acropachy (Graves' disease) is by far the commonest and is linked in some fashion to immunological disturbances against the thyroid (see Dr Doniach's paper). The disease is very common, there being about 500 new cases per million population per year in the West of Scotland. Toxic multinodular goitre, not associated with extrinsic thyroid stimulation by LATS or similar immunoglobulins, is, by contrast, rare in this country. There is evidence, however, that this type of thyrotoxicosis is not uncommon in areas where simple nodular goitre is endemic and due to iodine deficiency (Connolly et al, 1970). Whether thyrotoxicosis supervening on a background of long-standing nodular goitre, but without extrathyroidal manifestations, is a variant of Graves' disease has yet to be clarified. Other varieties of thyrotoxicosis are rare.

SELECTION FOR RADIOACTIVE IODINE (^{131}I) THERAPY

Experience during the 1900-1940 era showed that two-thirds of patients failed to recover from thyrotoxicosis and suffered either chronic relapsing morbidity or death; a third ran a fluctuating course and eventually became euthyroid (Havard, 1969). The choice of treatment was basically between antithyroid drugs for up to 2 years, antithyroid drugs and then operation or radioactive iodine (^{131}I) therapy. When ^{131}I became generally available in 1946 for the treatment of thyrotoxicosis its efficacy and simplicity was quickly appreciated (Chapman & Evans, 1946). There were, however, fears that the irradiation used might:

1. Shorten the life-span of the treated person by some unknown mechanism
2. Have a somatic effect on tissues leading to thyroid and other malig-nancies
3. Lead to unfavourable reproductive events and/or genetic abnormalities in the children born of treated patients.

As a consequence ^{131}I therapy was rightly confined by the majority of physicians to the following groups of patients:

1. Those over 40 years of age and only in the infertile or when pregnancy was deliberately avoided.

2. Patients less than 40 years of age in whom the life span seemed to be limited. This group included patients with diabetes and rheumatic heart disease.

3. Those patients who were less than 40 years of age in whom other treatments for thyrotoxicosis had been tried but were unsuccessful, dangerous or unacceptable. This group, who comprised in the UK about 10% of all patients treated with ^{131}I in the interval 1950-1970, included patients who had an undesirable reaction to or poor control with anti-thyroid drugs. It also included those who refused or were for some good reason not fit for operation. In addition those patients with thyrotoxicosis who had recurred after surgery were treated with [131]I.

In this country ^{131}I therapy was very seldom used in patients less than 25 years of age and only exceptionally in children (MacGregor, 1957). In the USA, however, some physicians did treat children and young fertile women and men. As a consequence they have been able to report on their experience in relation to clinical outcome, reproductive events, and genetic effects on living offspring (Starr et al, 1969; Hayek et al, 1970; Chapman, 1971; Becker & Hurley, 1971).

TREATMENT PHILOSOPHIES

[131]I (physical half-life 8.03 days) was chosen because it seemed the most appropriate on physical and radiobiological grounds; in early trials it was effective. It had been released for general use and was available in large amounts at acceptable prices. [131]I decays with the emission of energetic beta rays which travel up to 2,200 μm (average 500 μm) in thyroid tissue. The beta rays which have a finite path constitute more than 95% of the radiation energy deposited within the thyroid. Moreover, the radiation doses immediately outside the gland fall off sharply. This means that the radiation doses to tissues adjacent to the thyroid are exceedingly small in comparison to those within the gland itself. Doses given to the marrow, blood and gonads are roughly equal and are about 20 rads in average effective therapy (Green et al, 1961). Radiation to salivary glands, stomach and kidneys is likewise small, representing only a tiny fraction of that within the thyroid tissue which during effective therapy receives an average of 10,000 rads. [131]I also emits gamma rays which travel many centimetres through tissues and out of the body, but the contribution to thyroid or body dose is negligible compared to the beta radiation. They are of course the radiation used for diagnostic tracer tests but this is a different matter.

Pioneers were cautious in the use of ^{131}I therapy, starting with small single doses which were repeated until the patient became euthyroid. It soon became apparent, however, that the best philosophy was to attempt control of the thyrotoxicosis with a single drink of ^{131}I and thus within three to four months to shrink the thyroid, and to avoid hypothyroidism if possible. It was assumed that damage in the thyroid depended on the total radiation energy deposited there: the absorbed dose (rads).

The rad dose is dependent on a number of variables:

1. amount of ^{131}I given (MCi dose)
2. proportion of ^{131}I taken into the gland (uptake)
3. mass of the gland and to some extent shape (grams)
4. stay of ^{131}I in the gland (biological half-life)
5. distribution of ^{131}I throughout the tissue and cells.

The net damage within the thyroid from a given radiation dose in rads depends on distribution and on cell and tissue radiosensitivity (Greig, 1965).

Dose prescription procedures had in common measurement of a tracer uptake, measurement of gland mass by palpation (or, more recently, by scanning) and some empirical estimate of biological half-life, distribution and radiosensitivity. Some clinicians attempted to be precise and deposit a stated radiation dose in rads within the thyroid; a typical dose was 7,000 rads (Blomfield et al, 1959). Others accepted that this could not be possible because of uncertain variables and aimed at being accurate at getting a given amount of ^{131}I into the thyroid; a typical regime was 150 μCi per gram thyroid (Chapman & Maloof, 1955). Yet others prescribed ^{131}I on an empirical basis having gained clinical and therapeutic experience with a more rational approach such as that of Blomfield et al (1959). This experience allowed them to adjust amounts of ^{131}I for the size and nodularity of the thyroid with adjustments for factors such as the urgency for rapid control (MacGregor, 1957). It is now known that any one of these three methods gives similar results (Becker & Hurley, 1971).

EFFICACY

In the early 1960s the progress of 242 patients from the start of therapy (time 0) through 8 years of complete follow up was described (Greig, 1963). The regime had been to titre the amount of ^{131}I given in order to deliver about 7,000 rads to the thyroid (Crooks et al, 1960). Results are summarised in Figure 1. Sixty per cent of patients were rendered euthyroid within three to four months with one dose but a further 25% required a second dose and the remainder responded to a third dose. All patients were eventually rendered euthyroid within a year and there were no true recurrences of thyrotoxicosis. Others have reported a similar experience (McGirr et al, 1964). However, after patients became euthyroid, more and more developed hypothyroidism with progressive follow-up until after 8 years 41.3% were in this state and

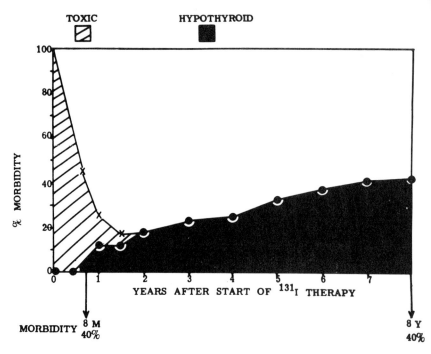

Figure 1. Summary of progress of 242 patients treated with a conventional single [131]I
dose regime – patients followed from time of treatment (0) through to full control and
on to 8 years (from Greig, 1963)

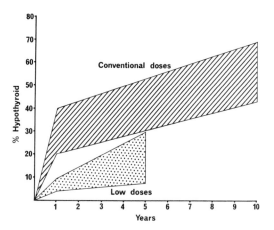

Figure 2. Graph summarising rates of increase in incidence of hypothyroidism after [131]I
therapy. Conventional doses are effective and of the order of 10,000 Rads; low doses
are of the order of 3,500 Rads. Sixty per cent of patients treated with low doses also
need antithyroid drug treatment for some time but the risk of late hypothyroidism is
not abolished.

only 52.5% were euthyroid (the remaining 6.2% were lost to follow-up). In the same study (Greig, 1963) a review of 134 patients who had ^{131}I therapy after antithyroid drugs and 59 patients who had ^{131}I therapy for post-operative recurrence of thyrotoxicosis was also reported. The clinical outcome in both groups of patients was substantially the same as in those treated with ^{131}I from the time of initial presentation.

These data highlight two of the outstanding problems of conventional ^{131}I therapy; these are the slow rate of control and, after a variable interval of euthyroidism, a progressive risk of thyroid failure. It is now established that ^{131}I used alone to control thyrotoxicosis will ultimately cure the condition in every case, but the amount of isotope given nearly always leads to hypothyroidism; the rate is 80% after a 15-year follow-up. If the initial dose prescription philosophy is set back at a low range, the rate of control will be unacceptably slow due to a slow response and the frequent need for multiple doses. Adjuvant therapy will then be required (Figure 2). If the initial dose prescription philosophy is set at a very high range, rapid cures will be obtained in the majority of patients but the same patients will become hypothyroid at a faster rate than with conventional doses. The dosimetric and radiobiological aspects of these observations are discussed below.

SAFETY — EARLY EFFECTS

A few minor radiation effects are occasionally encountered. Radiation thyroiditis is rare and seldom is there more than slight discomfort; the gland may be tender — exceptionally the pain may be severe. It occurs within a few days of treatment, and settles spontaneously or very quickly with a short course of prednisone. Radiation sialitis producing pain and swelling in the submaxillary and parotid glands is very rare, seldom requires medication and subsides quickly.

An exacerbation of thyrotoxicosis is difficult to measure so that its true frequency is not known. Thyroid crisis when it does occur usually does so in people who are severely thyrotoxic before therapy.

SAFETY — LATE EFFECTS

Late effects, other than those of hypothyroidism, are directly concerned with the risks of thyroid cancer, leukaemia or undesirable genetic consequences.

Thyroid Cancer

Thyroid cancer was a real possibility on general grounds when ^{131}I therapy commenced in the 1940s. This fear was further justified when it was shown that incidental external irradiation to children's thyroids during treatment of enlarged thymus glands or tuberculous lymph nodes led to a progressive

incidence of up to 30% of thyroid nodules and a 3% incidence of cancer after
a latent interval of many years (Hempelmann, 1968). Likewise it was shown
that children from Hiroshima (Wood et al, 1969) and more recently from the
Marshallese Islands, whose thyroids were irradiated externally by gamma
rays and internally by radioactive ^{131}I, ^{132}I, ^{133}I and ^{135}I were also developing
thyroid neoplasms (Conard et al, 1970). Nevertheless, X-irradiation of the
neck for thyrotoxicosis in the 1920s did not appear to be associated with
thyroid cancer (De Lawter & Winship, 1963). Yet, as a result of the observations in children and because of the enormous numbers of patients treated
with ^{131}I for thyrotoxicosis, the United States Public Health Thyrotoxic
Follow Up Study (USPHS) was started in 1961. This has reported on the incidence of thyroid cancer in 22,000 patients treated over the years with ^{131}I
and they have similar data from 11,000 thyrotoxic patients treated by surgery.
There was no difference in the thyroid cancer rate, it being negligible in both
groups (Sheline et al,1969; Becker & Hurley,1971). It would thus appear
that the 10 cases of thyroid cancer in the literature in association with ^{131}I
treated thyrotoxicosis represent remote and incidental cases (McDougall et
al,1971a and b). It has been pointed out, however (Becker & Hurley,1971),
that most of the patients examined by the Thyrotoxicosis Follow Up Study
were over 40 years of age at the time of ^{131}I treatment and the average
follow-up was only 10 years. It is known that the latent interval for radiation
induced thyroid cancer may be as long as 20 years and children and young
adults receiving ^{131}I therapy are at slightly greater risk than older people.
Thus although it would seem that radioiodine treatment for adults less than
40 years of age is safe, some caution is necessary.

Leukaemia

Leukaemia was one of the somatic radiation effects feared by those pioneering
^{131}I therapy (Stanbury, 1970). In the USPHS data from 22,000 ^{131}I treated
patients gave a patient follow-up of 119,000 years; 17 patients developed
leukaemia. In 14,000 thyrotoxic patients treated by surgery there were
114,000 years of patient follow-up and 16 cases of leukaemia (Saenger et
al,1968). Pochin (1960) found 18 cases of leukaemia in a total of 59,200
patients treated with ^{131}I in this country. It would appear that the incidence
of leukaemia is not increased in ^{131}I treated patients compared either to
surgically treated patients or to the general population (Becker & Hurley,
1971).

Chromosome Abnormalities

These are found in the peripheral lymphocytes of ^{131}I treated patients
(Speight et al,1968) but not in surgically treated patients. The lymphocyte
cells carrying these abnormalities persist in the circulation for many years

but do not appear to represent clones of leukaemic cells (Boyd et al, 1973).

Genetic and Related Effects

Genetic effects were another major concern of the pioneers. This aspect was not evaluated in the USPHS because of the difficulty in obtaining control data. Although the Atomic Bomb Casualty Commission surveys showed no demonstrable increase in major congenital abnormalities (Hollingsworth, 1960), stillbirths or infant mortality in persons born of parents exposed to radiation doses much greater than those from ^{131}I therapy, the safety of the latter in fertile women and men had to be established. Hayek et al (1970), Chapman (1971) and Starr et al (1969) have gone a long way to providing the necessary data. Table I demonstrates that reproductive events such as fertility, pregnancy and its outcome are not influenced by ^{131}I therapy.

Table I. Reproductive history of 103 women treated with ^{131}I

	Full-term children	Premature	Miscarriages
Before ^{131}I	174	11	28
After ^{131}I	142	10	27
(from Chapman, 1971)			

The dose to the ovaries after successful ^{131}I therapy is about 17 rads (Weijer, 1964). Two hundred and nineteen children above 3 years of age, born of parents (male or female) treated with ^{131}I, have been seen and the incidence of disease determined (Table II). These data analysed against the actuarial risks of congenital abnormalities, which for the whole population seem to be about 4% of all live births, show a miniscule increase in the risk of birth defects which might be attributed to ^{131}I therapy. This reassuring information is similar to that reported for treated girls (Hayek et al, 1970); 12 given ^{131}I therapy before the age of 18 gave birth to 18 normal children. Starr et al (1969) treated 73 children with ^{131}I many years ago and now find that those who were female (numbering 28) eventually gave birth to 52 normal children. Einhorn et al (1972) examined peripheral lymphocyte chromosomes in 33 children born to mothers treated with ^{131}I. The prevalence of chromosome abnormalities did not differ from that expected in a non-irradiated population; there was only one exception — a child whose parent received ^{131}I therapy during pregnancy.

It thus appears that the reproductive history and outcome is not adversely affected by ^{131}I therapy.

45

Table II. Ultimate health of children born to ^{131}I treated parents

A. **Fathers** - 20 children - 18 healthy - 1 urethral stricture, 1 congenital heart disease

B. **Mothers** - 199 children - 190 healthy - 2 congenital heart disease, 1 mongol, 1 club foot, 1 congenital deafness, 1 bilateral hernia, 1 XYY karyotype, 1 hydrocephalus, 1 mental retardation

Karyotypes determined in only 41
Aminoacid defects not found in 61 tested

Data shown indicate miniscule increases in congenital abnormalities due to ^{131}I.

(from Chapman, 1971)

The effects of ^{131}I therapy on germ cells of individuals or the population as a whole can be looked at in another way. The International Commission on Radiological Protection (ICRP) estimated in 1966 that for each rad of parenteral gonad radiation above background, the risk of producing a child with a transmissible trait is 1.6 per 100,000 live births. When patients are rendered euthyroid with ^{131}I the ovaries receive on average 17 rads. Now the spontaneous incidence of these anomalies is about 0.8% so that ^{131}I therapy will increase the risk by not more than 0.025% (Becker & Hurley, 1971).

Most mutations are, however, recessive and are not expressed in the first generation. The concept 'genetic death' is used to evaluate the effects of mutations on future generations. Genetic death is 'the extinction of a gene lineage through the premature death or reduced fertility of some individual carrying the gene' (Crow, 1957). It is estimated that if each member of the parental generation received one rad to both gonads there would be an increase of 0.1% in the genetic deaths occurring in each generation for the next 10 generations (ICRP, 1966). Means et al (1963) hold that the incidence of hyperthyroidism is 0.02% per year or 1.4% in a normal life-time. If 50% of thyrotoxicosis occurred during child-bearing years and if all these subjects received ^{131}I therapy, the average gonadal dose to the population would be 0.014 x 0.5 x 16.6 = 0.116 rads. This would increase the incidence of genetic death by roughly 0.01% per generation. Radiation from natural background is about 100 milli rads per year and X-rays add another 55 milli rads to this (Brown et al, 1968). It would thus appear that the use of ^{131}I therapy in younger people is unlikely to increase the prevalence of transmissible genetic defects in succeeding generations.

46

Effects arising from ^{131}I given during pregnancy should, of course, not be amenable to study since pregnancy is an absolute contraindication to this treatment. Nevertheless the population currently receiving therapy are predominantly female, some are fertile, and occasionally pregnant, and do not know it. Foetal hypothyroidism has been reported on six such occasions (Pfannensteil et al, 1965; McDougall, 1972). Usually, however, the baby is otherwise perfectly healthy (Silver, 1968). More often than not the baby is completely unaffected although one would presume that if the foetal thyroid was irradiated there would be an increased risk of thyroid cancer in later life.

Abnormalities of Calcium Metabolism

Damage to thyroid 'C' cells has been suspected after ^{131}I therapy. Certainly such cells resident in the thyroid must be destroyed in the long term as the gland atrophies. ^{131}I treated patients tend to dispose of an intravenous calcium load at a slower rate than normals or untreated thyrotoxics (Williams et al, 1966) and the effects seem to increase as the thyroid atrophies. Nevertheless, plasma calcitonin levels are normal in those without thyroid tissue (Gudmundsson et al, 1969) and in untreated and treated thyrotoxics serum calcitonin levels are the same as in healthy people (Fraser & Wilson, 1971).

Damage to the parathyroids is a possibility during ^{131}I therapy. Very rarely, relative hypocalcaemia, spontaneous or induced by stress tests (Better et al, 1969) has been reported and these effects have been attributed to radiation loss of parathyroid reserve (Eipe et al, 1968). In practice, however, neither blood calcium levels nor bone density seems to be any different in age and sex matched patients treated by ^{131}I therapy compared to those treated with antithyroid drugs (Fraser et al, 1971).

It can be stated that ^{131}I destruction of the thyroid does not result in significant abnormalities of calcium metabolism.

RADIOACTIVE IODINE (^{131}I) THERAPY
THE CURRENT POSITION

The choice between antithyroid drugs, surgery and ^{131}I therapy must depend on a variety of factors both medical and administrative and on the patient's own temperament and social circumstances. It is now known that ^{131}I therapy is safe, effective, convenient, cheap and simple. This applies to all patients over 25 years of age, provided pregnancy can be excluded. If enough ^{131}I is given, rate of control of symptoms is rapid and recurrence rate negligible. The debit side of ^{131}I therapy is the inevitable, climbing

47

incidence of hypothyroidism. Are there, therefore, any ways by which ^{131}I therapy can be optimised? By this I mean prescription of a single drink, all patients being made euthyroid by that, and for life, and none becoming hypothyroid. The initial response to therapy is unrelated to age, sex, degree of thyrotoxicosis or serum antithyroid antibody status (Irvine et al, 1962). Braverman et al (1969) have shown that patients euthyroid after ^{131}I treatment develop hypothyroidism more quickly if they receive stable iodide either as a therapeutic measure or if it is inadvertently administered. The post-irradiation thyroid remnant is particularly sensitive to the effects of stable iodide. The answer to the problems of ^{131}I therapy really lies in more fundamental aspects, namely the dosimetric and radiobiological events taking place at cellular level. It is therefore worthwhile recalling the structure and function of the untreated thyrotoxic gland, and considering what happens in the cells (Greig, 1965).

STRUCTURE, MICRODOSIMETRY AND RADIOBIOLOGY

In classical thyrotoxicosis there is an increase in the number of follicular cells (often in mitosis) and in the vascular network; there is a diminution in the proportion of the gland which is colloid. The apical ends of follicular cells (at which thyroglobulin secretion, iodination and resorption occurs) are in a state of very active pinocytosis in untreated thyrotoxicosis (Heimann, 1966).

Spontaneous thyrotoxicosis cannot be induced in animals but the functional and histological changes in the thyroid can be mimicked in rats given an iodine deficient diet or goitrogens. When the microdosimetry of ^{131}I and the radiobiological effects consequent upon it are carefully studied in animals whose thyroids are induced to undergo accelerated hormonogenesis and hyperplasia, a picture of what probably happens during ^{131}I therapy can be obtained (Greig, 1966).

^{131}I in the colloid homogeneously irradiates surrounding follicular cells (Figure 3). This is because the path lengths of the beta rays from ^{131}I are on average 500 μm and up to 2,200 μm. These dimensions are vastly in excess of the average length of a follicular cell, which is 15 μm. There is also mutual irradiation between contiguous follicles with crossfire through the interfollicular stroma. Thus the radiation dose from ^{131}I is relatively uniform throughout the gland, except for a small peripheral margin. If the gland is very nodular, however, there will be macroscopic inhomogeneity of the dose.

Therapeutic doses of ^{131}I kill cells outright by action on the nuclei or damage them so that they cannot multiply but they can function, or shorten their life span. If the vascular and stromal network is also disorganised there will be a slow, irreplaceable loss of cells (Greig, 1965; Philp, 1966).

48

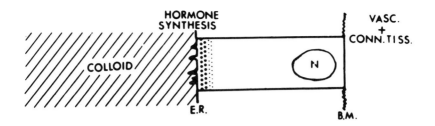

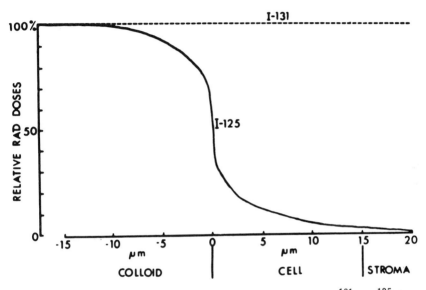

Figure 3. Relative radiation dose rates arising from equal amounts of ^{131}I and ^{125}I in an average thyrotoxic thyroid. Ninety per cent of nuclides are in colloid. Note that ^{131}I irradiates the hormone synthesising part of the surrounding cells and their nuclei (N) and basement membrane (BM) with equal intensity. [125]I, in contrast, delivers less irradiation to the cell nuclei, basement membrane and vascular or connective tissue (CT). ER = Ergoplasmic reticulum

In treated hyperthyroidism, the gland shrinks and the residual population of cells are abnormal since they are reproductively crippled. They may function, since hormonogenesis is radioresistant, but they have a limited life span, either by virtue of damage to the nuclei or because their nutrition is impaired. If such a population is under extrinsic stimulation by say LATS the number of thyroid cells and therefore the total hormonogenetic capacity of the tissue will fall slowly to euthyroid levels. If the population diminishes further due to the radiation effect on the reproductive integrity when accelerated cell turnover is needed, marginal hypothyroidism will ensure. At this point additional stimulation from pituitary TSH will be superimposed and it might be envisaged that the population would, from that point on, rapidly depopulate and frank, clinical hypothyroidism ensue. It follows from these considerations that the rate of control of thyrotoxicosis with ^{131}I must, and is, related to the total radiation dose given (Smith & Wilson, 1967) but the higher the doses the more rapidly do patients develop hypothyroidism. The only exception to this is when the thyroid is unusually nodular.

What are the implications of these points? Implied in the above is the acceptance of the principle that a dose of ^{131}I which is sufficient to control thyrotoxicosis in a reasonable time without other treatment inevitably results in hypothyroidism. The rate of onset of the latter is related to the initial radiation dose, the number of cells surviving the radiation onslaught and probably the mean cell life. It seems impossible to use a dose of ^{131}I which would produce permanent euthyroidism and no hypothyroidism (Greig, 1966; Greig et al, 1973). This hypothesis also implies that small doses which do not quickly control thyrotoxicosis may exert a progressive effect for some considerable time. Some workers have tried small doses of ^{131}I and have given those patients who were not euthyroid at 3-4 months, either potassium iodide (Hagen et al, 1967) in doses of about 90mg per day or antithyroid drugs (Smith & Wilson, 1967) such as Carbimazole. On cessation of such therapy many patients remain euthyroid. Propranolol, which has a peripheral action, has also been used in this context (Hadden et al, 1968) but not all the effects of thyrotoxicosis are relieved by this drug. It has the advantage that it does not affect thyroid function or measurements of hormone levels in blood.

It is wise to recall, however, that patients given small doses of ^{131}I are not in the long term immune from hypothyroidism; it seems that it is merely delayed for longer than in those treated with conventional doses (Werner, 1971). Also it is not in principle very satisfactory to embark on policies whereby a patient receives two types of therapy, since many of the advantages of ^{131}I therapy are lost.

IS THERE A PLACE FOR TRYING OTHER RADIOACTIVE ISOTOPES OF IODINE?

From a microdosimetric and radiobiological standpoint, ^{131}I is far from ideal (Rhodes & Wagner, 1971; Greig, 1968). Its location in the colloid confers no radiobiological advantages since its beta rays are so energetic they spray the surrounding cells, across the stroma and throughout the gland. Hertz and Roberts (1942) have used ^{130}I (Table III) and Berman et al (1957) treated some patients with ^{133}I. Goolden et al (1963) have shown that ^{124}I is an effective isotope for destroying thyroid tissue. I and others think that ^{125}I may have several advantages (Greig, 1968; Lewitus et al, 1971; McDougall et al, 1971a; Greig et al, 1973). ^{125}I has a physical half-life of 60 days and has a complex decay pattern which takes place in two steps, firstly by electron capture to Te^{125m} and subsequently to the ground state either by internal

Table III. Radioactive Isotopes of Iodine (^{127}I) of Therapeutic Interest (all emit 'B Rays')

Isotope	Half-life		Distribution of radiation in thyroid
^{124}I	4.2	D	Uniform
^{125}I	60.0	D	Very non-uniform
^{126}I	13.3	D	Almost uniform
^{129}I	16×10^6	Y	Almost uniform
^{130}I	12.5	H	Uniform
^{131}I	8.0	D	Almost uniform
^{133}I	21	H	Uniform

D = Days; H = Hours; Y = Years

conversion or by X-ray emission (Gillespie et al, 1970). Resulting from this decay, a rich cascade of low energy conversion and Auger electrons are emitted in addition to the electromagnetic irradiation. The majority of the latter pass through the gland without depositing energy and they account for about 20% of the total energy but the great proportion of the absorbed radiation dose within the thyroid is due to the low energy electrons. The majority

Table IV. Principal Emissions from ^{125}I and Approximate Ranges in Tissue

Number per 100 disintegrations	Mean Kev per disintegration	Approximate range in tissue (μm)
X and γ Rays		
23	0.2	100
112	30.6	30×10^3
24	7.4	50×10^3
7.3	2.5	70×10^3
Electrons		
376	2.4	0.02
78	2.9	0.30
156	6.2	0.40
15.4	3.5	12.00
8.8	1.8	15.00
12.0	3.7	22.00
3.7	1.3	26.00

Note the extremely short paths of the electrons (from Gillespie et al, 1970)

of these electrons travel no more than a few microns in tissues (Table IV). Thus the radiation dose rate from a source of ^{125}I in colloid falls over the short width of the colloid follicular cell apical border. In the treatment of thyrotoxicosis, 90% of ^{125}I is in the colloid and there is also a fall off in dose rate from ^{125}I across a follicular cell, whereas ^{131}I irradiation is uniform throughout the cell (Figure 3).

In thyrotoxicosis the proportion of the gland volume that is colloid is on average 15%; the remainder of the gland being follicular cells, stroma and vasculature. The follicular cells are about 15 microns in length and their nuclei lie about 10 microns from the apical margin (Heimann, 1966). During the passage of ^{131}I or ^{125}I from the circulation to the colloid, and vice versa, approximately 10% or less of radionuclides lie within follicular cells. It can be calculated (Gillespie et al, 1970) that the rad dose to the nuclei of follicular cells from ^{125}I is about 80% less than the rad dose to the apical margins of the same cells. Expressed in another way, it may be said that for equal concentrations of radionuclides in the thyroid, the dose rate from ^{131}I to the nucleus is very much greater than from ^{125}I for the same dose to the apical ends of the cells. Iodination of thyroglobulin, an important step in hormone synthesis, takes place at the apical border probably in close relationship to the microvilli (Stein & Gross, 1964). Pinocytosis of thyroglobulin, the essential starting point for hormone release, also occurs at the same site. It is conceivable, therefore, that hormone synthesis and release are preferentially reduced by therapeutic doses of ^{125}I but that nuclear integrity, responsible for cell replacement and vitality, is left relatively intact because the nucleus lies in a zone of low irradiation (Gillespie et al, 1970; Lewitus et al, 1971).

RADIOBIOLOGY OF ^{125}I

The hypothesis of selective reduction of hormonogenesis and retention of cell viability after ^{125}I compared to ^{131}I has been tested in animal experiments. In euthyroid rats fed equivalent doses of ^{125}I or ^{131}I, structural damage is much less extensive with ^{125}I than with ^{131}I; to induce the same degree of damage to rat follicular cell nuclei 20 times more ^{125}I is required (Vickery & Williams, 1971). Further proof that ^{125}I spares follicular cell nuclei is found in the retention of the capacity of the rat thyroid cell population to under go hyperplasia and hypertrophy when challenged to do so by goitrogenic stimulation. ^{131}I irradiated rats lose these aspects of cell viability much more readily than ^{125}I treated rats (Gross et al, 1968; Greig et al, 1970). The former authors showed that ^{125}I had a greater effect on hormone secretion than ^{131}I for the same degree of damage to nuclei. When the radiobiological effects of ^{125}I and ^{131}I are compared in rats pre-treated with an iodine deficient diet to mimic human thyrotoxic gland, the differences are accentuated (Vickery & Williams, 1971). In these circumstances sixty times more ^{125}I is required compared to ^{131}I to produce the same degree of damage to cell multiplication.

Also relevant are experiments assessing the effects of irradiation on cell function as distinct from cell multiplication. Munro (1970) showed that fibroblasts which had their cytoplasm selectively irradiated were highly resistant to the lethal effects of irradiation. Similarly the iodide concentrating capacity of single follicular cells in vitro was retained after as much as 50,000 rads of external irradiation (Dworkin & Carroll, 1968). Barzelatto et al (1962) showed that iodide incorporation into proteins, leucine incorporation into thyroglobulin and oxygen utilisation by thyroid tissue in vitro were highly radioresistant. It is of interest, however, that the different metabolic functions had different radiosensitivity, leucine incorporation into thyroglobulin being the most radiosensitive; this was reduced by 50% following 75,000 rads of gamma irradiation. Similarly Hall and Grand (1962) showed that it took 50,000 rads of external irradiation to reduce formate incorporation into protein by 50% in thyroid slices irradiated in vitro. Interestingly enough, a dose as small as 3,500 rads diminished formate incorporation into purines by 50%. It thus appears that thyroid cells have highly radiosensitive nuclei but relatively radioresistant cytoplasm. In the treatment of thyrotoxicosis we have in ^{125}I an irradiation whose microdosimetry is such that the cytoplasm of the cells receives much more irradiation than the nuclei. For this reason it seemed appropriate to try it in the treatment of thyrotoxicosis.

RESULTS USING ^{125}I IN THE TREATMENT OF THYROTOXICOSIS

Iodine-125 was first used in the treatment of thyrotoxicosis in August 1968. Ten elderly patients received therapy doses calculated to deposit about 10,000 rads at a distance of 10 microns from the colloid cell interface (Greig et al, 1969). This rad dose is similar to that deposited by conventional doses of ^{131}I. All ten patients treated with ^{125}I became euthyroid in a mean time of 8.5 weeks and none required more treatment. As expected, however, from the high nuclear doses, 30% have now become hypothyroid. The uniformity and speed of response suggested that lower doses would be equally effective and we thereafter embarked on extended trials, using different doses of ^{125}I (McDougall et al, 1971a and b; McDougall, 1972; Greig et al, 1973).

A total of 260 patients have now been treated and followed for an average time of 20 months (3-42 months). There were 7 groups who received differing mean doses of ^{125}I per gram thyroid (Table V and Figure 4). When 400 μCi of ^{125}I was administered per gram of thyroid, 88% were euthyroid, 10% hypothyroid and only 2% persistently thyrotoxic. At an average of 2 years follow-up, doses smaller than this lower the proportion of hypothyroid patients but increase the number who remain thyrotoxic and require further treatment. Larger therapy doses, presumably because of the higher nuclear rad doses, cause a progressively greater increase in hypothyroidism. With total doses

Table V. Results from Treatment of ^{125}I of 260 Thyrotoxic Patients at the Royal Infirmary, Glasgow

Group	Total mean dose (+1 SD) MCi	Dose given per gram thyroid (µCi)	Number of patients	Average follow-up (months)	Results per cent			
					Euthyroid	Hypothyroid	Thyrotoxic	Equivocal
1	6.9 +− 2.6	200	45	10.4	57.8	8.9	26.7	5.6
2	11.7 +− 3.6	300	61	11.3	67.2	4.9	24.6	3.3
3	16.6 +− 4.0	400	48	24.6	87.5	10.4	2.1	0
4	19.6 +− 4.6	500	32	25.3	65.6	22.9	6.3	5.2
5	22.7 +− 6.8	600	35	22.7	65.7	31.4	0	2.9
6	24.5 +− 6.8	700	22	22.4	63.4	31.8	0	4.8
7	32.2 +− 12.0	1000	17	29.4	58.8	29.4	5.9	5.9

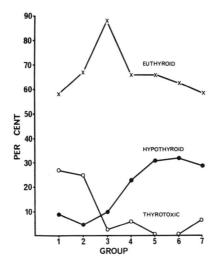

Figure 4. To be read with Table V. Graphs showing percentage of patients euthyroid, thyrotoxic or hypothyroid at about 2 years after different doses of ^{125}I. In group 3 who received 400 μCi per gram thyroid the results are very promising

greater than 25 MCi a rapid one dose cure is virtually guaranteed.

In a two centre trial in New York and Amsterdam, Werner et al (1970) found paradoxical results between two groups of patients who were treated with very similar doses of ^{125}I (10 MCi). Hypothyroidism was not found in 7 patients in Amsterdam but in New York 5 out of 6 became hypothyroid. Extension of the follow-up showed that 3 of the 5 hypothyroid patients were, however, only temporarily affected. Using similar doses (6.0 MCi), the incidence of hypothyroidism was reduced to 6%. Lewitus et al (1971) have argued that very small doses of ^{125}I are required to control thyrotoxicosis because of the intense apical irradiation but they have encountered recurrence of symptoms after initial control with doses as low as 2.5 to 3.0 MCi. This group now advocate the prescription of larger doses (5.0 to 6.0 MCi) or paradoxically a combination of small doses of ^{125}I with equal doses of ^{131}I (approximately 2.5 MCi plus 2.5 MCi). Since a surprisingly high incidence of hypothyroidism occurs after small doses of ^{131}I alone the results will probably be disappointing.

^{125}I THERAPY — THE CURRENT POSITION

In general the results of ^{125}I have been superior to those of ^{131}I therapy in several respects (McDougall et al, 1971a and b; Greig et al, 1973). The response to a single dose of 400 μCi per gram thyroid seems to be highly satisfactory. It is our clear impression that the rate of symptomatic response to ^{125}I is quicker than with ^{131}I, especially when account is taken for an equivalent hypothyroid rate at one year.

55

A preliminary plot of the time of onset of hypothyroidism in relation to time of ^{125}I therapy suggests that it may not continue to rise. We are not yet in a position, however, to recommend ^{125}I as a substitute for ^{131}I. We have found it to be extremely effective and the incidence of early side-effects appears to be just as negligible as with effective ^{131}I therapy. We have looked for thyroid nodules and carcinoma and found none and we have tested para-thyroid reserve and found it normal. We have calculated the radiation doses given to the marrow and blood and find they are not higher than those from ^{131}I (Gillespie et al, 1970). We are, however, reluctant to say that ^{125}I therapy is safe (New England Journal of Medicine, 1971) which we know ^{131}I therapy to be. Certainly until we know more about the state of the patients in the next few years we consider that the study is still a therapeutic trial.

^{131}I THERAPY — THE CURRENT POSITION

^{131}I is still the isotope of choice. Recent evidence shows it has no side-effects even when used in young adults, apart from the inevitable hypothy-roidism. This being so, several questions should now be posed and answered:

Which patients should be treated with ^{131}I?

What should the dose philosophy be?

What steps should be taken to supervise follow-up?

When is a patient hypothyroid?

What is the treatment for hypothyroidism?

WHICH PATIENTS SHOULD BE TREATED WITH ^{131}I?

All patients over 40 years of age should continue to have ^{131}I therapy by choice and without doubt the elderly, frail, and those with associated disorders such as atrial fibrillation and cardiac failure. The size and nature of the thy-roid should not influence this decision except that operation might be consi-dered when the goitre is exceptionally large or retrosternal. It is probable, however, that even the largest glands will shrink provided enough ^{131}I is given (Hamburger & Paul, 1968). There is no doubt that ^{131}I therapy is indi-cated for post-operative recurrence of thyrotoxicosis (McLarty et al, 1969) irrespective of the patient's age, sex or fertility, provided that pregnancy is excluded and avoided for one year after control. There is also much less reluctance to use ^{131}I therapy in young patients who have experienced a reac-tion to initial drug therapy. The presence of significant titres of serum anti-thyroid antibodies is no contraindication to ^{131}I therapy and, in fact, probably makes the case for it stronger; it is known that serological evidence of auto-immune thyroiditis increases the risk of post-operative hypothyroidism by a substantial fraction (Irvine et al, 1962). Similarly, patients who are not ob-taining control from drug therapy or who relapse after a course of antithyroid drugs given for 1-2 years (50% relapse) should have ^{131}I therapy rather than operation, in my opinion.

Patients less than 40 years of age with a large gland have in the past been treated, in this country, by surgery but this approach is not universal. Some clinics in the USA seldom refer any thyrotoxic patients for surgery and have experience of either controlling patients with antithyroid drugs on a long-term basis or referring them for ^{131}I therapy (Hershman et al, 1966). Certainly, the total morbidity from surgery may add up to as much as 50% (McNeill & Thomson, 1968; British Medical Journal, 1970) and perhaps if antithyroid drugs and ^{131}I therapy had been introduced in the 1920s surgery would seldom have been indicated in the management of thyrotoxicosis.

There are now very few absolute contraindications for ^{131}I therapy. Thyrotoxicosis at birth or shortly afterwards and thyrotoxicosis in pregnancy should not be treated with radiation. Similarly thyrotoxicosis in children and young adults should first be treated with antithyroid drugs and if this is not satisfactory by surgery or ^{131}I therapy. It is well to remember, however, that the results of surgery in children are not very good (Havard, 1969) and there is a place for ^{131}I therapy here too (see above).

WHAT SHOULD THE DOSE PHILOSOPHY BE?

The details of treatment are, of course, the province of the specialist in Nuclear Medicine or Radiotherapy working in close collaboration with an Endocrinologist. ^{131}I therapy should be organised on a regional basis with a central facility for patient assessment, dose calculation and prescription and follow-up.

In the elderly, frail and those with diabetes, rheumatic heart disease, rheumatoid arthritis, atrial fibrillation and cardiac failure, a large dose designed to quickly destroy the gland should be given. I now use doses twice those advocated by MacGregor (1957, 1963). If there is some risk of increasing the severity of the hyperthyroidism a course of carbimazole in a dose of 15mg every six hours can be given for a few weeks. This has the merit of initiating some control and depleting the gland of hormonal stores. The technique is to stop the carbimazole for one week, measure thyroid uptake by tracer, assess thyroid mass, and prescribe a large amount of ^{131}I. Some loading of the dose is probably necessary in this category of patient (Crooks et al, 1960; Goolden & Fraser, 1969). Carbimazole can be recommenced one week after the ^{131}I has been given in an amount of about 5mg every six hours but a careful watch must be kept for the rapid onset of hypothyroidism. Deliberately large doses of ^{131}I should also, in my opinion, be prescribed for younger patients who have suffered prolonged or fearsome morbidity due to post-operative recurrence, drug reaction, and poor control with or relapse after a long course of drugs.

How should we use ^{131}I in patients who have uncomplicated thyrotoxicosis? This group comprise mainly the relatively fit thyrotoxics in the 40-60 year age range or, indeed, young patients, depending on treatment philosophy. Most of these patients have moderately enlarged glands. There are two possible approaches, and each has its supporters. They may be summarised as:

1) Give large doses of ^{131}I from the start, anticipate hypothyroidism and either give replacement therapy at about 1-2 months or when the criteria for hypothyroidism are satisfied (see below).

2) Give small doses of ^{131}I and expect only a small proportion to become euthyroid at 3 months. If at 3 months the patients are still thyrotoxic, and on the assumption that ^{131}I will gradually create a progressive effect and the disorder will remit, give non-destructive antithyroid drugs or symptomatic therapy. In practice, this means adding either carbimazole in a dose of say 5mg three or four times a day or iodides in a dose of potassium iodide of 30mg three times a day or propranolol in a dose of about 20mg four times a day provided there are no contra-indications.

Of the three adjuvant treatments my preference is for carbimazole. Smith and Wilson (1967) used carbimazole in this way. They found, however, that 64% of patients treated with 3,500 rads from ^{131}I required drug treatment for a few months but 5 years later, when all drugs had been discontinued, only 7% were hypothyroid. It is interesting that no case given ^{131}I therapy and drugs became hypothyroid. The approach of Smith and Wilson (1967) could be combined with the suppression test described by Alexander et al (1967). If, after a small dose of ^{131}I followed by carbimazole for some months, thyroid uptake suppressibility returns, there might be a case for stopping the antithyroid drugs with a reasonable expectation of a permanent remission. The approach outlined does reduce the incidence of hypothyroidism to very low levels; the relapse rate is also less than that encountered in surgical cases (Wilson, 1967).

WHAT STEPS SHOULD BE TAKEN TO SUPERVISE FOLLOW-UP, DIAGNOSE HYPOTHYROIDISM AND TREAT IT?

It is obvious that enormous numbers of patients whose thyroid function is unstable require long term supervision if medical care is to be optimum. The problems raised here are formidable but as Philp et al (1968) and Hedley et al (1970) have shown, they are not insurmountable with present day technology. In the North East of Scotland thyrotoxic patients from a wide geographical area are treated at one centre, the Royal Infirmary. The physicians have kept track of ^{131}I treated and surgically treated patients by means of a computer-assisted follow-up register. When the patient has received primary treatment she is provisionally registered by the hospital doctor on a special register. After the clinical situation is stable, in order to minimise the number of patients attending hospital and to allow the general practitioner to participate in care, the patient is discharged from the clinic. When, however, the state of the patient is to be ascertained there is an automatic name recall and a follow-up kit is sent to the family doctor. This kit consists of a clinical hypothyroid index (Billewicz et al, 1969) and an iodine free bottle and syringe. The family doctor interviews and examines the patient and completes the hypothyroid index. He then takes a sample of venous blood and returns the clinical index and blood to the hospital laboratory. The protein bound iodine is estimated by autoanalyser. The clinical and laboratory data are processed by computer which segregates the information into normal results and abnormal results. If the results are normal, this information is automatically communicated to the family doctor and the patient re-registered for recall at pre-determined intervals.

Abnormal results are, however, scrutinised personally by the clinic doctor. If in his opinion no further investigation is needed, automatic follow-up continues. If it is needed, the patient is called to the clinic and re-management is initiated. After stabilisation, the patient's name and details return to the automatic recall system and follow-up at home continues; 94% of the family doctors in the region have collaborated, and the advantages are obvious. A much simpler, but less efficient method is described by Barker and Bishop (1970). The system described by Hedley et al (1970) has the advantage of flexibility. Thus, there is no reason why the hypothyroid index could not be modified, or a thyrotoxic index added (Crooks et al, 1959). In addition the serum sample could be used to estimate serum total thyroxine and T3 resin in addition to serum protein bound iodine (PBI). This point is of importance since a serum PBI is alone not a reliable measure of thyroid status (see also the contributions by Professors Landon and Hall).

SPECIAL PROBLEMS

1) Poor Thyroid Uptake of Therapy Dose

Potassium perchlorate stops iodide trapping so that the occasional patient who is taking the drug temporarily as a substitute for one of the thiouracils or imidazolines must stop it for at least a week before ^{131}I therapy is planned.

Patients who have taken stable iodides or iodine either intentionally or accidentally pose a special problem, because the thyroid uptake of tracer and therapeutic dose is blocked. The degree of blockage and the time it takes for recovery obviously depends on the amounts, character, route and duration of the iodide excess. Although the therapeutic dose can be adjusted to take account of very low thyroid uptakes, there is not much point in using this therapy unless the thyroid takes up at least 25% of the dose. There is no easy way of discharging stable iodide from the gland but in thyrotoxicosis the best that can be done is to prescribe antithyroid drugs and at a later date these can be stopped. If, after a week, the radioiodine tracer uptake is 25% or more, ^{131}I therapy can be prescribed.

2) Very Large Goitres

A very big thyroid is not a contraindication to ^{131}I therapy but treatment of such patients raises two issues — the amount of the therapy dose and the risk of an exacerbation of thyrotoxicosis due to the bulk of the tissue being irradiated and the possibility of releasing stored hormone into the circulation. A nodular thyroid of 100 grams in an ill patient might require 50 MCi of ^{131}I or more. There is not much to be gained from pre-treatment with drugs in this situation since the gland may increase in size and the drugs may at any rate induce relative radioresistance (Crooks et al, 1960). In this situation it is important to ensure that any complications such as atrial fibrillation and cardiac failure are firmly treated before ^{131}I is given. Similarly, propranolol may be prescribed (if there are no contra-indications) to subdue any slight exacerbation of hyperthyroidism. If there is a serious risk of exacerbation of thyrotoxicosis, there is no reason why the therapy cannot be divided into, say, two doses of 25 MCi separated by an interval of one month.

3) Radiation Risks to Others

Some ill patients are treated in hospital and they should be placed in a side-room and the advice of the Radiation Safety Officer sought. In general though, simple precautions suffice. These include a radiation sign on the door, lead aprons, and advice that the patient flushes the toilet several times. After a week no special precautions are required; no children should be allowed to visit during that week. If the patient has urinary incontinence she should be catheterised. If the patient vomits or soils the bedclothes these should be collected by the Radiation Safety Officer for incineration.

The radiation hazard to relatives and the public arising during ^{131}I therapy of an outpatient has been discussed by the ICRP (1966) and more recently by Buchan and Brindle (1971) and Pochin (1972). It is estimated that a husband might be expected to receive about 30 rads to his neck for every millicurie of ^{131}I given to his thyrotoxic wife; children receive much less. A working rule is that a patient receiving more than 30 MCi ^{131}I should be in hospital in a special hospital room for up to one week; thereafter she may return home. No special precautions are required at home but in general the patient should avoid contact with pregnant contemporaries and with young children for the first week.

4) Exophthalmos

The link between thyrotoxicosis due to Graves' disease and exophthalmos has not been fully identified. The balance of opinion is against an association with LATS (Munro, 1971) but Kriss et al (1967) studied the progress of eye signs in patients treated with ^{131}I. Serial serum LATS titres and serum antithyroglobulin antibody titres showed a rise in those whose eye signs deteriorated following this therapy. Others, however, have not found this (Munro, 1971). Kriss (1970) believes that energetic ^{131}I therapy does tend to lead to a deterioration in the ophthalmopathy when it is significant at the start of treatment. The mechanism for this, he believes, may lie in some common immunological link between thyroid antigen and an antigen in one or all of the extraglobal intraorbital tissues.

In practice, ^{131}I therapy given to people with uncomplicated moderate exophthalmos leads to a slight increase in this during initial control and is similar to the increase following antithyroid drugs (Greig et al, 1965). In the small minority of patients, however, whose eye signs are severe or progressive it is probably wise to avoid ^{131}I therapy because of the anxieties expressed by Kriss (1970). Certainly the induction of hypothyroidism in this group of patients has a deleterious effect on the ocular signs; flexible antithyroid drug treatment is preferable. Incidentally it was at one time thought that total thyroid destruction by removing some speculative but unknown antigen in the thyroid might lead to an improvement in severe ophthalmopathy. This theory has now been discounted in practice as shown by studies of Boyle et al (1969) and Volpe et al (1969). The specific management of the eye signs is, of course, a special problem and a decision about corticosteroid therapy or orbital decompression must in general be taken independently of the treatment for the hyperthyroidism.

ACKNOWLEDGMENTS

I wish to thank Dr I R McDougall for allowing me to use some of his data and Miss Joyce Muir for secretarial help.

REFERENCES

Alexander, W. D., Harden, R. McG., Shimmins, J., McLarty, D. and McGill, P. (1967) Journal of Clinical Endocrinology, **27**, 1682
Astwood, E. B. (1943) Journal of the American Medical Association, **122**, 78
Barker, D. J. P. and Bishop, J. M. (1970) British Journal of Preventive and Social Medicine, **24**, 193
Barzelatto, J., Murray, I. P. C. and Stanbury, J. B. (1962) Endocrinology, **70**, 328
Baumann, E. (1895-96) Physiological Chemistry, **21**, 319
Becker, D. U. and Hurley, J. R. (1971) Seminars in Nuclear Medicine, **1**, 442
Berman, M., Becker, D. U. and Benua, R. S. (1957) Journal of Clinical

Endocrinology, **17**, 1222

Better, O. S. , Garty, J. , Brautbar, N. and Barzilac, D . (1969) Israel Journal of Medical Sciences, **5**, 419

Billewicz, W . Z. , Chapman, R. S. , Crooks, J. , Day, M. E. , Gossage, J. , Wayne, Sir Edward and Young, J. A. (1969) Quarterly Journal of Medicine, **38**, 355

Blomfield, G . W. , Eckert, H. , Fisher, M. , Miller, H. , Munro, D . S. and Wilson, G. M. (1959) British Medical Journal, **1**, 63

Boyd, E. , Ferguson-Smith, M. A. , McDougall, I. R. and Greig, W.R. (1973) to be published

Boyle, I. T. , Greig, W. R. , Thomson, J. A. , Winning, J. and McGirr, E. M. (1969) Proceedings of the Royal Society of Medicine, **12**, 13

Braverman, L. E. , Woeber, K. A. and Ingbar, S. H (1969) New England Journal of Medicine, **281**, 816

British Medical Journal (1931) **2**, 760

Brown, M. L. , Roney, P. L. and Hilberg, A W (1968) American Journal of Public Health, **58**, 2267

Buchan, R. C. T. and Brindle, T. M. (1971) British Journal of Radiology, **44**, 973

Chapman, E. M. (1971) Missouri Medicine, page 21

Chapman, E. M. and Evans, R. D . (1946) Journal of the American Medical Association, **131**, 86

Chapman, E. M. and Maloof, F . (1955) Medicine, **34**, 261

Conard, R. A. , Dobyns, B. M. and Sutow, W. W. (1970) Journal of the American Medical Association, **214**, 316

Connolly, R. J. , Vidor, G. I. and Stewart, J. C. (1970) Lancet, i, 500

Crile, G. C. and Crile, G. C. Jr. (1935) Cleveland Clinical Quarterly, **2**, 23

Crooks, J. , Murray, I. P. C. and Wayne, E. J . (1959) Quarterly Journal of Medicine, **28**, 211

Crooks, J. , Buchanan, W. W. , Wayne, E. J. and Macdonald, E . (1960) British Medical Journal, **1**, 151

Crow, J. F. (1957) Eugenics Quarterly, **4**, 67

DeLawter, S. De W. and Winship, T. (1963) Cancer, **16**, 1028

Dworkin, H. J. and Carroll, M. (1968) Journal of Nuclear Medicine, **9**, 313

Einhorn, J. , Hulten, M. A. J. , Lindsten, J. , Wicklund, H. and Zetterquist, P. (1972) Acta Radiologica, **2**, 193

Eipe, J. , Johnson, S. A. , Kiamko, R. T. and Bronsky, D . (1968) Archives of Internal Medicine, **121**, 270

Fermi, E. (1934) Nature, **133**, 757

Fraser, S. A. and Wilson, G. M. (1971) Lancet, i, 725

Fraser, S. A. , Smith, D. A. , Anderson, J. B. and Wilson, G. M. (1971) Lancet, i, 981

Gillespie, F. C. , Orr, J. S. and Greig, W. R. (1970) British Journal of Radiology, **43**, 40

Goolden, A. W. G. , Fowler, J. F. and Matthews, C. M. E. (1963) British Journal of Radiology, **36**, 356

Goolden, A. W. G. and Fraser, T. R. (1969) British Medical Journal, **3**, 442

Green, M. , Fisher, M. , Miller, H. and Wilson, G. M. (1961) British Medical Journal, **2**, 210

Greig, W. R. (1963) MD Thesis, University of Aberdeen

Greig, W . R. (1965) Journal of Clinical Endocrinology, **25**, 1411

Greig, W. R. (1966) Scottish Medical Journal, **11**, 307

Greig, W. R. (1968) British Medical Journal, **3**, 250

Greig, W. R. , Mohammed, S. D. , Aboul-Khair, S. A. and Crooks, J. (1965) British Medical Journal, **2**, 509

Greig, W. R. , McDougall, I. R. and Halnan, K. E . (1973) British Medical Bulletin, **29**, 63

Greig, W. R. , Smith, J. F. B. , Gillespie, F . C. , Thomson, J. A. and McGirr, E. M. (1969) Lancet, ii, 1368

Greig, W. R., Smith, J. F. B. , Orr, J. S. and Foster, C. J. (1970)

British Journal of Radiology, **43**, 542

Gross, J., Ben-Porath, M., Rolin, A. and Bloch, M. (1968) in 'Thyroid Neoplasia'. (Ed) S. Young and D. R. Inman. Academic Press, London. Page 291

Gudmundsson, T. U., Galante, L., Woodhouse, N. J. Y., Matthews, E.W., Osafo, T. D., McIntyre, I., Kenny, A. D. and Wiggins, R. C. (1969) Lancet, i, 443

Hadden, D. R., Shanks, R. G., Montgomery, D. A. D. and Weaver, J. A. (1968) Lancet, **ii**, 852

Hagen, G. A., Quellette, R. P. and Chapman, E. M. (1967) New England Journal of Medicine, **277**, 559

Hall, R. and Grand, R. J. (1962) Endocrinology, **71**, 914

Hamburger, J. I. and Paul, S. (1968) New England Journal of Medicine, **279**, 1361

Havard, C. W. H. (1969) Abstracts of World Medicine (Review), **43**, 629

Hayek, A., Chapman, E. M. and Crawford, J. D. (1970) New England Journal of Medicine, **283**, 949

Hedley, A. J., Scott, M. A., Weir, R. D. and Crooks, J. (1970) British Medical Journal, **1**, 556

Heimann, P. (1966) Acta Endocrinologica (Kbh.), **53**, suppl. 110

Hempelmann, L. H. (1968) Science, **160**, 169

Hershman, J. M., Givens, T. R., Cassidy, C. E. and Astwood, E. B. (1966) Journal of Clinical Endocrinology, **20**, 803

Hertz, S. and Roberts, A. (1942) Journal of Clinical Investigation, **21**, 624

Hollingsworth, J. W. (1960) New England Journal of Medicine, **263**, 481

International Commission on Radiological Protection Committee (1966) Health Physics, **12**, 239

Irvine, W. J., MacGregor, A. G. and Smart, A. E. (1962) Lancet, **ii**, 843

Krisch, R. E. (1972) International Journal of Radiation Biology, **21**, 167

Kriss, J. P. (1970) Advances in Internal Medicine, **16**, 135

Kriss, J. P., Pleschakou, U., Rosenblum, A. L., Holderness, M., Sharp, G. and Utiger, R. (1967) Journal of Clinical Endocrinology, **27**, 582

Lewitus, Z., Lubin, E., Rechnic, J., Laor, Y., Ben-Porath, M. and Feige, Y. (1971) Hormones, **2**, 115

McDougall, I. R. and Greig, W. R. (1971) Scottish Medical Journal, **16**, 519

McDougall, I. R., Greig, W. R. and Gillespie, F. C. (1971a) New England Journal of Medicine, **285**, 1099

McDougall, I. R., Kennedy, J. S. and Thomson, J. A. (1971b) Journal of Clinical Endocrinology, **33**, 287

McDougall, I. R. (1972) PhD Thesis, University of Glasgow

McGirr, E. M. (1972) in 'Modern Trends in Endocrinology', Volume 4. (Ed) F. T. G. Prunty and E. Gardiner-Hill. Butterworth, London. Page 221

McGirr, E. M., Thomson, J. A. and Murray, I. P. C. (1964) Scottish Medical Journal, **9**, 505

MacGregor, A. G. (1957) British Medical Journal, **1**, 492

MacGregor, A. G. (1963) in 'Thyroid and Its Diseases'. (Ed) A. Stuart Mason. Pitman Medical, London. Page 19

McLarty, D. G., Alexander, W. D., Harden, R. McG. and Clark, D. H. (1969) British Medical Journal, **3**, 200

McNeill, A. D. and Thomson, J. A. (1968) British Medical Journal, **3**, 643

Means, J. H., DeGroot, L. J. and Stanbury, J. B. (1963) in 'The Thyroid and its Diseases', 3rd Edition. McGraw-Hill, New York. Page 232

Munro, D. S. (1971) Current Topics in Experimental Endocrinology, **1**, 175

Munro, T. R. (1970) Radiation Research, **42**, 541

Murray, G. R. (1913) British Medical Journal, **2**, 163

New England Journal of Medicine (1971) **285**, 1142

Pfannensteil, P., Andrews, G. A. and Brown, D. W. (1965) in 'Current Topics in Thyroid Research'. (Ed) C. Cascand and M. Andreolic.

Academic Press, New York. Page 749

Philp, J. R . (1966) Postgraduate Medical Journal, **42**, 437

Philp, J. R. , Duthie, M. B. and Crooks, J. (1968) Lancet, **ii**, 1336

Pittman, H. S. (1934) New England Journal of Medicine, **210**, 912

Plummer, H. S. (1923) Journal of the American Medical Association, **80**, 1955

Pochin, E. E. (1960) British Medical Journal, **2**, 1545

Pochin, E . E. (1972) British Journal of Radiology, **45**, 391

Rhodes, B. A. and Wagner, H. N. Jr. (1971) in 'The Thyroid'. (Ed) S. C. Werner and S. H. Ingbar. Harper and Row, New York. Page 163

Saenger, E. L. , Thoma, G . E. and Tompkins, E. A. (1968) Journal of the American Medical Association, **205**, 845

Sheline, G. L. , Dobyns, B. M. , Workman, J. B. , Tompkins, E. A. , McConahey, W. M. and Becker, D. U. (1969) Program for 118th Annual Convention American Medical Association, New York City

Silver, S . (1968) in 'Radioactive Nuclides in Medicine and Biology', 3rd Edition, Volume 2. Lea and Febiger, Philadelphia. Page 144

Smith, R. N. and Wilson, G. M. (1967) British Medical Journal, **1**, 129

Speight, J. W. , Smith, E. , Baba, W. I. and Wilson, G. M. (1968) Journal of Endocrinology, **42**, 277

Stanbury, J. B. (1970) Journal of Nuclear Medicine, **11**, 586

Starr, P. , Jaffe, H. L. and Oettinger, L. J. (1969) Journal of Nuclear Medicine, **10**, 586

Stein, O. and Gross, J. (1964) Endocrinology, **75**, 787

Vickery, A. L. and Williams, E. D. (1971) Acta Endocrinologica, **66**, 201

Volpe, R. , Desbarats-Schonbaum, M. , Schobakm, E. , Row, U. V. and Egrin, C . (1969) American Journal of Medicine, **46**, 217

Weijer, D. L. (1964) Journal of Canadian Association of Radiology, **15**, 153

Werner, S. C. (1971) in 'The Thyroid', 3rd Edition. (Ed) S. C. Werner and S. H. Ingbar. Harper and Row, New York. Page 697

Werner, S. C. , Johnson, P. M. , Goodwin, P. N. , Wiener, J. D. and Lindeboom, G . A. (1970) Lancet, **ii**, 681

Williams, G. A. , Hargis, G. K. , Galloway, W. B. and Henderson, W. J. (1966) Proceedings of the Society of Experimental Biology and Medicine, **122**, 1273

Wilson, G. M. (1967) Royal College of Physicians, Edinburgh. Publication No. 33, page 51

Wood, J. W. , Tamagaki, H. , Neriischi, S. , Sato, T. , Sheldon, W. F. , Archer, P. G. , Hamilton, H. B. and Johnson, K. G. (1969) American Journal of Epidemiology, **89**, 4

PART II

RHEUMATOLOGY
Chairman: Dr E G L Bywaters

Immunological Factors in Systemic Lupus Erythematosus

G R V HUGHES

Systemic lupus erythematosus (SLE), although a relatively uncommon disease, has gained increasing recognition during recent years as a model of immune complex disease. It is characterised by widespread and profound immunological abnormalities. While some of these abnormalities may have little clinical relevance, others have important pathogenetic and clinical implications.

The discovery of the LE cell in 1948 led to a wider recognition of the disease and to the discovery of a large number of circulating antibodies. These antibodies, while not the primary aetiological factor in the disease, may result in further tissue damage, either directly, eg haemolytic anaemia, thrombocytopenia or circulating anticoagulants, or through the formation of immune complexes.

While abnormalities of humoral immunity have been reasonably well-defined in SLE, evidence for cellular immune defects is scanty at present. Some of the major immunological abnormalities in SLE are listed in Table I. The present discussion is intended to have clinical emphasis, and will concentrate on selected aspects, in particular on anti-DNA antibodies and their clinical and pathogenetic relevance.

LE CELL TEST

Hargraves et al (1948) demonstrated, in incubated bone marrow and in clotted blood, polymorphs with large homogeneous basophilic inclusion bodies. It was subsequently shown that LE serum when incubated with normal bone marrow gave rise to LE cells and that the 'LE factor' was an IgG antibody to DNA-nucleoprotein. DNA alone does not absorb LE cell activity from the serum (Glynn & Holborow, 1965).

Antibodies do not enter living cells. Thus the reaction is predominantly an in vitro event, involving firstly the reaction of antibody with the damaged nucleus, and secondly, the phagocytosis of the altered nucleus by polymorphs, a reaction known to require complement. In vivo LE cell formation may

Table I. Immunological abnormalities in SLE

ANTINUCLEAR ANTIBODIES (ANF)

Double stranded DNA
Single stranded DNA
Nucleoprotein (LE cell test)
Nucleolar RNA

Histone
Histone-DNA complexes
Nuclear glycoprotein (Sm antigen)

ANTICYTOPLASMIC ANTIBODIES

RNA, Mitochondria, Ribosomes, etc

RHEUMATOID FACTORS

IgG or IgM

CRYOGLOBULINS

False positive serological tests for syphilis (STS)
Circulating anticoagulants
Antiviral antibodies
Antibodies against collagen
Organ specific antibodies
RBC, WBC, lymphocytotoxins, platelets, etc

---

occasionally be demonstrated in pleural or pericardial fluid.

LE cell preparations are positive in 70-80% of SLE cases and in other 'connective tissue diseases', especially Sjøgren's syndrome (Hughes & Whaley, 1972; Whaley et al, 1973) and rheumatoid arthritis (in up to 10% of cases: Lenoch & Vojtisek, 1967). Some 10-15% of patients with chronic active hepatitis demonstrate LE cell formation — this subgroup being given the confusing label 'lupoid hepatitis'.

Positive LE cell tests are occasionally seen in discoid LE and are a prominent feature of drug induced lupus having been found in 60 out of 66 patients with procainamide-induced lupus (Condemi et al, 1970). While the LE cell test is more specific for SLE than immunofluorescent testing for antinuclear factor (ANF), it is time consuming. Attempts to correlate positive results with the clinical picture are of little practical value. Nevertheless, the test continues to provide the cornerstone of diagnosis, its diagnostic significance being enhanced if the strong reactions (more than 5-10% of cells involved in an indirect test) are separated from the remainder.

ANTINUCLEAR ANTIBODIES

Antinuclear factors (ANF) are most commonly IgG although IgM and IgA (Barnett et al, 1964) as well as 7S IgM and even IgD ANFs have been reported. Although most ANFs are non-species specific, occasional sera react only with human tissue. Cryostat sections of either human thyroid or rat liver are the commonly used substrates.

A variety of nuclear immunofluorescent patterns have been described although there has been, if anything, a tendency to over-emphasise their importance in differential diagnosis. The commonest is the so-called 'diffuse' staining pattern which is usually associated with antibody to DNA nucleoprotein. The 'rim' or 'peripheral' pattern correlates best with raised anti-DNA titres (Luciano & Rothfield, 1972).

ANF testing gains in sensitivity at the loss of specificity. Thus its main value clinically is as a screening procedure. The diagnosis of active SLE is virtually untenable if this test is negative (patients with severe uraemia being a possible exception). Positive ANF tests, on the other hand, are found in a seemingly endless list of conditions, including up to 60% of patients with systemic sclerosis (Rothfield & Rodnan, 1968), rheumatoid arthritis, Sjøgren's syndrome, fibrosing alveolitis, Addison's disease, thyroiditis, myasthenia, leukaemia, pregnancy and burns. Positive results are more frequent with increasing age (Alarçon-Segovia et al, 1970) and in relatives of patients with SLE (Dubois, 1966).

ANTI-DNA ANTIBODIES

Anti-DNA antibody measurements using the Farr techniques have been shown to be the most specific and sensitive guide to diagnosis and to disease activity in SLE (Hughes, 1971). These antibodies were reported almost simultaneously by a number of groups in 1957 (Robbins et al, 1957; Seligmann, 1957; Miescher & Strassle, 1957; Cepellini et al, 1957).

Early studies used native (double-stranded) DNA as the antigen, but it was subsequently found that many SLE sera reacted more effectively and even exclusively with heat denatured (single-stranded) DNA (Barbu et al, 1960; Stollar & Levine, 1961; Arana & Seligmann, 1967). A variety of methods have been used in the studies of Anti-DNA antibodies, including gel diffusion, complement fixation, passive haemagglutination and radioimmunoelectrophoresis. With the application of the Farr ammonium sulphate technique (Wold et al, 1968) to the measurement of anti-DNA antibodies a clinically useful aid in SLE became available (Pincus et al, 1969; Hughes et al, 1971a; Hughes, 1971; Pincus et al, 1971).

The method is based on the precipitability of DNA/anti-DNA complexes by 50% saturated ammonium sulphate. A considerable amount of data on the methodology of the test has now been collected (Pincus, 1971; Hughes, 1973).

The most satisfactory results are obtained using internally labelled DNA, prepared by the addition of labelled thymidine to cell tissue culture; $0.1\mu gm$ of DNA (obtainable from Amersham Radiochemicals, Amersham, Bucks) is added to 5 μlitres of test serum. The addition of saturated ammonium sulphate in equal volume results in the precipitation of any DNA/anti-DNA complexes formed. A comparison of radioactivity in supernate and precipitate gives the so-called 'DNA binding' activity. Values of under 20% (at the present time, values of under 30% are for reasons to be discussed later) considered normal. Sera from patients with active SLE may give 100% binding values. In such cases up to 10-fold dilution may be required to attain a binding value below 100%.

CLINICAL STUDIES WITH DNA ANTIBODIES

In our initial studies, 83% of SLE sera had anti-DNA activity. In patients with clinical evidence of disease activity, this figure was 100% (Hughes et al, 1971a). Patients with other diseases in which the ANF test was positive did not have anti-DNA antibodies (Hughes, 1971). Since the introduction of the test to this country two years ago, over 2,000 anti-DNA estimations have been performed in this laboratory. The current data confirms the initial findings regarding the specificity and reproducibility of the test and will be presented in part below.

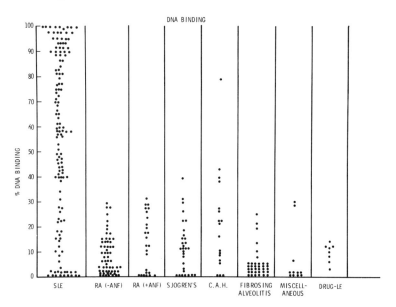

Figure 1. DNA binding in 262 ANF positive sera. A control group of rheumatoid arthritis patients with negative ANF tests is shown in column 2. Values of <30% are seen in all but seven of the nonSLE sera. Evidence of circulating complexes is shown by C_1q reactions and anticomplementary titre measurements

In an analysis of the patients studied at Hammersmith Hospital raised anti-DNA antibody titres correlated with a clinical diagnosis of SLE, as defined by the American Rheumatism Association (these detailed results will be presented elsewhere).

Of particular interest has been the value of the test in conditions in which positive ANF immunofluorescent tests had been obtained. Figure 1 shows the results obtained in 262 such sera. The data on chronic hepatitis patients was obtained in collaboration with Dr Deborah Doniach, Middlesex Hospital, that in fibrosing alveolitis with Professor Margaret Turner-Warwick, Brompton Hospital and the Sjøgren's data in collaboration with Dr Keith Whaley, University of Glasgow. A control group of RA patients with negative ANFs are shown in a separate column. It can be seen that with the exception of 7 patients, values in conditions other than SLE were below 30%.

In routine testing negative values have been uniformly found following viral infections, drug reactions and in a wide variety of conditions. In a collaborative study with Dr T Pincus, NIH, Bethesda, on 100 sera from children with juvenile rheumatoid arthritis and a variety of renal diseases only the SLE patients had raised anti-DNA antibody titres (Pincus et al, 1971).

From a clinical viewpoint, the superiority of anti-DNA measurements over previous tests has been in the assessment of progress and treatment. Of particular interest has been the observation that a rising anti-DNA antibody titre may precede clinical evidence of disease exacerbation (Hughes et al, 1971a). Such a case is shown in some detail in Figure 2.

A 31-year old woman developed SLE in 1971 during her first pregnancy with arthritis, skin rash, alopecia, mouth ulcers and thrombocytopenia. She was found to have a DNA-binding value of 87%, and low C3, C4 and CH_{50} levels, (the C3 levels only are plotted in Figure 2). With the institution of corticosteroid therapy she improved and the DNA binding value fell. During mid-1972 she was completely asymptomatic, but DNA antibody titres started rising and for the second half of the year remained persistently elevated at over 90%. In December 1972 she again became acutely ill with arthritis, pulmonary infiltrates and alopecia. At no time during the illness had there been clinical evidence of renal disease, although circulating complexes as detected by C_1q precipitation and anti-complementary activity (see later) were detected.

Lightfoot (1972) in a careful study of the prognostic value of such measurements attempted a correlation of clinical course with changes in haemolytic complement (CH_{50}) and DNA-binding. In 28 clinically well SLE patients in whom persistent elevations of DNA-binding were noted, 21 went on to a flare-up of disease. Abnormally low serum complement levels were somewhat less predictive, approximately half being followed by disease exacerbations.

71

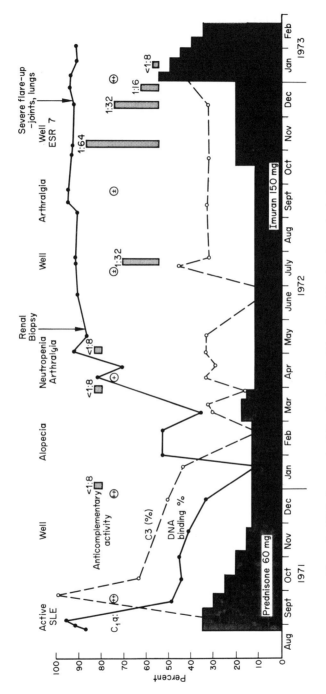

Figure 2. Clinical course in SLE patient. The DNA antibody titre (continuous line) after an initial fall to normal levels, became abnormal, despite the absence of clinical evidence of disease activity. The C3 levels (dotted line) after an initial rise to normal, remained persistently low

IMMUNOLOGY OF ANTI-DNA ANTIBODIES

Both complement fixation and agarose gel precipitation methods have been used to show that anti-DNA antibodies are a heterogeneous group, combining with a variety of sites on the DNA molecule. The details of these reactions have been reviewed in detail elsewhere (Arana & Seligmann, 1967; Stollar, 1968; Cohen et al, 1971). The majority of anti-DNA antibodies are IgG, particularly γG1 and γG3, ie those most strongly associated with low serum complement levels and active lupus nephritis (Schur et al, 1972). The antibody class bears no relationship to the property of precipitation of native vs denatured DNA (Cohen et al, 1971).

In view of the high binding of denatured DNA seen with many non-lupus sera, it is imperative to ensure that the radiolabelled DNA is in 'native' form. Methods of assessing and improving the nativity of DNA have included complement fixation tests using anti-nucleoside antisera (Cohen et al, 1971) or fractionation on methylated albumin Kieselguhr columns (Tan & Natali, 1970). Until more widespread standardisation of the antigen is achieved, it is safer to regard DNA-binding values below 30% as being within normal limits.

AETIOLOGY OF DNA ANTIBODIES

The factors leading to the development of anti-DNA antibodies in patients with SLE are unclear.

Experimental attempts to induce anti-DNA antibodies in a variety of species have had limited success. Christian et al (1965), using a complement fixation procedure, found that approximately 15% of sera of rabbits hyperimmunised to E. coli or S. typhimurium exhibited anti-DNA antibodies at serum dilutions of 1:100 or higher. These antibodies cross-reacted with DNAs from a variety of sources but were non-reactive with native DNA, ie they reacted only with heat denatured DNA. This finding was compared with production of rheumatoid factor — also produced by chronic immunisation and showing specificity for denatured products.

In attempts to induce antibodies by immunisation, two methods have largely been used — immunisation with intact DNA, and immunisation with a nucleotide or nucleoside covalently linked to a carrier protein or polypeptide. Using the former approach, it has been difficult to remove small traces of protein, leading to doubt concerning the specificity of the antibodies produced. Using purified DNA several workers have failed to induce antibody formation. In studies employing hyperimmunisation of animals with whole bacteria (Lackman et al, 1941; Christian, 1963), therefore, it is probable that protein-nucleic acid complexes were the immunogens. That this is the case is further suggested by the work of Plescia et al (1964) who found negatively charged DNA, complexed to positively charged methylated

73

bovine serum albumin effectively induced anti-DNA antibody formation.

Using the second approach Erlanger and Beiser (1964) have described the preparation and use of protein-nucleoside and protein-nucleotide conjugates, capable of producing anti-DNA antibodies, and Butler et al (1962) have produced anti-DNA antibodies by coupling purinoyl derivatives to proteins.

Using these and other methods, it has been found that experimentally induced antibodies have varying specificity, depending on the method used. In the case of conjugates of DNA with purines or pyrimidines the antibodies are quite specific for the base used, but cross-react extensively with nucleic acids from numerous sources which contain that individual base. In all of these experiments, it has been found that experimentally induced antibodies react either exclusively or preferentially with denatured DNA.

SOURCE OF DNA ANTIGEN IN SLE

Thus at the present time no experimental model has been devised for the production of antibodies to native DNA.

In SLE, the source of the antigen is unknown. Tan et al (1966) demonstrated free circulating DNA in the sera of some patients with SLE at times when anti-DNA antibodies were absent. This raised the possibility that DNA and anti-DNA could coexist, giving rise to potentially harmful antigen/antibody complexes. It was subsequently shown (Hughes et al, 1971b) that DNA release is not confined to SLE but occurs under a variety of conditions leading to cell death. In non-SLE patients thus studied, circulating DNA did not lead to antibody production.

It may be that further structural alteration of the DNA is required to render it more immunogenic. One interesting mechanism is that of ultraviolet irradiation. Tan (1968) found that in contrast to native DNA, UV-irradiated DNA (thereby altered to the form of thymine dimers) is a potent immunogen, and pointed out the relevance to human SLE, where the disease is often precipitated by sun exposure.

OTHER ANTIBODIES

RNA ANTIBODIES

Antibodies reacting with double stranded RNA have been demonstrated by agar gel diffusion and haemagglutination tests (Koffler et al, 1969; Schur & Monroe, 1969). Recently a Farr type immunoassay for the detection of these antibodies using a ^{14}C-labelled synthetic polynucleotide (Poly I:C) has been described (Warren et al, 1972). Antibodies against double stranded RNA have provoked the suggestion that the RNA antigen in question might be of viral origin (Talal, 1970). However, despite their prevalence in SLE and relationship to disease activity, double stranded RNA antibodies are not specific for SLE, being found for example in 15% of RA sera (Koffler et al, 1971).

74

EXTRACTABLE NUCLEAR ANTIGEN

Of possible clinical importance is the recent development of the haemagglutina-tion-inhibition assay for the measurement of antibodies to saline-extractable ribonucleoprotein (extractable nuclear antigen or ENA — Sharp et al, 1972). This antibody, while detectable in SLE, has been associated in particular with 'mixed connective tissue disease' — a syndrome resembling sclero-derma with some of the immunological characteristics of SLE.

While most studies have been concerned with DNA and nucleoprotein as the nuclear antigens, a third system appears to involve an acidic carbohydrate and protein containing antigen — the 'Sm antigen', this antigen occurring in about 75% of SLE sera (Tan & Kunkel, 1966).

FALSE POSITIVE TESTS FOR SYPHILIS AND CIRCULATING ANTICOAGULANTS

Perhaps the earliest recognised immunological abnormality in SLE was the presence of false positive serological tests for syphilis (STS). This finding may precede the other clinical manifestations of SLE by months or years. The incidence of biological false positive reactors who subsequently develop SLE is higher than might be expected from a random population (Harvey & Shulman, 1966).

A point of clinical importance is the association between false positive STS in SLE and the presence of circulating anticoagulants (German, 1958) especially against factor VIII. Fortunately, haemorrhagic problems in such cases are rare.

RHEUMATOID FACTORS AND CRYOGLOBULINS

Anti-IgG antibodies (rheumatoid factors) are found in approximately one-third of patients with SLE. The exact role, if any, played by such rheumatoid factors in the disease is unclear, though specific reactions between rheuma-toid factors and gamma-globulin complexes have been demonstrated. This interaction may occasionally be manifested clinically as cryoglobulinaemia (Agnello et al, 1971). While it is possible that rheumatoid factor in SLE may protect against immune-complex mediated renal damage, present clini-cal evidence does not support such a contention (Estes & Christian, 1971).

VIRAL ANTIBODIES

Following the report by Phillips and Christian (1970) of raised haemaggluti-nation-inhibition antibody titres to two paramyxoviruses (Measles and Para-influenza type I) in patients with SLE, raised antibody titres to Epstein-Barr (EB) virus were also noted (Evans et al, 1971). It is now known that a variety of antiviral antibody elevations are seen in this disease. Such findings are consistent with the existence of immunologically hyper-reactive state in SLE and do not necessarily carry aetiological implications (Hollinger et al, 1971).

ORGAN SPECIFIC ANTIBODIES

Despite the abundance of non-organ specific antibodies in SLE, organ specific antibodies are relatively uncommon. The most important are those against blood constituents although the action against platelets and leucocytes may in some cases reflect the secondary adherence of immune complexes rather than a direct autoantibody effect. The immune haemolytic anaemia which occurs in about 5% of patients with SLE is considered to be the direct result of the antibody on the cell surface.

SERUM COMPLEMENT IN SLE

As indicated in the opening paragraph, serum complement estimations have become extremely useful in the management of the SLE patient. There are eleven complement components plus inhibitors. In total these normally constitute together approximately 10% of the serum globulin fraction. Activation of complement occurs after an immune complex of the complement-fixing antibody and its specific antigen has formed. This leads to a complement reaction sequence or cascade and in turn to secondary actions such as those on cell membranes, the chemotaxis of neutrophils, enhanced phagocytosis, smooth muscle contraction and increased capillary permeability. It is these reactions which lead in immunopathological processes to tissue damage,

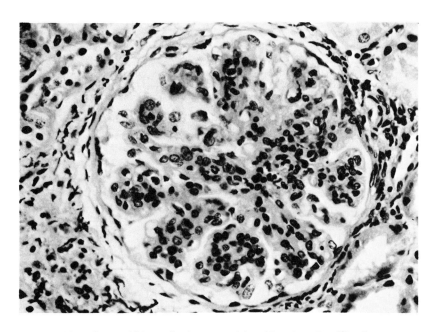

Figure 3. Renal biopsy showing mesangial proliferation. Renal function tests and urinanalysis continue to remain normal

particularly in blood vessels, or in the glomerulus, with its limited repair mechanisms.

Total haemolytic complement levels are depressed at some time in most patients with SLE, while normal levels are generally found in discoid lupus. Comprehensive complement profiles are, from the clinical management viewpoint, unnecessary. More important is the knowledge that in all but a minority of SLE patients low total complement levels reflect the presence of circulating immune complexes, and therefore, potentially of renal damage. In practice, serum complement estimations have proved by far the most sensitive guide to the presence of renal disease in SLE. Figure 3 is the renal biopsy of the patient discussed in Figure 2, in whom there was no evidence to suggest renal disease other than lowered CH_{50} levels and C3 and C4. With the use of such measurements, it is becoming clear that the incidence of renal involvement in SLE approaches 100%.

Recently low levels of C4 have been formed in the CSF of patients with cerebral lupus (Petz et al, 1971) although the diagnostic value of such measurements awaits confirmation (Bennett et al, 1972).

IMMUNOLOGICAL FACTORS IN THE PATHOGENESIS OF SLE

IMMUNE COMPLEXES AND NEPHRITIS

Evidence that the nephritis of SLE is immune complex mediated comes from a variety of sources (Table II).

Table II. SLE and immune complexes

SERUM

Low serum complement and nephritis
Anticomplementary activity of serum
Density gradient studies (+ DNase treatment)
C_1q precipitation
Rheumatoid factor precipitation
Anti-DNA ABs

RENAL

Glomerular lesions resemble serum sickness
Elution of anti-DNA antibodies
Elution of DNA from glomeruli
Distribution of DNA, antibody and C

EXPERIMENTAL

DNA injection into NZB mice
UV DNA nephritis in rabbits

Firstly there is clear association between lowered serum complement levels and renal involvement in the disease as discussed above. The serum of SLE patients may in turn show marked anticomplementary activity – itself a pointer to the presence of circulating immune complexes. Secondly, the glomerular lesions of SLE closely resemble those of the experimental serum sickness syndrome (Dixon et al, 1961; Germuth et al, 1957; Pincus et al, 1968) in which a small percentage of animals immunised daily with heterologous serum proteins develop chronic nephritis, with glomerular deposition of immune complexes.

That DNA/anti-DNA complexes might be of pathogenic importance in SLE nephritis is suggested by the high specificity of anti-DNA antibodies for SLE and the close correlation of the titre of these antibodies with clinical activity (Hughes et al, 1971a). The situation whereby DNA and anti-DNA antibodies may coexist in serum has been discussed earlier.

In addition, Koffler et al (1967) have eluted anti-DNA antibodies from isolated glomeruli by treatment with deoxyribonuclease. Quantitative immunochemical studies indicated that these eluted antibodies were present at significantly higher concentration per milligram of gamma globulin than in serum suggesting concentration and deposition of these complexes in the glomerulus. That this process was selective was suggested by the absence of other antibodies such as blood group antibodies in the glomerular eluate.

Direct evidence that the antigen (DNA) itself was also deposited in the glomerulus was obtained using fluorescein-labelled anti-DNA antibodies. The distribution of glomerular DNA by immunofluorescence was similar to that of gamma globulin and of complement (Freedman & Markowitz, 1965; Lachmann et al, 1962). Possibly one of the earliest changes in the kidney in SLE is the finding that fluorescein-labelled antibodies to pyrimidine bases of DNA become bound to the glomerular capillary walls, suggesting the presence of denatured DNA in these granular lesions (Andres et al, 1970).

Finally, in the New Zealand hybrid mouse strain, which mimics the human spectrum of SLE, daily injections of DNA into mice with antinuclear antibodies led to the deposition of immune complexes in the glomeruli. When anti-DNA complement fixing antibodies were present, the injection of DNA produced or aggravated an existing immune glomerulitis (Dixon, 1968).

Natali and Tan (1972) in a series of elegant experiments have recently provided an experimental model for the study of DNA/anti-DNA immune complex renal disease. By immunising rabbits with UV-irradiated DNA, antibodies were readily produced. The further IV injection of antigen resulted in immune complex nephritis.

SEROLOGICAL STUDIES
Apart from the indirect evidence of circulating complexes provided by serum complement estimations, more direct methods are available. The best

method involves the use of sucrose density gradient with ultracentrifugation. In such studies, heavy sedimenting gamma-globulin may be detected. Treatment with the enzyme DNAse shows shifting of the 'shoulder' of heavy sedimenting immunoglobulin to lighter portions of the gradient, suggesting that at least a considerable fraction of the globulin was complexed to DNA (Natali & Tan, 1972).

Two further methods for the measurement of immune complexes have recently been described in Kunkel's laboratory at the Rockefeller University — precipitation against the first component of complement (C_1q) in low ionic strength agarose (Agnello et al, 1969) and the agarose gel precipitation against monoclonal rheumatoid factor (Winchester et al, 1971). In the studies of Agnello, 23 out of 83 SLE sera gave precipitin reactions with C_1q. All were in hypocomplementaemic sera. In our own experience, the correlation between C_1q precipitability and disease activity or DNA antibody titres is variable.

THE AETIOLOGY OF SLE

While the aetiology of SLE is unknown, two aspects have recently received increasing attention — viral and genetic factors.

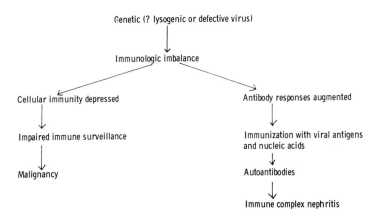

Figure 4. Pathogenesis of autoimmunity and malignancy in New Zealand mice (Talal, 1970)

Talal, using data obtained from the studies of the animal SLE model, the NZB mouse, has proposed a scheme by which such factors could interact (Figure 4) and has discussed their relevance to human SLE. A number of examples of viral infection in animals has been shown to contribute to tissue injury through the mediation of virus-containing immune complexes (Oldstone & Dixon, 1970). In the NZB mouse, where genetic factors are paramount, depressed cellular immunity may be an important factor in the persistence of viraemia (Leventhal & Talal, 1970). In human SLE, while the similarities with the disease of NZB mice are striking, no direct evidence for a viral infectious aetiology exists at the present time.

CONCLUSIONS

While some of the immunological findings described above seem far removed from the clinical arena, they may provide a theoretical basis for new approaches to therapy.

From the more immediate standpoint of practical therapeutics, the introduction of a sensitive assay for the measurement of anti-DNA antibodies, together with the use of serum complement estimations, have already begun to contribute to more precise management of this disease.

ACKNOWLEDGMENTS

I would like to thank Dr Charles Christian, New York and Professor E G L Bywaters for their help and advice. I am grateful to Dr D Brown, Department of Immunology, Hammersmith Hospital for antinuclear factor tests, Dr W Doe, Department of Gastroenterology for C_1q precipitation analyses and Miss Brenda Atkins for technical assistance.

Figure 4 is published by kind permission of Dr N Talal and the editor of 'Arthritis and Rheumatism'.

REFERENCES

Agnello, V., Eisenberg, J. W., Koffler, D., Winchester, R. J. and Kunkel, H. G. (1971) Arthritis and Rheumatism, **14**, 147 (Abstract)

Agnello, V., Winchester, R. J. and Kunkel, H. G. (1969) Arthritis and Rheumatism, **12**, 654

Alarçon-Segovia, D., Fishbein, E., Alcala, H., Olguin-Palacios, E. and Estrada-Parra, S. (1970) Clinical and Experimental Immunology, **6**, 557

Andres, G. A., Accinni, L., Beiser, S. M., Christian, C. L., Cinotti, G. A., Erlanger, E. F., Hsu, K. C. and Seegal, B. C. (1970) Journal of Clinical Investigation, **49**, 2106

Arana, R. and Seligmann, M. (1967) Journal of Clinical Investigation, **46**, 1867

Barbu, E., Seligmann, M. and Joly, M. (1960) Annales de l'Institut Pasteur, 99, 695

Barnett, E. V., Condemi, J. J., Leddy, J. P. and Vaughan, J. H. (1964) Journal of Clinical Investigation, **43**, 1104

Bennett, R. M., Hughes, G. R. V., Bywaters, E. G. L. and Holt, P.J.L. (1972) British Medical Journal, **2**, 342

Butler, V. P., Beiser, S. M., Erlanger, B. F., Tanenbaum, S. W., Cohen, S. and Bendich, A. (1962) Proceedings of the National Academy of Sciences of the USA, **48**, 1597

Cepellini, R., Polli, C. and Celada, F. (1957) Proceedings of the Society for Experimental Biology and Medicine, **96**, 572

Christian, C. L. (1963) Journal of Experimental Medicine, **118**, 827

Christian, C. L., Abruzzo, J. L., De Simone, A. R. and Howes, E. L. (1965) Annals of the New York Academy of Science, **124**, 143

Cohen, S. A., Hughes, G. R.V., Noel, G.and Christian, C. L. (1972) Clinical and Experimental Immunology, **8**, 551

Condemi, J. J., Blomgren, S . E. and Vaughan, J. H. (1970) Bulletin of the Rheumatic Diseases, **20**, 604

Dixon, F. J. (1968) Proceedings of the 5th International Symposium of Immunopathology. Punta Ala, 1968. (Schwabe)

Dixon, F. J., Feldman, J. D. and Vasquez, J. J. (1961) Journal of Experimental Medicine, **113**, 899

Dubois, E. L. (1966) Lupus Erythematosus. Discoid and Systemic. McGraw-Hill, New York

Erlanger, B. F. and Beiser, S. M. (1964) Proceedings of the National Academy of Sciences of the USA, **52**, 68

Estes, D. C. and Christian, C. L. (1971) Medicine, **50**, 85

Evans, A. S., Niederman, J. C. and Rothfield, N. F. (1971) Lancet, **i**, 167

Freedman, P. and Markowitz, A. S. (1965) Journal of Clinical Investigation, **44**, 1657

German, J. L. (1958) Journal of Experimental Medicine, **108**, 179

Germuth, F. G . Jr., Flanagan, C .and Montenegro, M. R. (1957) Bulletin of the Johns Hopkins Hospital, **101**, 149

Glynn, L. E. and Holborow, E . J. (1965) 'Autoimmunity and Disease'. Blackwell, Oxford

Hargraves, M. M., Richmond, H. and Morton, R. (1948) Proceedings of the Staff Meeting at the Mayo Clinic, **23**, 25

Harvey, A. M. and Shulman, L. E. (1966) in 'Dubois's Lupus Erythematosus'. McGraw-Hill, New York. Page 104

Hollinger, F. B., Sharp, J. T., Lidsky, M. D. and Rawls, W. E .(1971) Arthritis and Rheumatism, **14**, 1

Hughes, G. R. V. (1971) Lancet, **ii**, 861

Hughes, G. R. V. (1973) MD Thesis, London University

Hughes, G. R. V., Cohen, S. A. and Christian, C. L. (1971a) Annals of the Rheumatic Diseases, **30**, 259

Hughes, G. R.V., Cohen, S . A., Lightfoot, R. W., Meltzer, J. I. and Christian, C. L. (1971b) Arthritis and Rheumatism, **14**, 259

Hughes, G. R. V. and Whaley, K. (1972) British Medical Journal, **4**, 533

Koffler, D., Carr, R. I., Agnello, V., Feizi, T .and Kunkel, H. G. (1969) Sciences (Washington), **166**, 1648

Koffler, D., Carr, R. I., Agnello, V., Thoburn, R. and Kunkel, H. G. (1971) Journal of Experimental Medicine, **134**, 294

Koffler, D., Schur, P. H. and Kunkel, H. G. (1967) Journal of Experimental Medicine, **126**, 607

Lachmann, P. J., Muller-Eberhard, H. J., Kunkel, H. G. and Paronetto, F. (1962) Journal of Experimental Medicine, **115**, 63

Lackman, D., Mudd, S., Sevag, M. G., Smolens, J. and Weiner, M. (1941) Journal of Immunology, **40**, 1

Lenoch, F. and Vojtisek, O. (1967) Acta rheumatologica Scandinavia, **13**, 313

Leventhal, B. G. and Talal, N. (1970) Journal of Immunology, **104**, 918

Lightfoot, R. W. (1972) 36th Annual Meeting of the American Rheumatism Association, June 1972 at Dallas (Abstract)

Luciano, A. A. and Rothfield, N. F. (1972) Arthritis and Rheumatism, **15**, 118 (Abstract)

Miescher, P. and Strassle, R. (1957) Vox sanguinis, **2**, 283

Natali, P. G .and Tan, E. M. (1972) Journal of Clinical Investigation, **51**, 345

Oldstone, M. B. A. and Dixon, F. J. (1970) Journal of Experimental Medicine, **131**, 1

Petz, L. D., Sharp, G. C., Cooper, N. R. and Irvin, W. S. (1971) Medicine, **50**, 259

Phillips, P. and Christian, C. L. (1970) Science, **168**, 982

Pincus, T. (1971) Arthritis and Rheumatism, **14**, 623

Pincus, T., Haberkern, R. and Christian, C. L. (1968) Journal of Experimental Medicine, **127**, 819

Pincus, T., Hughes, G. R. V., Pincus, D., Tina, L. U. and Bellanti, J. A. (1971) Journal of Pediatrics, **78**, 981

Pincus, T., Schur, P. H., Rose, J. A., Decker, J. L. and Talal, N. (1969)

New England Journal of Medicine, 281, 701

Plescia, O. J., Braun, W. and Palczu, N. C. (1964) Proceedings of the National Academy of Sciences of the USA, 52, 279

Robbins, W. C., Holman, H. R., Deicher, H. and Kunkel, H. G. (1957) Proceedings of the Society for Experimental Biology and Medicine, 96, 575

Rothfield, N. F. and Rodnan, G. P. (1968) Arthritis and Rheumatism, 11, 607

Schur, P. H. and Monroe, N. (1969) Proceedings of the National Academy of Sciences of the USA, 63, 1108

Schur, P. H., Monroe, N. and Rothfield, N. (1972) Arthritis and Rheumatism, 15, 174

Seligmann, M. (1957) Comptes Rendus Hebdomadaires des Sances de l'Academie des Sciences, 245, 243

Sharp, G. C., Irvin, W. S., Tan, E. M., Gould, R. G. and Holman, H. R. (1972) American Journal of Medicine, 52, 148

Stollar, B. D. (1968) 'Nucleic Acids in Immunology'. (Ed) Plescia and Braun. Springer-Verlag, Berlin. Page 114

Stollar, B. D. and Levine, L. (1961) Journal of Immunology, 87, 477

Talal, N. (1970) Arthritis and Rheumatism, 13, 887

Tan, E. M. (1968) Science, 161, 1353

Tan, E. M. and Kunkel, H. G. (1966) Journal of Immunology, 96, 464

Tan, E. M. and Natali, P. G. (1970) Journal of Immunology, 104, 902

Tan, E. M., Schur, P. H., Carr, R. I. and Kunkel, H. G. (1966) Journal of Clinical Investigation, 45, 1732

Warren, R. D., Henry, P. H., Irvin, W. S. and Sharp, G. C. (1972) 36th Annual Meeting of the American Rheumatism Association, June 1972 in Dallas (Abstract)

Whaley, K., Webb, J., McAvoy, B. A., Hughes, G. R. V., MacSween, R. N. M. and Buchanan, W. W. (1973) Quarterly Journal of Medicine (in press)

Winchester, R. J., Kunkel, H. G. and Agnello, V .(1971) Journal of Experimental Medicine, 134, 2865

Wold, R. T., Young, F. E., Tan, E. M. and Farr, R. S. (1968) Science, 161, 806

Immunopathological Mechanisms in Rheumatoid Arthritis

I M ROITT

Rheumatoid arthritis is primarily an inflammatory disorder of joints, despite the variety of possible systemic manifestations. The infiltration of synovial tissue with mononuclear cells including plasma cells actively synthesising immunoglobulin, the formation there of lymphoid aggregates, and an ever increasing number of abnormal immunological findings have served to sustain and indeed to strengthen the now commonly held view that immunopathological processes directly underlie the development of joint lesions in this disease. I intend to review some of the evidence bearing on this question; no attempt has been made, however, to cover topics such as genetic influences and the effectiveness of immunosuppressive therapy.

ANTIGLOBULIN FACTORS

One of the most characteristic serological features is, of course, the presence of rheumatoid (or preferably 'antiglobulin') factors which are antibodies directed against the host's IgG. Classically these were recognised to be IgM antiglobulins detectable by the agglutination of sheep cells coated with rabbit antibody or latex particles bearing human IgG, but they can also be detected in other immunoglobulin classes. Because of their readiness to bind with IgG altered by heat aggregation or by formation of an immune complex, it has usually been considered that the stimulus for synthesis of antiglobulins has come from IgG which had undergone a structural change in vivo either through abnormal physical conditions or proteolytic enzyme action generated by inflammation or through complexing with an antigen. The latter view receives support from the high incidence of antiglobulins in chronic infective disorders (Williams & Kunkel, 1962; Bartfeld, 1969) and in hyperimmunized animals (Christian, 1963).

The antiglobulins in sera from rheumatoid arthritis show reactivity against a number of specificities in the IgG molecule (Kunkel & Tan, 1964; see Hood & Prahl, 1971) which amongst other considerations has helped to define genetic marker systems such as Gm and Inv (Grubb, 1970; Natvig & Turner, 1971). A reaction with native IgG as distinct from altered IgG can undoubtedly be shown as, for example, in the 22S IgM-IgG complexes of patients' sera (Schur & Kunkel, 1965), the inhibition of Gm agglutination reactions and the demonstration of some rheumatoid factor specificities hidden by complexing with autolous IgG (Allen & Kunkel, 1966). Thus, it has been suggested that the full determinants for reaction with rheumatoid factors are already present on native IgG and that precipitation does not occur with the native molecule perhaps because this behaves as a monovalent antigen; on this basis the apparent superiority of aggregated or complexed IgG as an antigen and the inability of native IgG to complete with it (Henney, 1969) is ascribed merely to the multivalence of the aggregated form. However, the affinity of rheumatoid factors for native IgG seems to be relatively weak (eg Cerottini & Grey, 1969) whereas the binding to aggregated IgG is particularly firm and, furthermore, the data on the cross-reactions with IgG of other species are indicative of specificities linked to determinants either 'buried' in the native molecule or formed by conformational changes associated with denaturation or complex formation (Glynn, 1968a). The high circulating concentration of native IgG throughout life would ensure the maintenance of immunological tolerance in the appropriate thymus-dependent (T) lymphocyte population and of those thymus-independent (B) lymphocytes (Roitt et al, 1969) with receptors of moderate to high binding avidity (Chiller et al, 1970). But the ease with which antiglobulins can be induced in normal individuals and experimental animals by immune responses involving prolonged exposure to complexes and, in fact, the presence of these factors (at low levels) in most human subjects (Torrigiani et al, 1970) indicates that tolerance to 'altered' IgG does not normally exist. Following an immunological response to the new configurations on altered IgG, antibodies with a weak avidity for native IgG could be obtained both through some structural similarity with the 'altered' configuration and also through the new determinant acting as a carrier for T-cell cooperation to promote the activation of those lymphocytes bearing weak affinity receptors for other parts of the molecule.

The relevance of the rheumatoid factors to the pathogenesis of the disease was thought to be weakened by the existence of a significant proportion of patients with negative results in the sheep cell and latex agglutination tests, the so-called seronegative individuals. Torrigiani et al (1970) have recently shown that the serum of these patients contains raised levels of IgG antiglobulins capable of binding firmly to horse IgG which has been converted to an insoluble immunosorbent by cross-linking with bis-diazobenzidine. These antiglobulins could be eluted with acid and a minimal estimate of their concentration made by single radial immunodiffusion using specific anti-immunoglobulin sera. IgG antiglobulins were similarly detected in children with Still's disease, the majority of whom are seronegative by the classical agglutination tests for rheumatoid factor (Torrigiani et al, 1969). It seems reasonable to conclude so far that antiglobulins occupy a central position in the disease and that their formation is probably provoked by alteration in host IgG.

THE ROLE OF COMPLEXES

Although purified rheumatoid factor preparations have long been known to be harmless on injection into normal subjects, there is now an increasing body of evidence to show that immunoglobulin complexes formed with antiglobulin factors are present in the joint and contribute, at least in part, to the development of inflammation.

Specific immunofluorescent staining procedures have demonstrated the presence of IgG, IgM, antiglobulin activity, and complement components, in differing proportions in the inclusion bodies of polymorphonuclear cells in the synovial fluids, within synovial phagocytic lining cells and deposited extracellularly in the synovium (Rodman et al, 1964; Rawson et al, 1965; Fish et al, 1966; Bonomo et al, 1968; Vaughan et al, 1968; Brandt et al, 1968; Kinsella et al, 1970; Tursi et al, 1970). These complexes of antiglobulin with IgG antigen and bound complement components are almost certainly generated within the joint. Not only is there local antiglobulin synthesis (Mellors et al, 1959; Smiley et al, 1968), but soluble aggregates of IgG can be detected in the synovial fluid by precipitation with IgM rheumatoid factor (Hannestad, 1967) or with C_1q (Winchester et al, 1969). The latter study also indicated that the aggregates could be composed of IgG and 7S antiglobulin. Other findings which indicate the presence in synovial fluid of material having the characteristics of immune complexes are (a) the frequent occurrence of cryoprecipitates (Barnett et al, 1970), (b) a high molecular weight histamine releasing factor (Baumer & Brodie, 1968), (c) a lowered complement level (Hedberg, 1964; Ruddy & Austen, 1970), and (d) a tendency to develop raised titres of immunoconglutinin (Bienenstock & Bloch, 1967).

Contrary to earlier views, it is now evident that the globulin-antiglobulin system itself can fix complement, a phenomenon which can more readily be demonstrated if one uses as antigen aggregated IgG, which has been reduced and alkylated to remove its inherent anti-complementariness (Zvaifler & Schur, 1968; Zvaifler, 1969; Tesar & Schmid, 1969; Davis & Noell, 1970). Several factors may influence the outcome of this interaction (Schmid et al, 1970).

Direct evidence that the inclusion bodies in synovial phagocytic cells are probably derived from these aggregates in the fluid was provided by the finding that addition of IgM rheumatoid factor to aggregated IgG (Parker &

Schmid, 1962) or to seronegative synovial fluid (Hurd et al, 1970) induced phagocytosis by polymorphonuclear cells; furthermore, normal polymorphonuclear leucocytes phagocytosed inclusion bodies staining for IgM, IgG and β_{1c} when placed in contact with synovial fluids from the majority of patients with IgM rheumatoid factors. The uptake of this material is accompanied by the release from synovial phagocytic cell lysosomes of a collagenase, neutral proteases able to split cartilage protein-polysaccharide, cathepsins capable of destroying basement membrane, cationic proteins which act to increase vascular permeability, and endogenous pyrogens, constituting a potent collection of mediators of joint inflammation and destruction (Hollander et al, 1965; Weismann, 1966; Weismann et al, 1969). It is likely, therefore, that the joint lesions in rheumatoid arthritis can be linked to a significant degree to a chain of events involving formation of an immunoglobulin complex with antiglobulin factor, activation of complement to generate chemotactic factors which attract polymorphonuclear cells, and uptake of complexes by synovial phagocytic cells to form intracellular inclusions with concurrent release of lysosomal components capable of prolonging the acute inflammatory reaction and of breaking down local connective tissue. But what is the antigen which initiates the formation of antiglobulin factors in the first place?

TRIGGERING MECHANISMS

It has long been postulated that the chain of events is triggered by the formation of autoantibodies to a joint constituent. Some hold that it might be nothing more than IgG itself. The fact that only 5% of the IgG synthesized by the rheumatoid synovium has antiglobulin specificity (Smiley et al, 1968) does not rule out this possibility since it is known that after injection of an antigen into a joint, only a small percentage of the local plasma cells which are present can be stained for specific antibody. However, the production of antiglobulins is not unique to rheumatoid arthritis patients; as mentioned above, all normal individuals have low levels, patients with gout slightly higher concentrations, and many with chronic infections high titres, yet they usually do not develop rheumatoid arthritis. Perhaps the arthritics have a cell-mediated hypersensitivity reaction to IgG? Their blood mononuclear cells show a greater tendency to form rosettes with human 0 Rh-negative erythrocytes coated with subagglutinating doses of a rabbit antiserum; thus 42% of patients formed more than 10 rosettes/1000 lymphocytes as compared with 3% of controls (Bach et al, 1970). However, it will not be possible to assess the significance of this finding in relation to cell mediated hypersensitivity until the proportion of rosettes formed by T lymphocytes can be established. The migration of patients' peripheral leucocytes from capillary tubes in vitro is sensitive to the presence of soluble aggregates of human IgG (Froland & Gaarder, 1971; now confirmed by ourselves). Previously, we had found no evidence for any exceptional reactivity of rheumatoids to intradermal injection of 'native' and heat-aggregated autologous IgG; the expected Arthus-type reaction produced was no more severe than in the controls and had largely resolved by 24 hours (Chamberlain et al, 1970; Runge & Mills, 1969).

A further point arises in that these observations do not accord with Glynn's hypothesis (1968b) that the chronic lesion in these patients is due to autosensitization to a product of the inflammatory response. This arose from earlier work on the induction of chronic arthritis in rabbits, previously sensitized with autologous fibrin in Freund's adjuvant, by intra-articular challenge with autologous fibrin (Dumonde & Glynn, 1962). Subsequent studies showed that a similar phenomenon could be induced by intra-articular installation of a range of different antigens to which delayed sensitivity had been established.

With respect to other autoantigens there is evidence for an increased incidence of antinuclear antibodies, mostly of low titre (Corbett et al, 1967) and for the presence of anticollagen antibodies (Steffen, 1970), but there is as yet no convincing demonstration of a response to a joint-specific autoantigen; unless intra-articular immunological reactions display some inherently characteristic feature which leads to chronic inflammation or some additional factor is operating, it is not clear why a response to materials widespread in the body such as nuclear antigens and collagen should produce lesions largely localised to the joint.

This difficulty gives more impetus to studies of an infectious aetiology, particularly in view of the production of diseases resembling rheumatoid arthritis by infectious agents such as Erysipelothrix Rhusiopathiae in swine and Mycoplasma Arthritidis in rats. There have been many conflicting reports of isolations of different microorganisms from the joints of arthritis patients (Hill, 1968; Duthie, 1971). It has recently been claimed that a transmissible form of polyarthritis can be induced in mice and their litters by injection of rheumatoid synovial tissue (Warren et al, 1969) and there is an intriguing report that synovial cells derived from patients with rheumatoid arthritis are resistant to infection with rubella virus (Grayzel & Beck, 1970), suggesting pre-infection with some agent. Duthie and his colleages (Duthie et al, 1967; Stewart et al, 1969) have consistently isolated diphtheroid organisms from these tissues, especially from patients with positive sheep cell agglutination tests. No characteristic immunological response to the diphtheroid organisms has yet been demonstrated in the patients and Duthie, while considering that the evidence is against their being contaminants, puts forward three possible interpretations of the findings: (a) the inflamed synovium is susceptible to infection by the diphtheroids which therefore play no part in the aetiology of the disease; (b) they may provide the initiating antigen

87

but the immunological response has not been detected for technical reasons; and (c) they may act like Corynebacterium Parvum in abrogating immunological tolerance to cellular antigens in the joint. In this connection it has been reported that tolerance to human albumin in rabbits can be abolished by one of the isolated diphtheroids (see Duthie, 1971).

M H Williams had had different experiences. Using equilibrium centrifugation in a sucrose density gradient in an attempt to concentrate any organisms and to separate them from the bulk of the fluid phase which might contain antibody and lysosomal hydrolases detrimental to growth, he reported the isolation of Mycoplasma Fermentans from approximately half of the fluids obtained from seropositive patients. Solubilised urea treated membrane preparations of M. Fermentans selectively inhibited the capillary tube migration of leucocytes from patients with seropositive rheumatoid arthritis (Williams et al, 1970) while further observations in collaboration with Dr Friedman (unpublished) indicate that the migration test returns to normal after patients have been treated with gold or chloroquine. Although there was a complete absence of correlation between the sheep cell agglutination titre and the degree of inhibition in the migration test, the possibility that migration inhibition is caused by residual small amounts of horse globulin (from the culture medium) in the antigen preparation has not yet been rigidly excluded, particularly since it has now been shown that aggregated IgG itself can cause migration inhibition.

A cautious attitude to these findings remains the rule and further studies are clearly warranted to establish their significance.

REFERENCES

Allen, J. C. and Kunkel, H. G. (1966) Arthritis and Rheumatism, **9**, 758
Bach, J-F., Delrieu, F. and Delbarre, F. (1970) American Journal of Medicine, **49**, 213
Barnett, E. V., Forsen, N. R., Bluestone, R., Cracchiolo, A., Mayor, H. and Goldberg, L. S. (1970) Immune Complex Diseases. Ciba Foundation Symposium. Page 152
Bartfeld, H. (1969) Annals of the New York Academy of Science, **168**, 30
Baumer, R. and Brodie, T. (1968) Clinical and Experimental Immunology, **3**, 555
Bienenstock, J. and Bloch, K. J. (1967) Arthritis and Rheumatism, **10**, 187
Bonomo, L., Tursi, A. and Gillardi, U. (1968) Annals of the Rheumatic Diseases, **27**, 122
Brandt, K. D., Cathcart, E. S. and Cohen, A. S. (1968) Journal of Laboratory and Clinical Medicine, **72**, 631
Cerottini, J-C. and Grey, H. M. (1969) Annals of the New York Academy of Science, **168**, 76
Chamberlain, M. A., Shapland, C. G. and Roitt, I. M. (1970) Annals of the Rheumatic Diseases, **29**, 173
Chiller, J. M., Habicht, G. S. and Weigle, W. O. (1970) Proceedings of the National Academy of Sciences of the United States, **65**, 551
Christian, C. L. (1963) Journal of Experimental Medicine, **18**, 827
Corbett, M., Downes, J. M. and Schmid, F. R. (1967) Annals of the Rheumatic Diseases, **26**, 487
Davis, J. S. and Noell, P. (1970) Clinical Research, **18**, 82

Dumonde, D. C. and Glynn, L. E. (1962) British Journal of Experimental Pathology, **43**, 373

Duthie, J. J. R. (1971) Modern Trends in Rheumatology, **2**, 78

Duthie, J. J. R., Stewart, S. M., Alexander, W. R. M. and Dayhoff, R. E. (1967) Lancet, **1**, 142

Fish, A. J., Michael, A. F., Gewury, H. and Good, R. A. (1966) Arthritis and Rheumatism, **9**, 267

Froland, S. S. and Gaarder, P. I. (1971) Lancet, **i**, 1071

Glynn, L. E. (1968a) in 'Clinical Aspects of Immunology'. (Ed) P. G. H. Gell and R. R. A. Coombs. Blackwell, Oxford. Page 848

Glynn, L. E. (1968b) Annals of the Rheumatic Diseases, **27**, 105

Grayzel, A. I. and Beck, C. (1970) Journal of Experimental Medicine, **131**, 367

Grubb, R. (1970) 'The Genetic Markers of Human Immunoglobulins'. Springer-Verlag, Berlin and New York

Hannestad, K. (1967) Clinical and Experimental Immunology, **2**, 511

Hedberg, H. (1964) Acta rheumatologica Scandinavica, **10**, 109

Henney, C. S. (1969) Annals of the New York Academy of Science, **168**, 52

Hill, A. G. S. (1968) Proceedings of the Royal Society of Medicine, **61**, 971

Hollander, J. L., McCarty, D. J., Astorga, G. and Castro-Marillo, E. (1965) Annals of Internal Medicine, **62**, 271

Hood, L. and Prahl, J. (1971) Advances in Immunology, **14**, 291

Hurd, E. R., LoSpalluto, J. and Ziff, M. (1970) Arthritis and Rheumatism, **13**, 724

Kinsella, T. D., Baum, J. and Ziff, M. (1970) Arthritis and Rheumatism, **13**, 734

Kunkel, H. G. and Tan, E. M. (1964) Advances in Immunology, **4**, 351

Mellors, R. C., Heimer, R., Carlos, J. and Korngold, L. (1959) Journal of Experimental Medicine, **110**, 875

Natvig, J. B. and Turner, M. W. (1971) Clinical and Experimental Immunology, **8**, 685

Parker, R. L. and Schmid, F. R. (1962) Journal of Immunology, **88**, 519

Rawson, A. J., Abelson, M. M. and Hollander, J. L. (1965) Annals of Internal Medicine, **62**, 281

Rodman, W. V., Williams, R. C., Bilka, P. J. and Müller-Eberhard, H. J. (1964) Arthritis and Rheumatism, **7**, 749

Roitt, I. M., Greaves, M. F., Torrigiani, G., Brostoff, J. and Playfair, J. H. L. (1969) Lancet, **ii**, 367

Ruddy, S. and Austen, K. F. (1970) Arthritis and Rheumatism, **13**, 713

Runge, L. A. and Mills, J. A. (1969) Arthritis and Rheumatism, **12**, 694 (Abstract)

Schmid, F. R., Roitt, I. M. and Roche, M. J. (1970) Journal of Experimental Medicine, **132**, 673

Schur, P. and Kunkel, H. G. (1965) Arthritis and Rheumatism, **8**, 468

Smiley, J. D., Sachs, C. and Ziff, M. (1968) Journal of Clinical Investigation, **47**, 624

Steffen, C. (1970) Zeitschrift für Immunitätsforschung und experimentelle Therapie, **139**, 219

Stewart, S. M., Alexander, W. R. M. and Duthie, J. J. R. (1969) Annals of the Rheumatic Diseases, **28**, 477

Tesar, J. T. and Schmid, F. R. (1969) Federation Proceedings (Federation of American Societies for Experimental Biology), **28**, 307

Torrigiani, G., Ansell, B. M., Chown, E. E. A. and Roitt, I. M. (1969) Annals of the Rheumatic Diseases, **28**, 424

Torrigiani, G., Roitt, I. M., Lloyd, K. N. and Corbett, M. (1970) Lancet, **i**, 14

Tursi, A., Trizio, D. and Bonomo, L. (1970) Clinical and Experimental Immunology, **6**, 767

Vaughan, J. H., Barnett, E. V., Sobel, M. V. and Jacox, R. F. (1968) Arthritis and Rheumatism, **9**, 127

Warren, S. L., Marmor, L., Liebes, D. M. and Hollins, R. L. (1969) Nature (London), **223**, 646

Weismann, G. (1966) Arthritis and Rheumatism, **9**, 834
Weismann, G., Spilberg, I. and Krakauer, K. (1969) Arthritis and Rheumatism, **12**, 103
Williams, M. H., Brostoff, J. and Roitt, I. M. (1970) Lancet, **ii**, 77
Williams, R. C. and Kunkel, H. G. (1962) Arthritis and Rheumatism, **5**, 126
Winchester, R. J., Agnello, V. and Kunkel, H. G. (1969) Annals of the New York Academy of Science, **168**, 195
Zvaifler, N. J. (1969) Annals of the New York Academy of Science, 168, 30
Zvaifler, N. J. and Schur, P. (1968) Arthritis and Rheumatism, **11**, 523

Sero-negative Rheumatoid Arthritis

E D R CAMPBELL

INTRODUCTION

Since the discovery of the rheumatoid factor by Waaler (1940) and later by
Rose et al (1948) it has been possible to distinguish a number of separate
entities which previously were described under the general title of rheumatoid
arthritis. This was one further stage in the history of the classification of
polyarthritis, which has been one of a gradual distinction of separate diseases
since the Hippocratic era when all types of arthritis were lumped together as
'gout', although even then rheumatic fever was considered a distinct variant
if not a separate entity. In the seventeenth century de Baillou differentiated
gout from other forms of polyarthritis and also first used the word 'rheumatism' specifically for joint disease. The term 'rheumatoid arthritis' was
introduced in the mid-nineteenth century by Sir Alfred Garrod; Still's disease
and ankylosing spondylitis were recognised at the end of the last century and it
was not until the very beginning of this century that degenerative joint disease
was separated from inflammatory polyarthritis. Until the 1950s, however,
the great bulk of polyarthritis remained under the title 'rheumatoid arthritis'.

Nowadays it is convenient to classify polyarthritis into two main divisons:
one usually or frequently associated with the rheumatoid factor — sero-
positive, and the other not — sero-negative.

The commoner members of the sero-negative group are given in Table I.
On the whole they present little difficulty in diagnosis, provided one is aware
of their existence, and although presenting many features of interest to the
rheumatologist, I propose to concentrate on those cases which at present are
classified as rheumatoid arthritis, but which lack the serum factor, and perhaps to suggest that there are still some distinct clinical entities lurking
under the cover of 'rheumatoid arthritis'.

SERO-POSITIVE RHEUMATOID ARTHRITIS

Like most serological tests, the Rose-Waaler test is neither 100% accurate

Table I. Sero-negative non-rheumatoid polyarthritis

UNKNOWN ↑	PSORIATIC ARTHROPATHY
	POLYARTHRITIS OF ULCERATIVE COLITIS
	ANKYLOSING SPONDYLITIS
	BEHÇET'S SYNDROME
	STEVENS-JOHNSON'S SYNDROME
	AORTIC ARCH ARTERITIS
AETIOLOGY	REITER'S SYNDROME
	HENOCH-SCHÖNLEIN SYNDROME
	ERYTHEMA NODOSUM
	SERUM SICKNESS
	SNAKE BITE
↓	RUBELLA
KNOWN	POLYARTICULAR GOUT

nor 100% specific. To make matters more complicated the clinical manifestations of rheumatoid arthritis are so varied and in some cases so slight that different observers were using different criteria for diagnosis until a standardised system was proposed by the American Rheumatism Association in 1956, and the 1958 revision of this classification is still generally accepted. This system lists eleven features of the disease; seven features label the disease as classical, five as definite, three as probable and two as possible rheumatoid arthritis.

The specificity of the Rose test varies depending on the types of rheumatoid arthritis tested; thus it is positive in 85% of cases with 'definite' rheumatoid arthritis and in 65% with 'probable' rheumatoid arthritis, but rises to over 90% if radiological erosions are present, and to nearly 100% if nodules are present also (Hill & Greenbury, 1965). Furthermore, the significance of the Rose test, like most serological tests, does not depend simply on the presence or absence of the rheumatoid factor, but rather on the concentration in the serum, and the test is not considered positive in most laboratories until the factor is present in titre greater than 1:32. From this it will be apparent then that the terms sero-positive and sero-negative rheumatoid arthritis have little absolute value; they may represent two ends of a spectrum of a single disease entity or they may represent different diseases within the same broad grouping, or even a mixture of each. The mere fact that rheumatoid factor is not positively demonstrated by the usual tests in routine practice does not ipso facto mean that the patient is in the sero-negative category, for Ziff et al (1956) have shown that an extra factor inhibiting the effective working of the test is present in a number of 'sero-negative' patients who, when this inhibiting factor is removed, become sero-positive.

The inhibiting factor is also present in many cases of Still's disease, thus accounting for its apparent sero-negativity. An alternative explanation is that the appropriate antigen is present in such profusion that all the available rheumatoid factor is thereby removed. Other patients, usually with long-standing disease, may convert from sero-positive to sero-negative, the reason for this conversion being unknown, and finally another group, quoted as up to 20% of sero-positive cases, may fluctuate between sero-positive and sero-negative at different times. Some of these are simply varying by one or two dilutions from time to time, so that their titres cross over the border line between normal and abnormal.

SERO-NEGATIVE RHEUMATOID ARTHRITIS

Excluding the groups just mentioned, there remains a sero-negative group which tends to be milder in degree, has a more favourable prognosis in terms of complete remission, and in which can be discerned the possibility of sub-groups. These are shown in the lower part of Table II: episodic rheumatoid arthritis, palindromic rheumatism and intermittent hydrarthrosis may all eventually develop into definite rheumatoid arthritis, but many cases remain distinct and these three are at present regarded as variants of rheumatoid arthritis. Palindromic rheumatism is interesting in a number of ways, first of all because of its name, which means running back and forth, a palindrome being a word or a sentence which reads the same forwards and backwards, such as 'marram', or 'able was I ere I saw Elba', as Napoleon might have said. In its clinical sense palindromic is merely a synonym for

Table II. Sero-negative 'rheumatoid arthritis'

TRUE	RHEUMATOID ARTHRITIS
↑	i) Sero-positive but serum inhibition factor present (10% of definite RA)
	ii) (Still's disease)
	iii) Conversion from sero-positive to sero-negative
	iv) Positive/Negative fluctuations (up to 20% of cases)
RA	EPISODIC RHEUMATOID ARTHRITIS
	PALINDROMIC RHEUMATISM
	INTERMITTENT HYDRARTHROSIS
↓	LARGE JOINT ONSET (USUALLY MALE)
FALSE	STREPTOCOCCAL DEPENDENT 'RHEUMATOID ARTHRITIS'

93

recurrent: attacks of arthritis occur which are sudden in onset and which may be severe in intensity, resembling an acute attack of gout. The episodes subside and in the interval between attacks the previously affected joints appear normal. In episodic rheumatoid arthritis the same joints tend to be involved each time and damage to the joint does eventually occur. Intermittent hydrarthrosis usually affects young women in whom recurrent effusions appear in large joints, particularly the knee.

Other sub-groups have less distinctive clinical features: one of these consists of male patients whose disease begins in large joints, such as the knee or shoulder, rather than in the classic small joints of hand or foot, and whose disease progresses much more slowly and with less disability than the classic form. A second sub-group of sero-negative cases has much greater clinical significance, however, because in these there is the prospect of cure or marked alleviation: such cases have raised titres of streptococcal antibodies and search will often disclose a source of streptococcal infection which when eradicated gives marked relief, if not complete resolution of the arthritic process. The usual laboratory test for streptococcal antibodies is estimated by the antistreptolysin O (ASO) titre, and, as in the past this test has had its main use in the diagnosis of rheumatic fever in children and adolescents, some comment on normal values is necessary. Many laboratories do not report the precise titre below 1:200 because in rheumatic fever the titres obtained are higher than this or rapidly become so as the disease becomes established: most clinicians therefore assume that 1:200 represents a normal value and this is not so. By usage a titre of 1:200 is expressed as 200 Todd units, 1:50 as 50 units etc.

A number of papers on ASO levels in patients with rheumatoid arthritis have been published since the test was introduced in 1932 and these have been reviewed by Francois (1965) who made a further study of the subject. However, of these papers only one (Otten & Westendorp Boerma, 1959) analysed sero-negative rheumatoid arthritis separately from the sero-positive group and here the results are interesting in that the control group and the sero-positive group were identical, whereas the sero-negative group had over twice the number of raised ASO titres (greater than 200) than the controls. This seemingly straightforward finding is complicated, however, because levels among the apparently healthy population vary with age, with a peak level around ten years, according to Rantz et al (1952) who give the mean 8-12 age level as 184 units, compared with a level of 46 units for over 40; furthermore, there is also a seasonal variation with higher 'normal' levels in the winter quarter. Finally, the ability to provoke ASO varies between different types of Group A streptococci, so that for full accuracy other streptococcal antibodies should be measured.

Such difficulties are high-lighted by the conflicting results in different

94

papers. Thus Muller et al (1969) in a study of 711 patients with definite rheumatoid arthritis found 27% sero-negative and this sero-negative group showed no difference in ASO levels from the sero-positive group. However, in this paper the exact levels are not given and even the upper limit of normal is not specified, so it is difficult to draw any conclusion from this. Furthermore, Francois (1965) showed that patients with established sero-positive rheumatoid arthritis have a higher acquisition rate of streptococcal infection than the normal population and so raised ASO levels may be expected in this group without necessarily having any relation to possible aetiology of the disease.

In order to identify the possibility that a portion of the sero-negative group may have a direct aetiological connection with streptococcal infection we decided to investigate patients attending the rheumatology clinic at the Royal Free Hospital who had an established diagnosis of sero-negative rheumatoid arthritis. Recognising the difficulties inherent in using ASO levels as the sole arbiter of streptococcal infection we attempted also to measure antibodies to group-specific streptococcal polysaccharides as described in animals by Erwa et al (1969). This work was never completed because of the untimely death of my collaborator, Professor N Crowley, but there are sufficient

Table III. ASO levels in four gradings of sero-negative rheumatoid arthritis

ASO levels	Classic	Grade of Rheumatoid Arthritis Definite	Probable	Possible
> 200	-	2 (*)	3 (**)	-
100-200	2	1	6 (**)	1
50-90	2	-	3	2 (*)
< 50	-	7	1	1
	4	10	13	4
			Total 31	

features of interest to warrant some discussion. Table III shows the ASO levels obtained in the four different gradings of sero-negative rheumatoid arthritis — 5 patients were in the age range 19-39, the remainder being over 40. Throat swabs were taken in all cases and in three streptococci of group A were isolated; these three patients had ASO levels of 440, 280 and 170; a further patient had beta-baemolytic streptococci, but not in groups A, C or G, and the ASO level was only 60. Two patients had respectively one and three infected teeth. These six patients were all treated with a 10-day course of phenethicillin 1G daily during which course the patients with infected teeth had those teeth removed; all six patients have had complete resolution, for at least eighteen months, of the signs of rheumatoid arthritis with an eventual fall of the ASO level to below 100. These patients are indicated in Table III by the symbol (*). One of these patients has persistent symptoms of diffuse aching in the limbs with no objective signs of any disease process. Two other patients have persistently raised ASO levels (280-700 units and 250-310 units) without the source of infection being discovered. In spite of courses of penicillin their ASO levels remain raised and their joint symptoms unabated.

As mentioned previously the investigation could not be completed in its intended form and clearly the figures are insufficient for any form of statistical analysis, but nevertheless it does appear that a small proportion of cases at present included under the omnibus title of sero-negative rheumatoid arthritis have a different aetiology and are capable of substantial relief with appropriate treatment.

ACKNOWLEDGMENTS

The original work mentioned was made possible by generous financial support from the Peter Samuel Royal Free Fund, and was undertaken in collaboration with the late Professor Nuala Crowley. The laboratory investigations were done by Mrs C James.

REFERENCES

Erwa, H. H., Maxted, W. R. and Brighton, W. D. (1969) Clinical and Experimental Immunology, **4**, 311

Francois, R. J. (1965) Annals of the Rheumatic Diseases, **24**, 369

Hill, A. G. S. and Greenbury, C. L. (1965) 'Progress in Clinical Rheumatology'. Churchill, London

Muller, W., Languess, U. and Petersen, K. F. (1969) German Medical Monthly, **14**, 329

Otten, H. A. and Westendorp Boerma, F. (1959) Annals of the Rheumatic Diseases, **18**, 24

Rantz, L. A., di Caprio, J. M. and Randall, E. (1952) American Journal of the Medical Sciences, **224**, 194

Rose, H. M., Ragan, C., Pearce, E. and Lipman, M. O. (1948) Proceedings of the Society for Experimental Biology and Medicine, **68**, 1

Waaler, E. (1940) Acta pathologica et microbiologica Scandinavica, **17**, 172

Ziff, M., Brown, P., Lospalluto, J., Bachin, J. and McEwan, C. (1956) American Journal of Medicine, **20**, 500

Biological False Positive Reactions and Systemic Disease

R D CATTERALL

One of the most important developments in medicine during the past decade has been the great progress in immunology, particularly in the demonstration, isolation and characterisation of antibodies. As a result of these advances there has been a better understanding of those immune reactions which can cause tissue destruction. It is now apparent that both humoral antibody production and cell-mediated immunity may be involved in the pathogenesis of immune injury. If the immune system is defective, the mechanisms that prevent immunocytes and antibodies from reacting with normal components of the body may break down and cause autoimmune disease. The aetiology of most immunopathological lesions is still unknown and the situation is frequently complicated by external or genetically determined alterations in responses to common antigens.

SEROLOGICAL TESTS FOR SYPHILIS

Throughout the whole of this century the long and close collaboration between venereologists and serologists has resulted in a detailed understanding of many immunological aspects of syphilis. Much of modern immunology began when Bordet (1898) discovered haemolysis and shortly afterwards Bordet and Gengou (1901) described the phenomenon of complement fixation. Employing these two discoveries, Wassermann et al (1906) introduced the Wassermann reaction (WR), the first satisfactory serological test for the diagnosis of human disease.

The antigen used by Wassermann was a saline extract from the livers of foetuses with congenital syphilis, as he believed that treponemal material was responsible for the apparent specificity of the test. However, it was soon demonstrated that the test was non-specific in the usual immunological sense, when Marie and Levaditi (1907) prepared a successful antigen from the livers of non-syphilitic, new-born babies. Michaelis (1907) showed that flocculation techniques could be used to demonstrate syphilitic antibodies in the serum.

The fact that saline or better still alcoholic extracts of normal tissue provide a satisfactory antigen for the Wassermann reaction is a paradox that has not been completely resolved. Over the years the Wassermann reaction and the Kolmer test have emerged as the most popular complement fixation procedures. The most commonly used flocculation tests are the Kahn, Price, Eagle, Hinton, Kline and Venereal Disease Research Laboratory (VDRL) tests. The complement fixation and flocculation tests have together become known as the standard serological tests for syphilis (STS). They are all based on the same immunological and physico-chemical processes and differ from one another only in certain technical details (Table I).

Table I. Standard serological tests for syphilis (STS)

COMPLEMENT FIXATION TESTS
Wassermann Reaction (WR)

FLOCCULATION TESTS
Venereal Disease Research Laboratory Test (VDRL)
Detect syphilitic reagin: employ lipoidal antigens

The antigens were formerly prepared by extracting ox heart muscle with ethanol and adding cholesterol as a sensitising agent. However, Pangborn (1941) extracted an acid phospholipid, called cardiolipin, which appears to be the active antigenic component of the extracts. This pure chemical substance is now widely used as the antigen, together with carefully adjusted proportions of lecithin and cholesterol, and it will fix complement or flocculate with syphilitic serum.

The antibody detected by these non-specific lipoidal antigens, syphilitic reagin, should not be confused with other types of reagin, which occur in atopic disease and belong to the IgE class of immunoglobulin. Syphilitic reagin is non-specific, is not directed solely against Treponema pallidum, and occurs with equal frequency in the other treponemal diseases, such as yaws, bejel and pinta.

Syphilitic reagin begins to appear in the serum one to two weeks after the development of the primary chancre and tests for its detection usually reach their maximum titre during the secondary stage of the disease. During the latent phase reagin diminishes to the point that in about a quarter of untreated cases it disappears from the serum, but in the majority it persists for the rest of the patient's life. Both IgM and IgG globulins are increased in early syphilis and IgA may be raised in the secondary stage (Laurell et al, 1968; Delhanty & Catterall, 1969). In late syphilis IgG predominates, but there may be high levels of IgM in some late cases of the disease (Aho, 1968).

In treated cases there is usually a rapid decline in titre in primary and secondary syphilis and the tests for reagin usually become negative after four to eight months. In late syphilis of all types, the usual effect of treatment is to reduce the titre of tests for reagin: a proportion of these cases become seronegative, but the majority remain positive.

The fact that some persons who have not been infected by treponemal disease have reagins in their serum in such quantities that the standard serological tests are positive has been a subject of investigation for many years. Such reactions were often called non-syphilitic or non-specific, but gradually the term 'biological false positive reaction' came to be used to distinguish them from false positive reactions due to technical variation or error.

Ever since serological tests were first used, attempts have been made to employ T. pallidum as the antigen. In 1949 Nelson and Mayer demonstrated that live, motile treponemes, mixed with human syphilitic serum and complement under strictly anaerobic conditions, were immobilised and killed, whereas with normal serum they remained actively motile. These observations formed the basis of the treponemal immobilisation test (TPI), which was the first practical, specific test for treponemal infections.

Absorption experiments have shown that immobilising antibody is distinct from reagin and the other antibodies detected by other tests. It does not occur in the serum of normal persons or in those suffering from non-treponemal disease, but occurs uniformly in cases of syphilis and the other related treponematoses. It does not occur in other spirochaetal diseases such as leptospirosis, relapsing fever, rat-bite fever or Vincent's infection.

In untreated syphilis immobilising antibody usually first appears in the serum late in the primary stage. It is almost invariably present during the secondary stage and is always present in the latent stage, when it is detectable at the highest titres. It is almost always present in cases of late symptomatic syphilis, except in some very longstanding cases, such as quiescent tabes dorsalis or congenital syphilis of the middle-aged or elderly.

Treatment seems to have little effect on the presence of immobilising antibody and, except in early infections, it tends to persist for the remainder of the patient's life. However, because of the expense and technical difficulties of the TPI procedure and the requirement that the test sera should be free of treponemicidal agents, many attempts have been made to develop tests which were equally specific, but without these disadvantages.

One of the most successful of these has been the fluorescent treponemal antibody absorbed test (FTA-ABS). Fluorescent techniques were first used in the serodiagnosis of syphilis in 1957 and Hunter et al (1964) developed the absorbed fluorescent treponemal antibody test or FTA-ABS. In this test the group reactive antibody is absorbed out from the test serum with a concentrated filtrate of the culture medium on which Reiter treponemes have been grown and called sorbent. The group reactive antibody can also be absorbed out with intact or ultrasonically disintegrated Reiter treponemes, but these are less satisfactory than sorbent.

The FTA-ABS test is carried out by applying the absorbed serum from the patient to T. pallida on a slide; then anti-human globulin, coupled with fluorescin isothiocyanate, is added and the treponemes are visualised microscopically under ultra-violet light.

In untreated primary syphilis the FTA-ABS test is the most sensitive available and becomes positive before the reagin tests. At all stages of syphilis it is reactive more frequently than the STS or the TPI test, and after treatment it appears to behave in a similar manner to the TPI test. In patients treated early in the disease reversal to negative may occur, but more slowly than with other tests, and when treatment is started late in the disease this test remains positive, frequently for the rest of the patient's life.

The specificity of the FTA-ABS has been the subject of much discussion. It may be reactive with sera containing abnormal globulins (Mackey et al, 1969), antinuclear factor (Jokinen et al, 1969) and rheumatoid factor (Wilkinson & Rayner, 1966). More recently Kraus et al (1970) have reported on the beaded appearance of the fluorescence of treponemes with sera from patients with systemic lupus erythematosus, which does not occur with syphilitic sera.

More recently a test based on haemagglutination has become increasingly popular and is now widely used throughout the world. The early work on this test was carried out in Copenhagen, but the techniques used currently were developed in Tokyo by Tomizawa and his colleagues (1969). Rabbit or fowl red blood cells are treated with tannic acid and then sensitised by exposure to a preparation of virulent treponemes which have been disrupted by ultra sound. The patient's serum and the sensitised red cells are brought together in haemagglutination trays. If the patient's serum contains antibody to T. pallidum the red cells are agglutinated and form a web-like mosaic at the bottom of the tube. If no antibody is present the red cells accumulate on the floor of the tube in a button-like configuration.

The treponema pallidum haemagglutination test (TPHA) is a sensitive test and in early infectious syphilis it is reactive shortly after the FTA-ABS test and just before the reagin tests. In late syphilis, either treated or untreated, it remains positive usually for the rest of the patient's life and the antibody it detects is even more persistent than those measured by the TPI and the FTA-ABS tests.

Specific serological tests for syphilis are summarised in Table II.

With the increasing use of automated techniques in all laboratories the types of serological tests performed are changing rapidly. It is probable that in future the routine screening tests for all sera will be the VDRL test,

Table II. Specific serological tests for syphilis

Treponemal Immobilisation Test (TPI)

Fluorescent Treponemal Antibody Test (FTA-ABS)

Treponema Pallidum Haemagglutination Test (TPHA)

---

measuring reagin, and the TPHA test, measuring agglutinating antibody.   In cases where these tests are reactive, but the diagnosis is still in doubt, the tests should be repeated and the FTA-ABS should be performed.   This combination of tests, together with a careful history and physical examination, should enable an accurate diagnosis to be made in the majority of patients. In a small number, where repeated investigation does not clearly establish the diagnosis, the TPI test will be necessary.   The complement fixation tests, including the Wassermann reaction which has served us so well for 67 years, will gradually disappear, victims of automation and the machine orientated age.

Screening procedure for treponemal disease is summarised in Table III.

Table III. Screening procedure for treponemal disease

---

1. All sera tested by both —
   Venereal Diseases Research Laboratory Test (VDRL)
   Quantitated if positive.
   Treponema Pallidum Haemagglutination Test (TPHA)

2. If diagnosis is not apparent —
   Fluorescent Treponemal Antibody Test (FTA-ABS)

3. If doubt still exists —
   Treponemal Immobilisation Test (TPI)

BIOLOGICAL FALSE POSITIVE REACTIONS

Although clinicians had long suspected that false positive reactions occurred in a proportion of patients with positive results to STS, little accurate information was available until the second world war.   During this period large numbers of American servicemen and women were investigated under conditions which were not possible in peace time.   Further large scale blood testing on demobilization indicated that biological false positive reactions were probably much more frequent than had been believed in the past.   The investigations of Moore and Mohr (1952) in Baltimore and the description of the TPI test in 1949 by Nelson led to the introduction of the concept of acute and chronic BFP reactions. Later Moore and Lutz (1955) showed that patients with chronic BFP reactions had a high incidence of autoimmune diseases, especially systemic lupus erythematosus, Sjögren's disease, autoimmune haemolytic anaemia, Hashimoto's thyroiditis, purpura and rheumatoid arthritis. Other less clear cut connective tissue diseases were found to develop in a proportion of the patients with the chronic reaction.

Chronic BFP reactions were commoner in women than in men and were frequently detected for the first time in women between the ages of 20 and 35 years. Haserick and Long (1952) showed that the chronic BFP reaction may occur many years before the onset of a collagen disease. A genetic factor may be involved in the development of the chronic reaction and Harvey and Schulman (1966) reported eleven patients with one or more close relatives with the BFP reaction, while Tuffanelli (1968) found a higher incidence of raised serum gamma globulin levels, antinuclear factors and rheumatoid factors in 199 relatives of 103 chronic BFP reactors than in a series of control patients.

Other abnormalities have been frequently found in the sera of patients with chronic BFP reactions, such as raised serum globulin levels, anaemia, a raised erythrocyte sedimentation rate (ESR), abnormal liver function tests, abnormal immunoglobulins, antinuclear, rheumatoid and LE-cell factors. Thyroid antibodies are often present in appreciable amounts and in a few there is a high level of circulating anticoagulant. The antibodies are usually IgM in type, but may also be of IgG type or a combination of the two (Delhanty & Catterall, 1969). Anticomplementary activity in complement fixation tests occurs in the presence of raised gamma globulins and when the serum contains antigen-antibody complexes such as cryoglobulins and rheumatoid factors (Lassus, 1969).

The antibodies responsible for the BFP reaction cross the placenta into the foetal circulation during pregnancy. These passively transferred antibodies disappear from the infant's serum within a few weeks.

THE PRESENT SERIES

All the patients described in this series have been seen personally during the past sixteen years. There were 76 patients in whom a diagnosis of an acute biological false positive reaction was made. They came from a variety of sources. Fifty-four were attending clinics for venereal diseases and were found to have positive STS on routine blood testing, 12 were referred from antenatal clinics, 6 came from the blood transfusion services and 4 were referred by other physicians.

A diagnosis of the acute BFP reaction was made only if there was no history of syphilis or other treponemal disease, physical examination did not reveal any signs suggestive of those diseases and the STS were positive on three or more occasions on different specimens of serum with negative results to the TPI and FTA tests. In all the cases the positive STS disappeared spontaneously within weeks or months — always less than six months — and the patients were followed for a further six to twelve months, and the STS remained negative throughout this period.

The acute BFP reaction could be shown to have occurred in association with a variety of events and diseases in 52 cases (Table IV). It followed

Table IV. Presumed causes of acute biological false positive reactions

Recent vaccination against smallpox	12
Infective hepatitis	6
Recent inoculation with TAB vaccine	5
Infectious mononucleosis	3
Virus pneumonia	3
Chickenpox	2
Measles	2
Virus encephalitis	1
Pregnancy only	18
Undetermined	24
	76

recent vaccination against smallpox in 12 patients and recent inoculation with TAB vaccine in 5. Infective hepatitis was present in 6 and infectious mononucleosis in 3. Virus pneumonia had occurred in 3, chickenpox and measles in 2 each, and virus encephalitis in one. The only unusual event in 18 young women was pregnancy: in all of these patients the STS became negative later in the pregnancy or after delivery and remained negative. All the babies were clinically normal and sero-negative at six weeks and three months of age.

The cause of the acute BFP reaction remained undetermined in 24 cases. There was no history of a possible precipitating factor and no abnormality on clinical examination; the serological tests became negative within six months and remained negative throughout the follow-up period.

There is general agreement that the acute BFP reaction is without serious significance to the patient and the greatest danger is that the reaction will be misdiagnosed as syphilis. It has been estimated that about 20% of the population are potential acute BFP reactors under appropriate circumstances. There are probably a large number of potential precipitating factors, but provided the diagnosis is clearly established, the patient can be safely re-assured that the reaction is without long term significance.

The situation with the patients diagnosed as having chronic BFP reactions is quite different. In the present series the chronic BFP reaction was diag-nosed only in those patients whose sera produced positive results to STS in repeated tests for a minimum period of one year, but in whom there was no past history of treponemal infection, no clinical evidence of syphilis on care-ful physical examination and negative results to the TPI and FTA-ABS tests, as well as negative tests of the cerebrospinal fluid and a normal chest X-ray. All the patients were investigated in great detail and the period of follow-up has varied from 2 to 14 years.

There were 134 chronic biological false reactors of whom 98 were women and 36 men. Of the 98 women, 95 were white, two of negro origin and one Indian. Of the 36 men, there were 33 of European origin, one Indian, one Chinese and one negro. The ages ranged from 17 to 74 years, but the majority were young and in the third or fourth decades of life.

Of these 134 chronic BFP reactors, 10 had systemic lupus erythematosus with LE-cells in the peripheral blood. Seven of them developed manifestations of the disease months or years after the discovery of the false positive reac-tion; the other 3 had the disease when the BFP reaction was first discovered. All 10 were women. Four have died of their disease and post mortem exami-nation in 2 has confirmed the diagnosis.

Six patients had rheumatoid arthritis and 6 had rheumatic heart disease, all with valvular damage. Six women had Hashimoto's thyroiditis and 6 pre-sented with a multiple sclerosis-like neuropathy and on investigation were found to have both the BFP reaction and evidence of a connective tissue disease probably in the form of SLE.

Six patients had possible connective tissue disease; all remain unwell and have a variety of symptoms and physical signs suggestive of a connective tissue disorder, as well as abnormal immunological and biochemical findings. It has not yet been possible to make an exact diagnosis in any of them and LE-cells have not been found in their peripheral blood. In some their disease is slowly progressive, but in others it appears to be stationary.

Discoid LE was found in 4 patients, one of whom had mild haemolytic anaemia. Hepatic cirrhosis occurred in 2 patients and 2 others had haemo-lytic anaemia of the autoimmune type, with a positive Coomb's test and the presence of cold agglutinins.

Two men were found to have polyarteritis nodosa and one of these has since died. Two women have Sjögren's disease. Two patients developed a well-defined psychotic illness during observation. Chronic nephritis was present in 2 patients.

There were 2 narcotic addicts in the series and both of them had been injecting themselves with heroin for a considerable period. It could not be established whether the chronic BFP reaction was related to the use of the narcotics themselves, to additives, or to inadequately sterilized needles and syringes.

One patient had obliterative vascular disease and died after a long and progressive illness. Systemic sclerosis was found in one woman, whose predominant symptom was dysphagia.

The associated disorders are summarised in Table V.

Table V. Principal disorders associated with 134 chronic biological false positive reactions

Systemic lupus erythematosus		10
Rheumatoid arthritis		6
Rheumatic heart disease		6
Hashimoto's thyroiditis		6
Multiple sclerosis-like neuropathy		6
Possible connective tissue disorder		6
Discoid lupus erythematosus		4
Hepatic cirrhosis		2
Haemolytic anaemia		2
Polyarteritis nodosa		2
Sjögren's disease		2
Psychotic illness		2
Chronic nephritis		2
Heroin addiction		2
Peripheral vascular disease		1
Systemic sclerosis		2
Undetermined	with symptoms	14
	without symptoms	60
		134

Of the remaining 74 patients, 14 have symptoms of disease and feel unwell, but no diagnosis has been possible up to the present time. The other 60 are symptom-free, but 8 have a persistently raised ESR and moderately severe anaemia. Thus, 52 of the 134 chronic BFP reactors have no clinical or laboratory evidence of disease up to the present time.

The majority, namely 62, of these patients were referred by other physicians and surgeons because of the finding of positive serological tests. Forty were first found to have the reaction when they attended a clinic for venereal diseases, 18 came from antenatal clinics and 8 from blood transfusion services. Four were discovered as a result of contact tracing and 2 because of family investigations.

Hypersensitivity to a variety of drugs had occurred in 26 of the patients, 24 of whom were women. A history of sensitivity to penicillin was obtained in 20 patients, 18 of whom were women. Six of these had suffered immediate reactions and in the other 14 the reaction was delayed. The onset of symptoms of autoimmune disease was related to the administration of penicillin in 5 patients.

Of the 6 youngish women who presented with symptoms and signs of a neurological disorder resembling multiple sclerosis, 5 had developed a progressive spastic paraplegia eight months to three years before they were found to have the chronic BFP reaction and other evidence of a connective tissue disease. The history and physical examination of all 6 patients had led to the clinical diagnosis of multiple sclerosis. The discovery of the BFP reaction was a marker which led to more detailed investigations. Some of these patients had noticed minimal joint stiffness and skin lesions during the course of the illness. A moderate elevation of the ESR was found in all of them and one had leucopenia. The gamma and alpha-2 globulins were raised and the serum IgM was very high. There were low titres of antinuclear factor and scanty LE cells were found in the peripheral blood of 5 of them. Other autoantibodies were also found in all these cases. The cerebrospinal fluids all showed moderate elevation of the protein content and a paretic type of Lange curve.

The following is a very brief case history of one of the patients:
The patient was a 35-year old secretary with a five year history of difficulty in walking. Weakness began in the left foot and leg, and then affected both legs, and urgency of micturition developed. She was diagnosed as having multiple sclerosis. She developed pain and swelling of the fingers, hands and wrists three years later, and one year later she had a pleural effusion and recurrent attacks of fever. Walking deteriorated and frequency and urgency of micturition recurred. There were signs of marked spastic paraplegia and tenderness of the small joints of the hands on examination. There was a BFP reaction, an ESR of 32mm in 1 hour, 50 mg of protein and a parapetic Lange curve in the CSF, antinuclear factor at a titre of 1 in 40, and other autoantibodies and LE-cells in the peripheral blood on two occasions.

This case history was typical of the six patients in whom the clinical picture of multiple sclerosis was associated with the BFP reaction and other laboratory findings suggestive of systemic lupus erythematosus. Several of the features were unusual for either disease. Nevertheless, there appears to be sufficient similarity between the six patients to suggest that they may form a distinct subgroup of the connective tissue diseases, the characteristics of which may be summarised as follows.

The patients are young women, who develop symptoms and signs resembling multiple sclerosis with minimal evidence of involvement of the other systems of the body, associated with the BFP reaction, moderate elevation of the ESR, weakly positive tests for antinuclear factor and other autoantibodies, raised serum IgM levels, moderate elevation of CSF protein levels, a paretic Lange curve and, in the majority, LE-cells in the peripheral blood (Table VI).

Table VI. Principal findings in six patients with 'lupoid' neuropathy

1. All young women
2. Symptoms and signs of multiple sclerosis
3. Minimal evidence of involvement of other systems
4. Chronic BFP reaction
5. Elevated ESR
6. Positive tests for antinuclear factor and autoantibodies
7. Raised IgM levels
8. Raised CSF protein
9. Paretic Lange curve
10. LE-cells in the majority

Although involvement of the central nervous system in SLE is well known, there has been no similar description of cases with the characteristics described and it could be that these patients do form a distinct group. For want of a better term, the name 'lupoid sclerosis' has been used to describe the condition, but further study is necessary before the syndrome can be fully understood.

IMMUNOLOGICAL INVESTIGATIONS

The standard serological tests for syphilis detect antibodies to cardiolipin, which is a complex of diphospholipids found mainly on the mitochondrial inner membrane. It is probable, but not fully proven, that Wassermann reagins are autoantibodies produced as a result of the adjuvant effect of treponemes in the body. Autoantibodies found consistently in patients with primary biliary cirrhosis, which react with a lipoprotein component of the mitochondrial inner membrane, but not with cardiolipin, have been described by Doniach and Walker (1969) and produce 'M' fluorescence with the Coon's technique.

Recently it has been possible to study 60 chronic BFP reactors at the Middlesex Hospital in collaboration with the Department of Immunology (Table VII). Of the 60 patients, 58 (96%) had one or more positive tests for autoantibodies. 'M' fluorescence, similar to that seen in primary biliary

Table VII. Autoantibodies in sixty patients with chronic BFP reactions

Antibodies	Number positive	Per cent
Mitochondrial fluorescence	34	56
CFT rat liver mitochondria	27	45
Nuclear fluorescence (ANA)	28	47
Smooth muscle	16	28
Rheumatoid factor latex FII	6	10
Thyroid specific	16	27
Gastric parietal cell	6/30	20
Total patients with one or more positive tests	58	96

cirrhosis, was found in 34 (56%) at titres varying from 1 in 5 to 1 in 50. The autoantibodies were mainly of the IgM class in ten cases, of both IgM and IgG classes in eight, and mainly of the IgG class in three. Non-organ specific complement fixation reactions were obtained with rat kidney homogenates in 27 cases. Antinuclear antibodies (ANA) were found in 28 patients (47%), 16 of whom had high titres. The ANA was predominately of the IgG class and of the so-called 'homogeneous' type, similar to that seen in SLE, 'lupoid' hepatitis, and other connective tissue disorders. Smooth muscle fluorescenc which is another antibody marker, was present in 16 cases (28%). This antibody is uncommon in patients who do not have liver disease. Rheumatoid antiglobulins and thyroid-specific antibodies had an incidence only slightly above that found in normal controls and organ-specific gastric parietal cell fluorescence was present in only 6 of the 30 patients tested.

The high incidence of tissue antibodies in this series of chronic BFP reactors appears to be related to the high incidence of systemic disease. The mitochondrial fluorescence was usually of low titre and the antibodies were present most frequently in the IgM immunoglobulins. The true pathological significance of this association is not understood, but both the cardiolipin antigen and the lipoprotein reactive in 'M' fluorescence are situated in close proximity on the mitochondrial inner membranes. Both these antibodies are uncommon in the normal population and they are both, therefore, useful markers of a special immunological abnormality related to the connective tissue diseases.

The majority of patients when found to have the chronic BFP reaction are healthy. However, in this group of patients, the presence of 'M' fluorescence usually indicated the development or actual presence of systemic disease. Tests for tissue antibodies and 'M' fluorescence may be helpful in detecting those patients who are likely to develop connective tissue disease and may, therefore, be important in the follow-up assessment of all patients with the chronic BFP reaction.

DISCUSSION

There are many difficulties in estimating the incidence of biological false positive reactions among the general population. In the United Kingdom at the present time, the majority of patients with syphilis present in the latent stage of the disease, and the commonest cause of positive STS is still syphilis, but the incidence of BFP reactions is sufficiently high to warrant careful investigation of all patients with positive serological tests before a diagnosis of latent syphilis is made and the antisyphilitic treatment is given. The differential diagnosis can be difficult in certain cases, even with modern serological aids. Studies indicate that the margin of error may vary from 2 to 10% and the most important methods of achieving accuracy in diagnosis are prolonged follow-up with repeated physical examinations as well as the use of specific serological tests and modern immunological techniques.

It is extremely difficult to predict the course of the condition in any individual patient after the discovery of the chronic BFP reaction. In many cases, in addition to the clinical progress of the diseases, there is a consistent sequence in the development of abnormal results to laboratory investigations. The chronic BFP phenomenon usually, but not invariably, appears first and is followed by an increase in the ESR. Frequently this situation does not change for many months or years, but in some patients a microcytic, hypochromic anaemia and a leucopenia develop, to be followed by abnormalities of the plasma proteins, especially of the gamma and to a lesser extent of the beta fractions. In some cases various autoantibodies and antinuclear factors appear at this stage, but the exact time at which they develop is as yet unknown. Later still LE-cells may be found. It is not yet known when mitochondrial antibodies of the IgM class first make their appearance in these patients, but their association with systemic disease and their relative infrequency in patients without systemic disease suggests that tests for their presence may prove useful in distinguishing between those who are likely to develop systemic illnesses and connective tissue disorders in the future and those in whom the condition is likely to remain benign and symptomless.

The high incidence of sensitivity to drugs and particularly to antibiotics is of great importance. There is abundant evidence that penicillin may be harmful to patients with autoimmune diseases and especially to chronic BFP reactors. There are serious dangers in the common practice of administering a course of penicillin to patients in whom the exact diagnosis is in doubt, 'just to be on the safe side', as this can precipitate severe illness and even, in occasional cases, death.

If evidence of systemic disease is found, or if it develops under observation, the question of prophylactic or symptomatic treatment should be considered. In practice, effective forms of treatment are restricted to corticosteroids and immunosuppressive drugs. Their use is usually limited because of the chronic and slowly progressive nature of most of the diseases associated with the chronic BFP reaction. With the corticosteroids the risk involved with prolonged treatment, in which the dose has often gradually to be increased, may be greater than the advantages to the patient. The toxic effects of the immunosuppressive drugs are such that they are probably indicated in only a few cases with severe and rapidly progressive symptoms. Experience with any form of therapy is at present too limited for any firm conclusions to be drawn.

The biological false positive reaction is an immunological phenomenon of considerable importance. The acute reaction is precipitated by a number of well recognised diseases and immunological procedures and is harmless to the patient, apart from the risk of misdiagnosis. The chronic reaction is associated with a wide variety of systemic diseases and has important prognostic implications in women. It offers an unusual and probably a unique situation in medicine, because it is possible to predict years in advance that a number of the patients with this reaction will later develop serious and occasionally fatal diseases. This fact gives us a special opportunity to study the presymptomatic stages, development and natural history of the autoimmune diseases, as well as the responsibility for developing safe and effective forms of preventive treatment.

REFERENCES

Aho, K. (1968) British Journal of Venereal Diseases, **44**, 49
Bordet, J. (1898) Annales de l'Institut Pasteur, **12**, 688
Bordet, J. and Gengou, O. (1901) Annales de l'Institut Pasteur, **15**, 289
Delhanty, J. J. and Catterall, R. D . (1969) Lancet, ii, 1099
Doniach, D. and Walker, J. G. (1969) Lancet, i, 813
Harvey, A. M. and Schulman, L. E . (1966) Medical Clinics of North America, **50**, 1271
Haserick, J. R. and Long, R. (1952) Annals of Internal Medicine, **37**, 559
Hunter, F. F., Deacon, W. E . and Mayer, P. E . (1964) Public Health Reports, **79**, 410
Jokinen, E. J., Lassus, A. and Linden, E . (1969) Annals of Clinical Research, **1**, 77
Kraus, S. J., Haserick, J. R. and Lantz, M. A. (1970) New England Journal of Medicine, **282**, 1287
Lassus, A. (1969) International Archives of Allergy and Applied Immunology, **36**, 515
Laurell, A. B., Oxeluis, V. A. and Rorsman, H. (1968) Acta dermato-venereologica, **48**, 268
Mackey, D. M., Price, E. V., Knox, H. M. and Scotti, A. (1969) Journal of the American Medical Association, **207**, 1683
Marie, A. and Levaditi, C. (1907) Annales de l'Institut Pasteur, **21**, 138
Michaelis, L. (1907) Berliner klinische Wochenschrift, **44**, 1477
Moore, J. E. and Lutz, W. B. (1955) Journal of Chronic Diseases, **1**, 297
Moore, J. E. and Mohr, C. F. (1952) Journal of the American Medical Association, **150**, 467

Nelson, R. A. Jr. and Mayer, M. M. (1949) Journal of Experimental
Medicine, **89**, 369
Pangborn, M. C. (1941) Proceedings of the Society for Experimental Biology
and Medicine, **48**, 484
Tomizawa, T. S. Kasamatsu, S. and Yamaya, S. (1969) Japanese Journal of
Medical Science and Biology, **22**, 341
Tuffanelli, D. L. (1968) Archives of Dermatology, **98**, 606
Wassermann, A., Neisser, A. and Bruck, C. (1906) Deutsche medizinische
Wochenschrift, **32**, 745
Wilkinson, A. E. and Rayner, C. F. A. (1966) British Journal of Venereal
Diseases, **42**, 8

The Pathogenesis of Rheumatoid Arthritis

D L GARDNER

"One word of truth outweighs the whole world"
Russian proverb, quoted by Alexander Solzhenitsyn in the Nobel Speech on Literature, 1970

INTRODUCTION

It is widely accepted that rheumatoid arthritis (RA) is a disease entity. Nevertheless, the 'disease' is seen as a symptom complex and no single feature affords the certainty of absolute diagnosis. It is therefore necessary to define the disorder by groups of arbitrary criteria that vary in severity and nature according to individual opinion (Tables I and II). This aspect of RA leads to considerable difficulty in analysing present views on pathogenesis: it is not clear which features reflect the primary disturbance and which are superimposed, secondary aspects of the disorder. The synovial tissues of the hands, feet, wrists and other diarthrodial joints appear, on the available evidence, to be the 'target' organs. But it is still quite possible that some

Table I. American Rheumatism Association criteria for rheumatoid arthritis; 3 or 4 points indicate 'probable', and $\geq$ 5 points 'definite' rheumatoid arthritis. (From Cathcart & O'Sullivan, 1970, New England Journal of Medicine)

Point	Criterion
1	Morning stiffness
2	Joint tenderness or pain on motion
3	Soft-tissue swelling of 1 joint
4	Soft-tissue swelling of 2nd joint (within 3 months)
5	Soft-tissue swelling of symmetrical joints (excluding distal interphalangeal)
6	Subcutaneous nodules
7	X-ray changes
8	Serum positive for rheumatoid factors

Table II. New York criteria for rheumatoid arthritis. Each joint group, for example, proximal interphalangeal, counted as one joint, each side being scored separately. (From Cathcart & O'Sullivan, 1970, New England Journal of Medicine)

Point	Criterion
1	History of episode of 3 painful limb joints
2	Swelling, limitation, subluxation or ankylosis of 3 limb joints:
	Must include hand, wrist or foot
	Must include symmetry of 1 joint pair
	Must exclude distal interphalangeal, 1st carpometacarpal, 1st metatarsophalangeal and hips
3	X-ray changes (erosions)
4	Serum positive for rheumatoid factors

widespread extra-articular disturbance antedates the joint disease, reflecting the activity of an, at present, unidentified aetiological agent.

These matters underline the great need to concentrate on early cases of RA in attempts to unravel its origins. In practice, however, it is unusual for patients with RA to seek advice and treatment during the first few months of illness. Consequently, by the time patients reach centres that provide special diagnostic and therapeutic facilities, a substantial variety of secondary inflammatory, mechanical and physical phenomena have generally been superimposed on the primary disturbances. There has been difficulty therefore in reaching the heart of the problem: the initial disorders are almost always obscured or distorted by epiphenomena.

Much has been learnt recently of the structure and physiology of normal joints and vigorous argument continues on crucial matters such as mechanisms of lubrication, intra-articular pressures, age-related physical and chemical changes in cartilage structure, the function and electron microscopic appearances of synovial cells, and joints as foci for immunological reactions.

Hyaline articular cartilage is avascular and aneural. Until 1968, this cartilage was thought to be 'strikingly smooth', a view disproved when the incident light- and scanning electron microscopes showed that the load-bearing surfaces are normally covered by a series of undulations corresponding in diameter to the size of the chondrocytes that lie only 3 - 5μm below the surface (Gardner & McGillivray, 1971a and b). It has been known since the time of Virchow that chondrocytes increase in size with age, and interferometric measurements are now available that prove a corresponding increase in the diameter and irregularity of the surface undulations (Longmore & Gardner, unpublished observations — Figures 1 and 2). The relationship between this surface structure and the normal mechanisms of lubrication

113

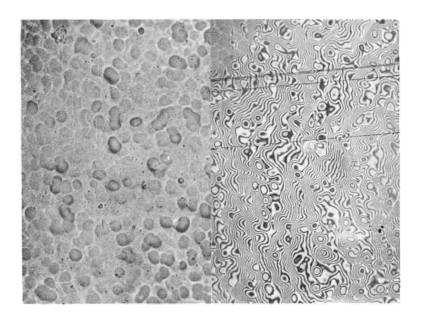

Figure 1. Normal articular cartilage surface from femoral condyle of stillborn child.
Left. Reflected light photomicrograph showing pattern of shallow undulations that increase in size and irregularity with age.
Right. Same field. Reflected light interference photomicrograph of same field, showing extent and height of contours. The two most widely separated reference lines, seen horizontally, are 100μm apart

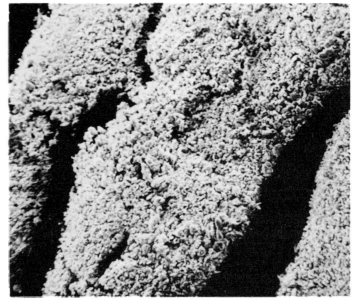

Figure 2. Normal synovial surface of human adult. Scanning electron micrograph.
x 300

during joint movement is not yet understood. The lubrication mechanism does not conform precisely with any recognised in engineering practice and the lubricant is several times more efficient than any known to tribologists.

Because of the lack of understanding that persists concerning these physiological mechanisms, there are great gaps in our knowledge of joint abnormalities in RA. The most difficult matter, in discussing the pathogenesis

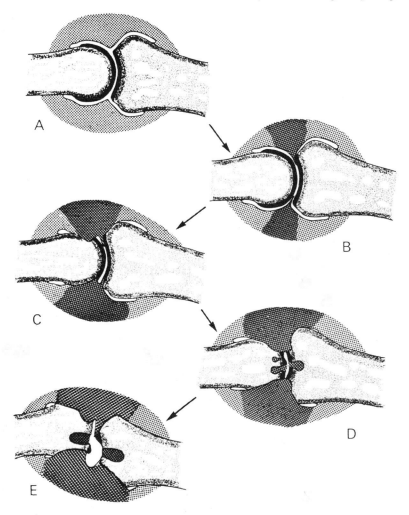

Figure 3. Pathogenesis of rheumatoid arthritis. A. Normal metacarpophalangeal joint. B. Early inflammation of synovia (dark stippling).   C. Marginal replacement of cartilage and bone with early superficial pannus. D. Pseudocyst formation with bone remoulding.   E. Late changes, with widespread inflammation, subluxation, partial loss of joint space and fibrous ankylosis.
(From Gardner, D. L., 1965. 'Pathology of the Connective Tissue Diseases'. Edward Arnold, London)

of the disease, is to know which of the observed disturbances is of a fundamental, primary character, which secondary, and thus probably inconse-
quential (Gardner, 1971).

The **established** clinical syndrome of RA is associated with inflammatory
articular changes that may affect any, or possibly all, of the 187 or so diarthrodial joints of the average human adult (Figure 3). The marginal
replacement of articular cartilage that is so characteristic a feature of the
early disease leads (Figures 4 and 5) to intra-articular fibrous adhesions,
progressing to fibrous but rarely to bony ankylosis. The vascular granulation tissue or pannus that forms in continuity with the synovial and periarticular connective tissues extends within nearby bone, predominantly at
the joint margin. Here, osteoclastic bony reabsorption appears to account
for the 'erosions' detectable clinically. Granulation tissue also extends
directly into zones of the articular surface where the pannus has focally
destroyed the whole thickness of the cartilage. In these latter situations it
is suspected that the very high pressures generated within flexed RA joints
play a part in causing granulation tissue to protrude, as radiolucent pseudo-
cysts, into the underlying cancellous bone.

The great extent to which the periarticular connective tissues, the

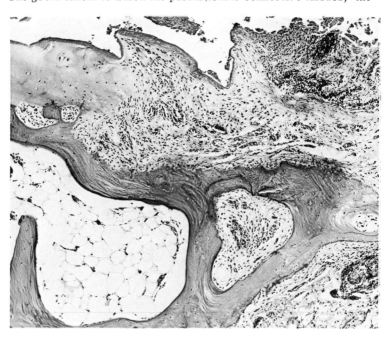

Figure 4. Marginal destruction of articular cartilage by extension of vascular
inflammatory tissue pannus. Remnant of normal cartilage seen, top left.
Note remoulding of bone (right). Haematoxylin and eosin.   x 60

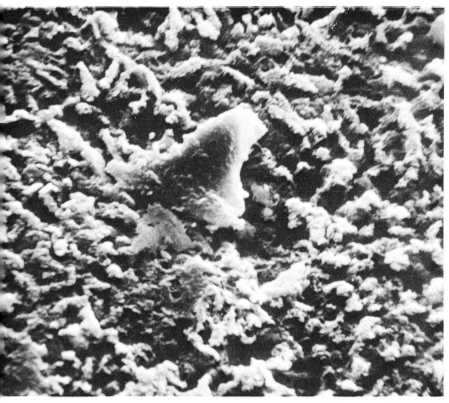

Figure 5. Synovial surface in rheumatoid arthritis. Note disorderly structure, with part of hypertrophic synovial cell (centre)   x 2530

tendons, ligaments and their sheaths, and the regional muscles are influenced by longstanding RA, is not always appreciated. There is ligamentous laxity with, presumably, a defect in collagenous cross-linkages in the component fibres; inflammation, weakness and even necrosis of tendons; and muscle wasting accompanied both by focal intramuscular collections of lymphocytes, recalling the appearances seen in myasthenia gravis, and by demonstrable increases in the levels of red cell cholinesterase and serum aldolase activities.

The clinical syndrome, the mirror of the pathological tissue changes that I have outlined, is the end result of molecular and cellular phenomena that have occurred at an earlier period. The clinical signs, in contemporary pathological terms, are relatively late. This viewpoint determines the philosophy of the investigator seeking to explore the mechanisms of tissue injury in RA: it is an aspect of the disease that may obscure the relevance of much contemporary laboratory research. The obligation is to seek,

117

necessarily, for sensitive and delicate biological indications relevant to the **initiation** of the polyarthritis.

The diseases of contemporary society that remain to be prevented appear to have a different form of origin from the environmental and infective disorders that have been brought under control during the past 30 years. In broad terms, conditions such as cancer, RA, arteriosclerosis and ageing can be said to have a genetic or genetic/somatic background (Burnet, 1971). Alternatively they may be caused by environmental agents that have not yet been discovered or, as was the case with asbestosis and with the aniline dyes, whose mode of action is so subtle or so prolonged, that proper understanding has been delayed.

It therefore seems logical in this lecture first to consider the possibility that RA is the result of a predisposing hereditary mechanism. Such a mechanism could be the result of a chromosomal anomaly; of the operation, in a Mendelian pattern, of a mutant gene of large effect; or of the interaction of a number of genes of less effect, on a multifactorial basis (Carter, 1969). I shall then consider the possible role of environmental agents which, with or without a genetic predisposition, may act to initiate the tissue changes. My account will lead to an analysis of the details by which tissue damage is mediated, and to an enquiry into the manner in which the pathological disturbances are promoted and perpetuated.

This lecture will deal in turn, therefore, with the **predisposition** to, **initiation, mediation** and **promotion** of RA.

PREDISPOSITION

There is little reason to suspect that ethnic origin determines the prevalence of RA (Table III).

The possible role of heredity has been the subject of much enquiry. Strict criteria are applied when a genetic mechanism in disease is suspected; much of the published evidence in relation to RA unfortunately is conflicting or inconclusive. It is reasonably clear that neither RA nor the presence of rheumatoid factor (RhF), is associated with the inheritance of blood group factors (Baxter et al, 1968), with the GM or InV groups (Fudenberg & Martensson, 1963), with haptoglobin types (Peacock & Alepa, 1966) or with the number and structure of the chromosomes. Thus, the dividing white cells of the peripheral blood of 5 patients with rheumatoid arthritis appeared, morphologically and in karyotype, to be similar to those of the cells of the normal human population (Bartfield, 1962).

These data provide limited indirect evidence against the role of heredity in RA. The question has been critically examined by Bennett and Burch (1968), by O'Brien (1967), by Meyerowitz et al (1968), by Whaley and Dick (1969) and by Lawrence (1970). Their views take account of the work of

Table III. Distribution of rheumatoid arthritis and rheumatoid factor in different ethnic groups. (From Lawrence, J.S. et al, 1966. Annals of the Rheumatic Diseases, **24**, 425)

Ethnic group	Region	Latitude	Number examined	Completion rate (%)	Age group	Definite rheumatoid arthritis* (%)	Rheumatoid factor	
							SCA test positive (%)	FII globulin test positive (%)
AMERINDIANS								
Haida	Queen Charlotte Islands	54°N	436	89	15+	1.4	3.1	8.3
Blackfeet	Montana	48°N	1,101	88	30+	1.8	5.8	5.5
Pima	Arizona	33°N	968	86	30+	2.4	9.2	20.5
NEGROES	Jamaica	18°N	536	89	35-64	1.7	1.6	7.6
CAUCASIANS								
German	Oberhorlen	50°N	421	95	15+	2.2	3.2	-
English	Watford	51°N	421	85	15+	0.5	1.0	0.0
English	Leigh	53°N	1,391	86	15+	1.1	4.9	-
English	Wensleydale	54°N	967	89	15+	1.4	2.2	6.7

* Criteria of the American Rheumatism Association

Harvald and Hauge (1956) who, surveying the 3,800 individuals comprising the twins born in Denmark between 1870 and 1910, discovered among them 76 cases of RA (2%). Sixteen of 47 monozygotic twins showed concordance for the disease but only 2 of 71 like-sex dizygotic twins and 8 of 70 different-sex pairs. Concordance in monozygotic twins was thus significantly higher than in dizygotic, suggesting the limited significance of genetic factor(s) in pathogenesis. Harvald and Hauge nevertheless considered that familial aggregation and the absence of dominant concordance among uniovular twin pairs were most easily explained by the concept that the disease results from environmental factors, operating in a familial manner. They proposed the intervention of climatic and nutritional conditions and infection, and emphasised that the disorder was sex-limited; this view agreed with their demonstration of greater concordance among binovular twins of the same sex than among binovular twins of different sexes. Similar observations were made by Lawrence (1970). In 20 monozygous twin pairs in which the index twin had seropositive polyarthritis, 65% displayed concordance for this condition, compared with a figure among dizygous co-twins of 16%. Of 18 monozygous and 51 dizygous twin pairs among whom one twin of each pair had sero-negative polyarthritis, no co-twin displayed evidence of RA.

In a further survey, Bennett and Burch (1968) studied the distribution of RA and RhF in two Indian tribes, the Blackfeet and the Pima, and proposed that there might be a familial aggregation of these factors in the latter tribe. There was no evidence of an hereditary transmission of the disease. Aggregation only showed, clinically, at about the age of 50. They suggested that RA and RhF may be caused by environmental agents operating maximally during infancy, childhood or adolescence; that is, factors likely to be transmitted from person-to-person before the family disperses at maturity. Generation-to-generation transmission was uncommon as shown by the lack of a significant difference between the prevalence of the disease in children of affected or unaffected parents.

One of the most interesting analyses is that of Meyerowitz et al (1968). They reviewed 8 proven monozygotic twin pairs of whom one had definite RA and collected a further 20 proven pairs from the literature. In only 3 of the 28 monozygous twin sets was there evidence of concordance. This, they concluded, argued strongly against the suggestion that heredity is an important factor in the development of RA. As an incidental observation they showed, among 4 of their own 5 adult twin pairs, the occurrence of a period of psychological stress preceding the disease onset, findings confirmed but less obvious in 2 of the 3 younger sets (Table IV).

It is apparent that there is a tendency for the syndrome of RA to aggregate in families but firm evidence to support the operation of even minor genetic predisposing factors is very slight indeed. The positive evidence that is available is limited to seropositive cases. The familial aggregation, more evident in the lateral than in the vertical axis, suggests the operation of an exogenous, transmissible agent of low infectivity. Activation is related to age and sex.

Table IV. Twin studies in rheumatoid arthritis. (From Lawrence, J. S., 1970. Annals of the Rheumatic Diseases, **29**, 357

Source	Authors	Date	Monozygous			Dizygous			MC/ DC
			Concordant No. Per cent		Discordant	Concordant No. Per cent		Discordant	
General Hospital and Department of Rheumatology	Claussen and Steiner	1938	6	35	11	2	13	14	3
Department of Rheumatism	Edström	1941	4	67	2	1	11	8	6
General Hospital	Brandt and Weihe	1939	2	40	3	2	29	5	1.4
Advertisement	Thymann	1957	3	50	3	1	17	5	3
Birth registrations	Thymann	1957	0	0	8	0	0	9	0
Birth registrations	Harvald and Hauge	1965	16	34	31	10	7	131	4.9
Various	Meyerowitz and Others	1968	0	0	8	-	-	-	-
Total			31		66	16		172	
Concordance			32 per cent***			9 per cent***			

*** P <0.001

INITIATION

Infection

The signs of rheumatoid arthritis may first appear following an episode of physical or mental stress. There is a growing suspicion, recalling views on pathogenesis expressed in the early years of the century, that such episodes serve to activate a microbiological infection. It is thought, for example, that a slow or latent virus may be provoked into activity. Whether this is so or not, the role of infection in the pathogenesis of RA is widely canvassed (Walton, 1968; Duthie, 1971).

The synovial fluid and synovial tissues in established RA are unusually susceptible to suppurative infection by agents such as staphylococci, haemolytic streptococci, Haemophilus, Escherichia coli, Proteus, Pasteurella and microaerophilic fungi (Kellgren et al, 1958; Gardner et al, 1962). The incidence of all forms of infection is significantly higher than in the general hospital population (Parker, 1965). These observations suggest that patients with RA have a diminished resistance to local and systemic bacterial and fungal infections. It is a reasonable assumption, not yet proven, that there may be a correspondingly diminished resistance to opportunistic viral agents. This contrasts with the demonstration of reticuloendothelial hyperactivity, shown by enlargement of the spleen and lymph nodes, and by an enhanced rate of clearance from the blood of particulate material, of high molecular weight dyes (Roy et al, 1955) and of oil/glycerine emulsions (Mills et al, 1964) and with the retention of more iron than normal within the reticuloendothelial system (Gardner & Roy, 1961; Muirden, 1966).

Suppurative but silent bacterial or fungal infections have usually been found in patients who have displayed lengthy clinical evidence of RA. It seems most unlikely that these superimposed infections bear any relationship to the origin of the disease. An entirely distinct primary microbiological cause for RA nevertheless appears probable. During the past 10 years many careful investigations have been made in order to search for previously unrecognised synovial microorganisms. These investigations have yielded conflicting evidence. This is not surprising in view of the different phases of the disease that have been studied, the variable quality of the studies and the fact that most of the organisms isolated have been of uncertain pathogenicity. Two principal problems emerge: first, if an organism is consistently isolated from a significant proportion of samples obtained under strict aseptic conditions, how can its role in RA be determined? It is no longer sufficient simply to satisfy Koch's postulates. Second, if a particular microorganism, such as the rubella virus, cannot be obtained on primary culture, how can its relationship to RA be established? The answer to the first question presupposes the possibility of indirect

tests for infection, such as those based on humoral or cellular allergic*
phenomena; the answer to the second may depend on demonstrating the activity, for example of interference phenomena.

Mycoplasmas have been isolated by tissue culture techniques from RA patients
(Bartholomew, 1965a and b) but also from patients with systemic lupus erythematosus (SLE) and with Reiter's syndrome. The organisms have been
obtained from synovial fluid, serum, kidney and bone marrow. Growth
inhibition is demonstrable against several known human mycoplasma strains
but the possibility that the organisms are contaminants remains high. Support
for the presence of mycoplasmas in RA was also gained by Marcolongo et al
(1969) and by Fraser et al (1971); the latter authors made their observations
with tissue culture and immunofluorescence techniques and concluded that
the 10 strains that they identified, of 2 main serological types, elicited no
host allergic response and were therefore unlikely to be related to the cause
of the disease. Jansson et al (1971) also ultimately isolated mycoplasmas
from 11 of 33 RA synovial fluids, either by direct primary culture or after
egg passage.

The significance of these results remains uncertain and is eagerly
debated. At the centre of the debate lies the work of Williams (1968 - Table
V) and of Williams et al (1970). Using sucrose density gradient centrifugation, Williams (1968) isolated Mycoplasma fermentans from 45% of 11 cases

Table V. Identification of mycoplasmas isolated from synovial fluids
(From Williams, M.H., 1968. Pfizer Medical Monograph
Number 3)

| Specimen | Number of mycoplasma isolates serologically related to | | |
	M. fermentans	M. hominis	Unidentified
All rheumatoid arthritics			
RA Seropositive	31	-	-
RA Seronegative	5	-	-
Controls	1	2	2
Various arthritides	2	1	-
Totals	39	3	2

(From Williams, M.H., 1968, Pfizer Medical Monograph Number 3,
University Press, Edinburgh)

of seronegative RA, and from 39% of 79 cases of seropositive RA. Subsequently it was shown that membrane preparations from M. fermentans
inhibited leucocyte migration in 67% of 45 patients, leading to the suggestion

---

*The convention is accepted that **allergy**, or altered reactivity, may be
manifested with benefit (as immunity) or with disadvantage (as hypersensitivity)

that mycoplasmas, whatever their possible action in initiating RA, might prolong the disease by provoking a cell-mediated allergic reaction with the liberation locally of lymphokine factors.

Bacterial 'L' forms have been recognised in the blood and joint fluid in RA but since these organisms have been identified in a wide variety of other tissues in a heterogeneous collection of diseases, their significance in RA must remain very doubtful.

Diphtheroids were recovered from the lymph nodes in RA many years ago (Cadham, 1932, 1942). Similar organisms were found by Duthie and his colleagues in RA synovial tissue and fluid: their most recent results showed that organisms could be obtained from 27% of RA synovial membranes (Stewart et al, 1969 - Table VI), a figure approximating to that gained by Hill et al (1967) in a small series and by Clasener and Biersteker (1969) whose careful studies eliminated any risk of contamination.

Table VI. Isolation rate of diphtheroid bacilli from synovial membranes
(From Stewart, Alexander & Duthie, 1969. Annals of the Rheumatic Diseases, 28, 477-487)

Diagnosis	Number of patients	Diphtheroids		Total number of membranes examined
		Isolated	Not isolated	
Rheumatoid arthritis	71	21 (27%)	57	78
Other conditions*	20	0	20	20
Total	91	21	77	98

(P<0.05)

*Diagnosis: Torn menisci and other internal derangements of the knee 15
Osteoarthrosis 4
Osteochondritis 1

(From Stewart, Alexander & Duthie, 1969, Ann. rheum. Dis., 28, 477-487)

The diphtheroids that have been isolated from synovial tissues in RA appear inert. They lie within cells, provoking no allergic reaction. Nevertheless, prepared from cultures and tested experimentally, they can be shown to have adjuvant properties (White & Gordon, 1970). It is therefore possible that their presence in RA is coincidental and that they are saprophytic passengers in abnormal cells whose protective mechanisms have become disordered; but that they may act synergistically, as adjuvants, boosting one or more of the tissue-damaging allergic responses described below.

There is no evidence that any **protozoon** is implicated in the pathogenesis of RA. However, the importance of known **viruses** such as rubella has been suggested. The possibility has also been raised that RA is caused by an unknown latent or slow virus the presence of which becomes evident, as

123

age advances, in response to an exogenous stimulus. Virus-like bodies have been found in synovial and other tissues in RA but their presence is not specific for this disease. No virus has been obtained by primary culture from RA synovium. However, rheumatoid synovial cells in culture cannot be infected by rubella virus, in contrast to the susceptibility of normal synovial cells (Grayzel & Beck, 1970). This cell resistance is presumably the result of interference phenomena; it is not caused by interferon production but can be interpreted as evidence that the RA cells are already hosts for another, unidentified virus. This does not, of course, establish that rubella virus is the cause of the disease. Indeed, negative evidence indicates that RhF is not present within 1 month of the onset of rubella synovitis (whether it is present later is not yet known) and patients with RA do not possess anti-rubella antibody (Ab) titres greater than normal. The data of Grayzel and Beck (1970), not yet confirmed, contradict the earlier views of Ford and Oh (1965) and of Barnett et al (1966). Both groups searched for viral agents in RA without success, by cell culture and by immunofluorescence techniques. The work of Ford and Oh (1965) in particular displayed no signs suggestive of a latent viral infection.

It is concluded that so far there is insufficient direct evidence to implicate viral infection in the pathogenesis of RA. Nevertheless, rapid advances in our understanding of persistent, latent and slow virus infections (Dick, 1972) and of the nature of the immune responses that they evoke (Allison, 1972) suggest that important new information is not likely to be long delayed.

MEDIATION

Lysosomal Activity

The signs of active inflammation that typify the acute onset of early RA are accompanied not only by soft tissue and synovial oedema with vascular congestion but, characteristically, by a series of changes in the volume, viscosity and constituents of the synovial fluid (Gardner, 1972). Perhaps the most interesting of these changes is the presence of a considerable variety of enzymes, some displaying proteolytic activity. It is probable that many of these enzymes are of lysosomal origin. The numerous synovial fluid polymorphs recognised in the active stages of the disease are a principal source. However, the high synovial fluid levels of polymorph lysosomal enzymes, such as acid phosphatase, are accompanied by raised lactate dehydrogenase levels. This argues against a simple primary lysosomal source since lactate dehydrogenase is of cytoplasmic origin. An alternative view suggests that these raised enzyme activities are incidental results of polymorph disintegration following a primary inflammatory reaction such as that caused, for example, by the phagocytosis of immune complexes, of exogenous infective agents or of the antigenic products of the inflammatory response. A further explanation could be a synovial cell or chondrocytic derivation.

Whichever view is taken of the origin of the lysosomal proteases, it is imperative to remember that the earliest inflammatory changes of RA appear, by inspection and by light microscopy, to be marginal: they are seen as a peripheral, vascular pannus; microscopically, the articular cartilage is degraded and replaced by vascular granulation tissue in a centripetal fashion. If the action of the lysosomal proteases referred to above is to bring about or, at least, to initiate, the degradation of the articular cartilage that is so characteristic of RA, it is quite uncertain why the initial degradation should be peripheral. All parts of the cartilage surfaces of the joint are presumably exposed to proteolytic activity simultaneously, under identical biological conditions. The explanation for the marginal response may be 1) that the techniques so far used to examine cartilage in early RA have been insufficiently sensitive to detect early degradation of cartilage in central zones; 2) that the peripheral cartilage may be more sensitive to early proteolysis, perhaps because of a different surface structure, permitting an unusually ready penetration by the relatively small molecules of proteolytic enzymes such as cathepsin D; 3) that the activity of the enzymes detected in synovial fluid may be largely irrelevant to the early progress of the disease, marginal cartilage destruction being the result of an entirely distinct mechanism; 4) that a protective mechanism guards central, weight-bearing cartilage zones against digestion by enzymes that readily degrade the histologically distinct marginal zones.

The first explanation for the centripetal loss of cartilage structure is improbable. Scanning electron- and light microscopic surveys have so far yielded no evidence in favour of this view. Admittedly, the volume of expert evidence is very small. The second explanation remains possible since it is clear from detailed scanning- and transmission electron microscopic studies that marginal articular cartilage, at least in small mammals, does not change abruptly to synovia but that there is a narrow, and possibly susceptible, intervening zone. The third explanation remains the most probable. The early inflammatory response in RA is in the vascular synovia, not in the avascular cartilage itself. The inflamed synovial fringe that borders the cartilage is almost certainly the source of agents that degrade marginal cartilage locally, exacerbated, no doubt, by the ready local availability of inflammatory factors brought to this cartilage zone by the synovial capillary meshwork. There is no evidence to support the fourth proposal, and, indeed, one would suppose that load-bearing, central articulating surfaces might be **more** susceptible to early degradation, not less.

The available data supporting the third proposal, advanced above, are now substantial. They may be traced back to the views of Dingle (1962)

125

Table VII. Measurements of "free" and "bound" naphthylamidase (as an index of lysosomal activity) in synovial lining cells of non-RA synovia (top) and RA synovia (bottom) expressed as relative absorption/unit field/30 min incubation, measured by scanning and integrating microdensitometry. (From Chayen et al, 1971 Beiträge zur pathologischen Anatomie und zur allgemeinen Pathologie, 142, 137)

Tissue	Number	Mean freely available activity ("free")	Activation conditions	Mean activated activity (total)	Ratio of bound * to total (%)
Non-rheumatoid	D2	48	5 min.acetate	-	-
	668	128	5 min.acetate	237	46
	782	96	5 min.acetate	190	48
	654	64.5	5 min.acetate	120	46
	686	68	5 min.acetate	131	48.5
	691	105	5 min.acetate	161	34.7
	776	35	5 min.acetate	51.2	31
	1025	123	5 min.acetate	205	40
	948	31.4	2 min.acetate	72	57
	782	45.5	0.05 mg/ml dicoumarin	92	51
Chondromalacia	981	154	-	-	-
	668	129	5 min.acetate	238	40
Non-rheumatoid, recent trauma	707	275	5 min.acetate	423	35
	820	332	5 min.acetate	488	32
	N	178	5 min.acetate	274	35
	N2	167	5 min.acetate	232	28
	N3	198	5 min.acetate	278	29
	825	172	5 min.acetate	264	28
	832	194	5 min.acetate	300	29

* Bound activity = "total" activity minus "free" activity

Number	Mean freely available activity ("free")	Incubation conditions	Mean activated activity ("total")	Ratio of bound * to total (%)
L1	735	5 min.acetate	decrease	0
L2	150	5 min.acetate	decrease	0
L3	173	5 min.acetate	decrease	0
L4	262	5 min.acetate	decrease	0
R1	215	5 min.acetate	-	-
530	205	5 min.acetate	192	0
534	320	5 min.acetate	336	5
535	390	5 min.acetate	369	0
840	182	5 min.acetate	192	2.4
841	191	5 min.acetate	187	0
834	147	5 min.acetate	164	5.2
835	363	5 min.acetate	376	2.8
970	272	-	-	-
972	320	-	-	-
923	780	-	-	-
931	239	-	-	-
951	80	2 min.acetate	61	0
952	68	2 min.acetate	45.5	0

deriving from the investigations made by Fell and her colleagues during 1952-1961 (Fell & Mellanby, 1952; Fell & Thomas, 1960; Lucy et al, 1961) on the ways in which cartilage matrix is degraded in cartilage rudiments maintained in organ culture. Numerous reports have now confirmed the presence of raised lysosomal enzyme activities in immediate relationship to the inflamed synovial tissues of RA. These high activities have been demonstrated in aliquots of homogenised tissue. They have also been recognised by subjective histochemical techniques and can be activated by allergic reactions involving complement (C'). The most convincing evidence specifically allocating the raised lysosomal enzyme activities to the hyperplastic synovial lining cells of RA while conclusively excluding the possibility that these high activities could derive from any other nearby cell type (except, perhaps, macrophages that have migrated into the synovia), is that of Chayen et al (1971 - Table VII). These authors identified and measured coloured enzyme reaction products by scanning and integrating microdensitometry; in this way they combined the exact anatomical localisation of enzyme activities with considerable biochemical precision that was, of course, of an indirect form.

Present opinion therefore favours the suggestion that centripetal cartilage degradation is one consequence of lysosomal proteases liberated from, and activated in the inflamed synovia. It is also suspected that the degradation may be sequential: one group of enzymes may depolymerise marginal cartilage proteoglycans, permitting subsequent disruption, by a second group, of cartilage collagen. Proteoglycans have a relatively short half-life and rapid turnover. They are readily replaced provided chondrocyte injury is not excessive. When collagen is destroyed, however, the results of injury are likely to be much more severe; the half-life of collagen is lengthy. Complete repair is in this way negated and the degraded cartilage is progressively replaced by vascular granulation tissue that, in turn, comes to resemble scar tissue.

Collagen Disorder

The destruction of collagen appears to be a prerequisite for complete cartilage loss in RA. The view that RA could be a primary diffuse, systemic disease of collagen (Klemperer et al, 1942) is now outmoded, but it remains possible that an early, **selective** injury to collagen or an impairment of collagen synthesis, can play a part in initiating the disease. Evidence to support this hypothesis has been gained from experiments in which a soluble antigen (Ag) was permitted to react with the appropriate precipitating Ab in the avascular rabbit cornea (Germuth et al, 1962; Mohos & Wagner, 1969). Corneal damage occurred where immune precipitates formed. In regions of Ag excess, ie where immune complexes were likely, Mohos and Wagner (1969) found polymorph degranulation (lysosomal enzyme activation) in zones engorged with immune precipitate. Where the precipitate lay in extracellular situations, it enclosed or surrounded collagen fibres: the fibres displayed reduced spacing and variable calibres, lying near the filopodia of phagocytes in which microvesicles abounded. Since these zones also showed the staining characteristics termed, simply for historical convenience, 'fibrinoid', it was deduced that 'fibrinoid' could represent evidence of collagen injury

127

and that immune complex formation, probably with the local adsorption and activation of C', could injure collagen directly.

To argue from this that direct injury to collagen may be a feature of early RA is debatable but the evidence presents a view that should continue to receive careful consideration.

PROMOTION

Allergy

The probability that the lymphoreticular tissues play an important part in the genesis of RA was raised by early descriptions of the lymphocytic foci that are a common feature of the synovial tissues in this disease. The variant of RA termed Felty's syndrome (Felty, 1924) was characterised by spleno- megaly, implicating the reticuloendothelial system. However, it was only when Cecil and his colleagues in the early 1930s demonstrated the presence of anti-streptococcal Ab in RA sera, paving the way for the development of the sheep cell agglutination test (Waaler, 1940; Rose et al, 1948) that it began to be suspected seriously that disorders of an allergic character could pro- mote or mediate the disease. This view was strongly reinforced when Fagraeus (1948) unravelled the key part played by plasma cells in Ab synthe- sis; it had been known from the earliest histological studies of RA that the inflamed synovia were widely interspersed with these cells. It immediately appeared probable that plasma cells might be engaged in the local synthesis of Ab protein and that this protein could cause tissue injury, or, perhaps respond to the local influence of a tissue-damaging Ag.

In RA, there is firm evidence that immunoglobulins, including autoanti- bodies, are often localised, both in or in relation to the plasma cell synovial infiltrate and, with C' components, in or on the synovial cells themselves. It is known, further, that the immune (Ag/Ab) complexes that are found in RA cells and free within the synovial fluid, are capable of attracting poly- morphs, by which they are phagocytosed, while simultaneously acting, with C', to promote inflammation. This evidence, the relatively low synovial fluid levels of C' and the influence of RhFs as autoantibodies, is quite suffi- cient to convince the most sceptical observer that allergic reactions are a characteristic feature of RA and to suggest that such mechanisms may play vital roles in pathogenesis. Two groups of critical questions remain unans- wered. First, are these allergic reactions an incidental part of a causative pathogenic stimulus, such as a viral infection; are they irrelevant to this mechanism; or are they themselves the pathogenic agent, directly causing tissue damage and cell injury? Second, assuming that allergic reactions are an essential part of the tissue-injuring mechanism in RA, how do they effect tissue damage, and is this reaction mainly a response to humoral Ab synthe- sised by plasma cells, or cellular allergic mechanisms, or, perhaps, to both?

128

Between 1950 and 1965 the view gradually gained support that the allergic responses in RA were causally related to the disease process, that RhF, IgM anti-immunoglobulin G Ab, were tissue-damaging autoantibodies, and that the key to a full knowledge of the pathogenesis of RA lay in understanding the nature of allergy. The evidence supporting this viewpoint was extensively reviewed by Glynn and Holborow (1965); it was based partly on the analysis of human material, partly on animal evidence. Thus, experimental arthritis, it was found, could be caused by an allergic reaction against heterologous or autologous fibrin, particularly when adjuvants were used to accentuate the allergic response; by the repeated local intra-articular injection of defined Ag, or by the local injection of Ag intra-articularly into animals already sensitised to the same Ag. Humoral allergic mechanisms were suspected in Aleutian disease of blue mink, a disease analogous with systemic lupus erythematosus (SLE), cellular mechanisms in mouse NZB disease and in the graft-versus-host reaction. In the latter there was a considerable resemblance to SLE and a less convincing resemblance to RA. Against the purely allergic viewpoint was, first, a growing body of evidence that virus-like agents could be seen in, or could be isolated from, the tissues in almost all these disorders, and second, the particularly intriguing demonstration that RA could occur in persons with hypo- or agammaglobulinaemia. Nevertheless, it remained a generally acceptable view that allergic disturbances were related to the pathogenesis of RA even if they could not be regarded as prime movers.

The manner in which allergic mechanisms injure tissues in RA has been the subject for detailed enquiry. Much of this work has centred on the possible part that the RhFs play in tissue injury. More recently, with the growth of interest in the role of macrophages and lymphocytes in cell-mediated immunity and hypersensitivity, the possibility that the tissues in RA are altered by cellular mechanisms has been increasingly considered.

The evidence that RhF can injure tissues directly, is conflicting. Seropositivity is common in severe cases of the disease, in those with nodule (granuloma) formation, in patients with vascular disease and in those with diffuse interstitial pulmonary fibrosis. Seropositivity is one index of continuous, active progressive disease and sero-positive patients have a poorer prognosis than sero-negative (Duthie et al, 1957). But this is a very different matter from being able to show that the factors themselves cause RA synovitis or the other associated lesions of the disease such as arteritis and pulmonary fibrosis. Additional indirect evidence of the pathogenic role of RhF has been obtained from the interation of RhF in synovial fluid with aggregated gammaglobulins to form Ag/Ab complexes that are quickly phagocytosed in vitro (Vaughan et al, 1969). This observation accords with the finding of Ag/Ab complexes and C' in the synovial fluid in vivo, and leads on to the suggestion of a possible mechanism by which such complexes could be phagocytosed by synovial fluid polymorphs, liberating lysosomal enzymes and degrading articular cartilage. A similar sequence is likely within marginal, synovial cells. Some limited, direct proof of the tissue-damaging actions of immune complexes in man was obtained by Hollander et al (1966): they showed that when altered IgG from a patient with RA was injected locally into the non-inflamed joint of another patient with the disease, local inflammation was produced, provided that the recipient had circulating RhF and that recipient and donor had in common at least two inherited Gm factors, genetically-determined antigens. Local inflammation could also be produced by the injection of autologous IgG or of the Fc fragment of IgG.

It remains possible that RhF acts, not directly, but synergistically, predisposing to injury in selected connective tissues, including the synovia. Evidence to support this concept was adduced by McCormick et al (1969); they demonstrated that nephrotoxic anti-kidney nephritis can be exacerbated when RhF is given simultaneously with nephrotoxic globulin. One of the few injurious actions directly attributable to the presence of high titres of RhF is the hyperviscosity syndrome (Jasin et al, 1970). The pathogenesis of this unusual syndrome, with high plasma viscosity, a bleeding diathesis and vasculitis, is, however, unlikely to determine the evolution of the synovial tissue injuries in the majority of cases of RA, but may explain certain of the systemic lesions.

The alternative view is that RhF formation is an incidental feature of RA, as it is in infective disorders such as subacute bacterial endocarditis, or that these immunoglobulins may even have a protective role, acting, for example, with the reticuloendothelial system to mediate against the ravages of an (unidentified) microorganism. Under certain circumstances, RhF inhibits C' fixation. Since the binding of C' to Ag/Ab complexes is a necessary preliminary to the cell damaging and inflammatory reactions in which C' plays a part, and since C' is so clearly shown in relation to the synovial cells and within phagocytosed synovial fluid Ag/Ab complexes in the active disease, there is a measure of support for a defensive role by RhF. It has, moreover, been shown that RhF may inhibit the lowering of serum C' levels that follows the experimental intraperitoneal injection of aggregated human gammaglobulin, in this way perhaps demonstrating a capacity for diminishing the local effects of an Ag stimulus. Nevertheless, aggregates of human gammaglobulin given intravenously do not apparently modify C' levels so that the explanation for this anti-Ag behaviour is not straightforward.

The view has been advanced that RhF may have a protective action mainly in extravascular sites such as the synovial and peritoneal spaces, limiting the damaging effects of Ag/Ab interactions and possibly assisting phagocytosis. Additional evidence that C' fixation is impaired by RhF derives from the demonstration that the factor prevents injury to C'-sensitive mitochondrial systems (Davis & Bollet, 1964; Gough & Davis, 1966).

It will be seen therefore that the significance of the RhFs, commonplace and characteristic of severe progressive RA but not found in the serum in the earliest stages of the disease, is not yet by any means clear. The synthesis of RhF may play no part in the genesis of the tissue lesions in RA. Alternatively, it still remains possible that in the nature and formation of RhF lies the key to some of the most important biological aspects of the disease.

Experimental Models

RA is not, apparently, reproducible in any animal species nor is the disorder transmissible from man-to-man, either by the transfusion of blood, by the injection of serum or by the implantation of viable synovial or white blood cells. Neither is RA encountered spontaneously in animals other than man. Having made these cautious comments, it is wise to balance them by drawing attention to a transmissible periarthritis of mice, to the natural infection of pigs caused by Erysipelothrix rhusiopathiae and to the polyarthritis caused by injecting adjuvants in rats. There is, in addition, an extremely large variety of other forms of arthritis that can be produced in a great diversity of animals by a bizarre range of techniques (Gardner, 1960 and 1965; Dumonde et al, 1973). As models, there are lessons to be learnt from all these animal studies that may aid in the elucidation of human RA.

It may not be entirely reasonable to expect the environmental agent(s) provoking rheumatoid arthritis in man to lead to exactly similar consequences in any animal species. Marked species differences are recognised in response to single damaging agents, or even to differing doses of a single agent. Taken in this light, the experiments of Warren et al (1969a and b; 1970) assume particular significance. Pooled RA synovial tissue was injected into inbred Swiss mice and the persistence of a transmissible agent demonstrated. The 'agent' could be recovered from inoculated mice after a periarthritis had been caused and homogenised material from the foot could be used to convey the 'infection' to further inbred animals. At the same time it was apparent that the 'agent' could be passed spontaneously through three generations by some, at present unidentified, congenital mechanism. The mode of action of this mechanism suggests a resemblance to the transmission of the Bittner mammary cancer virus, and it has been shown that the unidentified agent may be passed to cultured rabbit synovial cells. However, as yet, no microorganism has been isolated.

Erysipelothrix infection of swine, caused by an organism resembling the streptococcus, results in synovial tissue lesions that appear, by the crude criteria of light microscopy, to be identical with those of the synovia in

131

human RA. There is synovial cell hyperplasia, a widespread focal synovial lymphocytic infiltrate and progressive deformity. Although the disorder was at first thought to be a straightforward transmissible infective arthritis, a view supported by the ability to reproduce the disease in rabbits using the same microorganism, it was soon discovered that sensitisation by the repeated injection of the viable or non-viable Erysipelothrix could lead to the development of cardiac and of synovial lesions; the frequency and severity of the lesions were related to the levels of circulating complete Ab and to the extent of anaphylactic, dermal hypersensitivity to the bacterial Ag. It was then discovered that identical tissue changes could be produced in germ-free animals, using sterile Ag, and that the reaction could be transferred to non-immune animals by the passive use of immune sera.

A further model that has attracted much interest in recent years since the original descriptions of Stoerk et al (1954) and of Pearson (1956), is the polyarthritis caused in rats, but in no other animal, with the possible exception of the baboon, by the local intradermal injection of very small but measured quantities of Freund's incomplete adjuvant. The adjuvant mixture comprises very finely ground heat-killed Mycobacterium tuberculosis, or other acid-alcohol fast microorganisms, suspended in mineral oil; 0.05ml of this reagent given into the footpad or dorsal, cervical skin of the rat provokes an initial brisk, local inflammation. Different strains of rat display different susceptibilities. Nine to seventeen days later, a migratory sterile polyarthritis develops, affecting mainly the ankle, tarsal and metatarsal joints but also causing arthritis of the caudal joints with urethritis, conjunctivitis and ear nodules. The disease, transmissible to untreated syngeneic animals by means of lymphocyte suspensions but not by serum, can be suppressed by whole-body irradiation, by the use of radiomimetic or cytotoxic drugs or by the administration of rabbit anti-rat lymphocytic sera. There are obviously many features of the experimental disease that bear comparison with the problems of RA in man; adjuvant arthritis, as it has come to be called, has been used very extensively in the testing of anti-inflammatory and analgesic agents as well as in studies of the mechanisms of joint injury and their pathogenesis.

Chronicity

In microbiological disorders such as herpes simplex and tuberculosis, it is reasonably clear that the length of the disease is a result of a balance between the virulence and pathogenicity of the causal organisms, and the natural and acquired defence mechanisms of the host. A profitable host/parasite relationship is maintained by continual, but not excessive, viral or bacterial growth and multiplication. In RA, the reasons for the extended course of the disease are obscure. It is naturally possible that the characteristically

132

prolonged inflammatory response is the result of the survival and behaviour of a hitherto unidentified microorganism. A slow virus could be one such explanation. Another possibility is a progressive change in synovial and cartilage antigenic structure, with the formation and exposure of antigenic determinants that come to be treated by the patient as 'foreign'. Under these circumstances the immunological surveillance mechanism will activate T and/or B lymphocytes and a form of autoimmune (auto-allergic) reaction will develop. An alternative to this could be the emergence, on the basis of somatic mutation, perhaps in an X chromosome, of a clone of hitherto suppressed ('forbidden') immunocytes capable of perpetuating a longstanding inflammatory reaction against their own body tissues. These various explanations for the chronicity of RA have been discussed by Glynn (1968).

A view that has found favour in recent years, and that has received additional support from the work of Willoughby and Ryan (1970) on experimental granulomatous inflammation, is the concept that prolonged inflammation in RA is a consequence, not of a sustained allergic reaction against a foreign agent, or against altered somatic cell Ag, but against the **products** of inflammation themselves. Dumonde and Glynn (1962) demonstrated that a long lasting inflammatory reaction against heterologous, and in some cases, autologous fibrin, could be caused by the intra-articular injection of this Ag following intradermal sensitisation. The degree of the chronic reaction is influenced by the mechanism used to sensitise the animal; and the response is particularly prolonged when another Ag, to which the animal has previously been sensitised, is incorporated in the implanted fibrin. The chronic reaction is not, apparently, due to the persistence within the inflamed joint of the added Ag. It may be accompanied by the secretion of IgM RhF-like globulins but this form of response is by no means specific and is not necessarily relevant to the chronicity of the human disease.

CONCLUSIONS
(Figure 6)

The cause, or causes, of the clinical syndrome of RA remain unknown. There is still a great dearth of knowledge of the physiology, biophysics and metabolism of normal diarthrodial joints: the lack of understanding of the responses of joints to mechanical, inflammatory, allergic and chemical disturbances is correspondingly greater. These points, and the difficulty of gaining access to very early cases of the disease, all contribute to our ignorance of the true nature of RA and greatly restrict explanations of its pathogenesis.

The available evidence suggests that a genetic **predisposition** is not important; where heredity is implicated, the disease is of the more severe, seropositive type with a relatively poor prognosis. Any genetic factor must

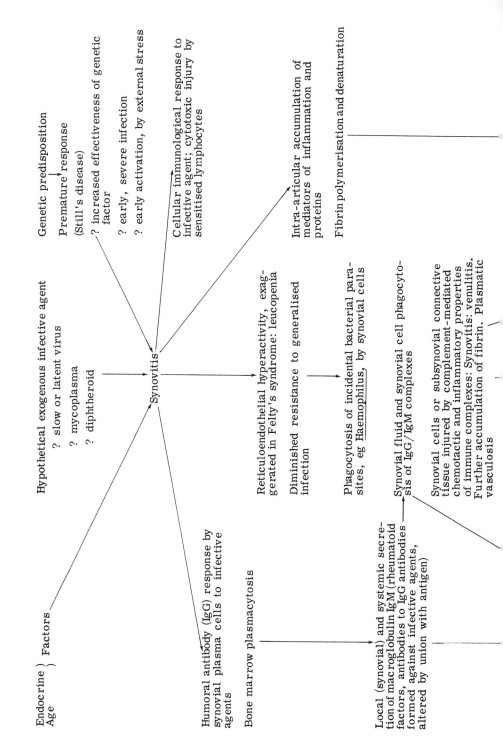

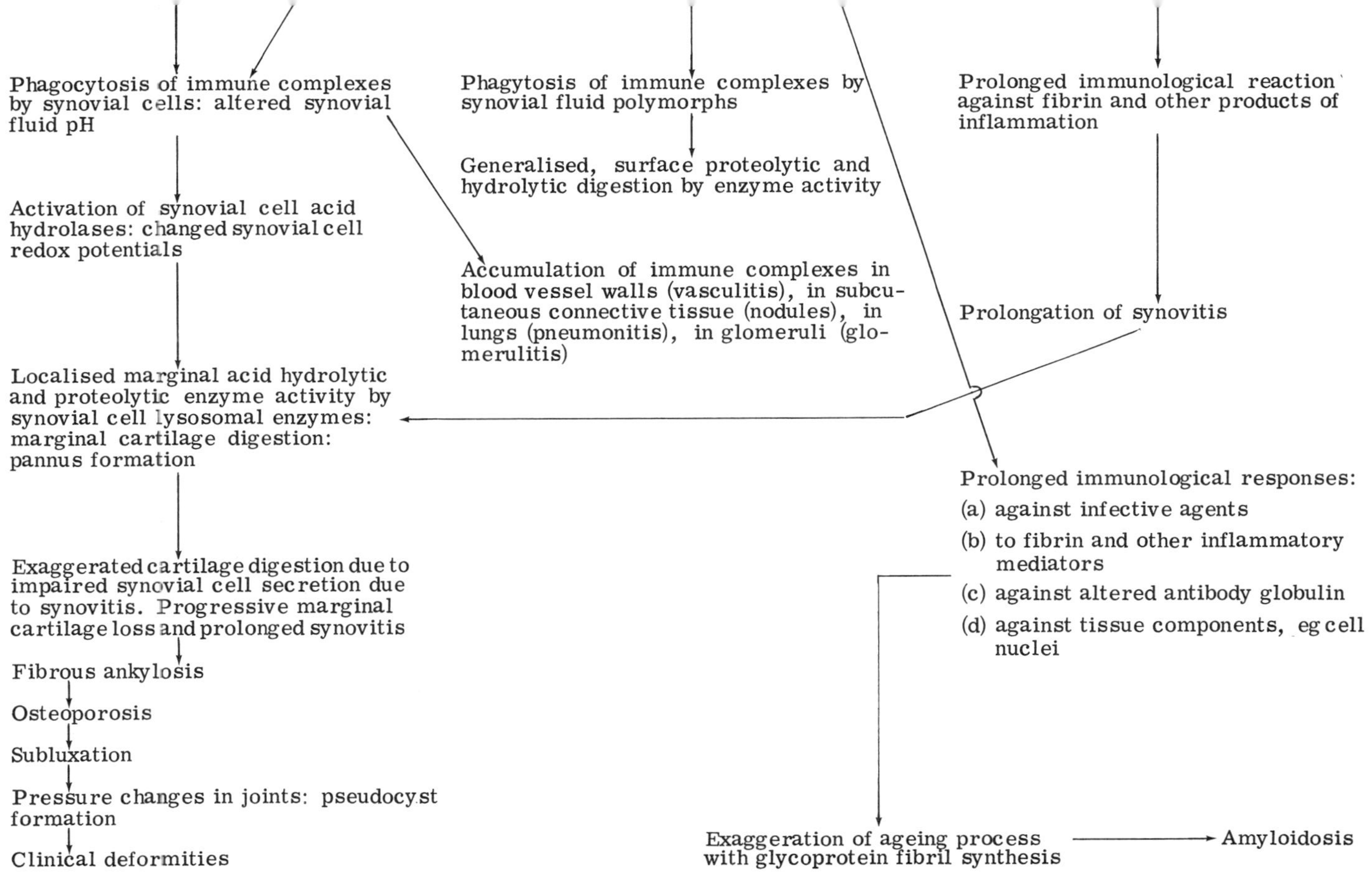

Prolonged immunological reaction against fibrin and other products of inflammation

Phagytosis of immune complexes by synovial fluid polymorphs

Generalised, surface proteolytic and hydrolytic digestion by enzyme activity

Accumulation of immune complexes in blood vessel walls (vasculitis), in subcutaneous connective tissue (nodules), in lungs (pneumonitis), in glomeruli (glomerulitis)

Prolongation of synovitis

Prolonged immunological responses:
(a) against infective agents
(b) to fibrin and other inflammatory mediators
(c) against altered antibody globulin
(d) against tissue components, eg cell nuclei

Phagocytosis of immune complexes by synovial cells: altered synovial fluid pH

Activation of synovial cell acid hydrolases: changed synovial cell redox potentials

Localised marginal acid hydrolytic and proteolytic enzyme activity by synovial cell lysosomal enzymes: marginal cartilage digestion: pannus formation

Exaggerated cartilage digestion due to impaired synovial cell secretion due to synovitis. Progressive marginal cartilage loss and prolonged synovitis

Fibrous ankylosis

Osteoporosis

Subluxation

Pressure changes in joints: pseudocyst formation

Clinical deformities

Exaggeration of ageing process with glycoprotein fibril synthesis ⟶ Amyloidosis

Figure 6. Scheme illustrating some of the possible mechanisms that may operate in the pathogenesis of rheumatoid arthritis. [From Gardner, D. L., 1972. 'Pathology of Rheumatoid Arthritis'. Edward Arnold, London]

be attributed to somatic mutation, probably of cells of the lymphoreticular system, and associated with one of the X chromosomes. A familial pattern of disorder, is, however, significantly frequent.

The most probable **initiating** agent leading to the clinical syndrome of RA, and occasionally manifest in childhood, when it accounts for what is termed Still's disease, is a microorganism. Investigations have suggested that streptococci, diphtheroids, mycoplasmas, bacterial 'L' forms, Bedsoniae and viral agents may be held responsible. But in no case is the evidence complete. For the most part, the recovery of any of these organisms from RA joints is inconstant, the results of different investigators conflicting. In all instances, there is a lack of direct evidence linking the common allergic phenomena of RA and the tissue lesions, with any identifiable microorganism.

The only reasonable possibility that remains open to analysis is that a persistent, slow or latent virus, within connective tissue cells, and normally evoking no allergic reaction, is activated by a variety of exogenous stimuli such as physical or mental stress, leading to selective inflammatory responses in susceptible tissues, in particular synovial joints. The inflammatory reactions progressively destroy cartilage by the marginal, centripetal action of synovial cells and histiocytes. The responses of these cells **mediate** the degradation of cartilage by the release and activation of lysosomal proteases: cartilage degradation probably occurs in a series of steps. The inflammatory changes detected in synovial fluid in RA are epiphenomena that have diverted much research effort from the marginal synovial cellular responses.

Whatever the initial disturbance, and the views expressed above should be seen as no more than working hypotheses, there is very general agreement that articular injury is **promoted** by allergic disorders that probably include humoral and cellular mechanisms. The synthesis of anti-IgG immunoglobulin M, RhF, a process that accounts for the clinical state of 'seropositivity' and which is linked with an adverse prognosis and the development of extra-articular disease, is an example of one humoral mechanism. It can be said to be of autoallergic ('autoimmune') character. There is disagreement as to whether the factor is injurious or protective. It may be coincidental to the disease. The lymphoreticular disorders of RA are shown by a frequent hyperplasia and overactivity of the cells of lymph nodes, spleen and bone marrow. The thymus does not appear to participate, but there is little evidence to substantiate this view.

Why RA follows such a prolonged course is obscure. There is evidence that the lengthy articular inflammatory reactions are allergic responses against products, such as fibrin, of the inflammatory changes themselves. In the context of the human disease, this is not yet proven. Alternatively, the long-standing changes that are so characteristic may represent reactions to a persisting, unidentified microorganism or be incidental consequences of the sequence of severe mechanical disturbances that are part of the clinical picture in the established disease.

ACKNOWLEDGMENTS

I am most grateful to Mrs Deirdri McCullagh for her help in the preparation of this manuscript.

My research continues to enjoy the generous support of the Arthritis and Rheumatism Council for Research and of the Nuffield Foundation, and has been aided by a grant from the Northern Ireland Hospitals Authority.

REFERENCES

Allison, A. C. (1972) Journal of Clinical Pathology, **25**, Suppl. (Royal College of Pathologists), **6**, 121

Barnett, E. V., Balduzzi, P., Vaughan, J. H. and Morgan, H. R. (1966) Arthritis and Rheumatism, **9**, 720

Bartfield, H. (1962) New England Journal of Medicine, **267**, 551

Bartholomew, L. E. (1965a) Arthritis and Rheumatism, **7**, 291

Bartholomew, L. E. (1965b) Arthritis and Rheumatism, **8**, 376

Baxter, A., Izatt, M. M., Jasani, M. K. and McAndrew, R. (1968) Acta rheumatologica Scandinavica, **14**, 79

Bennett, P. H. and Burch, T. A. (1968) Arthritis and Rheumatism, **11**, 546

Burnet, F. M. (1971) 'Genes, Dreams and Realities'. Medical and Technical Publishing Co. Ltd., Aylesbury

Cadham, F. T. (1932) Canadian Medical Association Journal, **26**, 287

Cadham, F. T. (1942) Canadian Medical Association Journal, **46**, 31

Carter, C. O. (1969) 'ABC of Human Genetics'. Lancet, London

Chayen, J., Bitensky, L., Butcher, R. G. and Cashman, B. (1971) Beiträge zur pathologischen Anatomie und zur allgemeinen Pathologie, **142**, 137

Clasener, H. A. L. and Biersteker, J. (1969) Lancet, **ii**, 1031

Davis, J. S. and Bollet, A. J. (1964) Journal of Immunology, **92**, 139

Dick, G. (1972) (Editor) Journal of Clinical Pathology, **25**, Suppl. (Royal College of Pathologists), **6**

Dingle, J. T. (1962) Proceedings of the Royal Society of Medicine, **55**, 109

Dumonde, D. C. and Glynn, L. E. (1962) British Journal of Experimental Pathology, **43**, 373

Dumonde, D. C., Steward, M. W., Glass, D. N. and Maini, R. N. (1973) British Journal of Hospital Medicine, **9**, 51

Duthie, J. J. R., Brown, P. E., Knox, J. D. E. and Thompson, M. (1957) Annals of the Rheumatic Diseases, **16**, 411

Duthie, J. J. R. (1971) in 'Modern Trends in Rheumatology' Volume 2. (Ed) A. G. S. Hill. Butterworth, London

Fagraeus, A. (1948) Acta medica Scandinavica (Suppl.), 204

Fell, H. B. and Mellanby, E. (1952) Journal of Physiology, **116**, 320

Fell, H. B. and Thomas, L. (1960) Journal of Experimental Medicine, **111**, 719

Felty, A. R. (1924) Bulletin of the Johns Hopkins Hospital, **35**, 16

Ford, D. K. and Oh, J. O. (1965) Arthritis and Rheumatism, **8**, 1047

Fraser, K. B., Shirodaria, P. V., Haire, M. and Middleton, D. (1971) Journal of Hygiene (Camb.), **69**, 17

Fudenberg, H. and Martensson, L. (1963) Bulletin of Rheumatic Diseases, **13**, 313

Gardner, D. L. (1960) Annals of the Rheumatic Diseases, **19**, 297

Gardner, D. L. (1965) 'Pathology of the Connective Tissue Diseases'. Edward Arnold, London

Gardner, D. L. (1971) Orthopaedics, Oxford, **4**, 1

Gardner, D. L. (1972) 'The Pathology of Rheumatoid Arthritis'. Edward Arnold, London

Gardner, D. L., Kreig, A. F. and Chapnick, R. (1962) Interamerican Archives of Rheumatology, 5, 561

Gardner, D. L. and McGillivray, D. C. (1971a) Annals of the Rheumatic Diseases, 30, 3

Gardner, D. L. and McGillivray, D. C. (1971b) Annals of the Rheumatic Diseases, 30, 10

Gardner, D. L. and Roy, L. M. H. (1961) Annals of the Rheumatic Diseases, 20, 258

Germuth, F. G., Maumenee, A. E., Senterfit, L. D. and Pollack, A. D. (1962) Journal of Experimental Medicine, 115, 919

Glynn, L. E. (1968) Annals of the Rheumatic Diseases, 27, 105

Glynn, L. E. and Holborow, E. J. (1965) 'Autoimmunity and Disease'. Blackwell Scientific, Oxford

Gough, W. W. and Davis, J. S. (1966) Arthritis and Rheumatism, 9, 555

Grayzel, A. I. and Beck, C. (1970) Journal of Experimental Medicine, 131, 367

Harvald, B. and Hauge, M. (1956) Danish Medical Bulletin, 3, 150

Hill, A. G. S., McCormick, J. N., Greenbury, C. L., Morris, C. J. and Kenningale, J. (1967) Annals of The Rheumatic Diseases, 26, 566

Hollander, J. L., Fudenberg, H., Rawson, A. J., Anelson, N. M. and Torralba, T. P. (1966) Arthritis and Rheumatism, 9, 675

Jansson, E., Vainio, U., Snellman, O. and Tuuri, S. (1971) Annals of the Rheumatic Diseases, 30, 413

Jasin, J. E., LoSpalluto, J. and Ziff, M. (1970) American Journal of Medicine, 49, 484

Kellgren, J. H., Ball, J., Fairbrother, R. W. and Barnes, K. L. (1958) British Medical Journal, 1, 1193

Klemperer, P., Pollack, A. D. and Baehr, G. (1942) Journal of the American Medical Association, 119, 331

Lawrence, J. S. (1970) Annals of the Rheumatic Diseases, 29, 357

Lucy, J. A., Dingle, J. T. and Fell, H. B. (1961) Biochemical Journal, 79, 500

McCormick, J. N., Day, J., Morris, C. J. and Hall, A. G. S. (1969) Clinical and Experimental Immunology, 4, 17

Marcolongo, R. Jr., Carcassi, A., Bianco, G., Bravi, A., Di Paolo, N. and Lunghetti, R. (1969) Bollatino dell'Istituto sieroterapico milanese, 48, 363

Meyerowitz, S., Jacox, R. F. and Hess, D. W. (1968) Arthritis and Rheumatism, 11, 1

Mills, D. M., Salky, N. K. and Diluzio, N. R. (1964) Arthritis and Rheumatism, 7, 331

Mohos, S. C. and Wagner, B. M. (1969) Archives of Pathology, 88, 3

Muirden, K. D. (1966) Annals of the Rheumatic Diseases, 25, 387

O'Brien, W. M. (1967) Clinical and Experimental Immunology, 2, 785

Parker, M. T. (1965) Journal of Hygiene (Camb.), 63, 457

Peacock, A. C. and Alepa, F. P. (1966) Annals of the Rheumatic Diseases, 25, 567

Pearson, C. M. (1956) Proceedings of the Society for Experimental Biology and Medicine (NY), 91, 95

Rose, H. M., Ragan, C., Pearce, E. and Lipman, M. O. (1948) Proceedings of the Society for Experimental Biology and Medicine (NY), 68, 1

Roy, L. M. H., Alexander, W. R. M. and Duthie, J. J. R. (1955) Annals of the Rheumatic Diseases, 14, 63

Stewart, S. M., Alexander, W. R. M. and Duthie, J. J. R. (1969) Annals of the Rheumatic Diseases, 28, 477

Stoerk, H. C., Bielinski, T. C. and Budzilovich, T. (1954) American Journal of Pathology, 30, 616

Vaughan, J. H., Jacox, G. A. and Clark, R. (1969) Annals of the NY Academy of Sciences, 168, 111

Waaler, E. (1940) Acta pathologica et microbiologica Scandinavica, **17,** 172
Walton, K. W. (1968) International Review of Experimental Pathology,
   6, 285
Warren, S. L., Marmor, L., Liebes, D. M. and Hollins, R. (1969a)
   Nature, **223,** 646
Warren, S. L., Marmor, L., Liebes, D. M. and Hollins, R. (1969b)
   Archives of Internal Medicine, **124,** 646
Warren, S. L., Marmor, L., Liebes, D. M. and Hollins, R. (1970)
   Clinical Orthopaedics, **70,** 217
Whaley, K. and Dick, W. C. (1969) British Journal of Hospital Medicine,
   2, 1916
White, R. G. and Gordon, J. (1970) Clinical and Experimental Immunology,
   7, 139
Williams, M. H. (1968) in 'Rheumatic Diseases'. (Ed) J. J. R. Duthie and
   W. R. M. Alexander. University Press, Edinburgh
Williams, M. H., Brostoff, J. and Roitt, I. M. (1970) Lancet, ii, 277
Willoughby, D. A. and Ryan, G. B. (1970) Journal of Pathology, **101,** 233

PART III

CLINICAL PHARMACOLOGY (I)
Chairman: Dr D G Grahame-Smith

CLINICAL PHARMACOLOGY (II)
Chairman: Dr A Goldberg

Recent Advances in Psychopharmacology
MALCOLM LADER

I intend to keep to my brief, that is to outline some of the areas in clinical psychopharmacology in which advances have occurred. I wish it were possible to say at this juncture whether these changes are really advances and not mere trends, but as will soon become apparent this area is so empirical that advances can only be detected from the vantage point of considerable retrospect. Some of the topics I shall discuss have little in common with others but some are interlinked, the common theme being drug metabolism and pharmacokinetics.

It is generally considered that the first modern psychotropic drug is chlorpromazine, introduced in France in 1952. Therefore, this year of 1973 is the 'coming of age' of modern psychopharmacology. But has it really grown up, ready to take its place as a discipline in its own right? Have any therapies been developed based on a rational approach rather than on empirical discoveries? Examination of the discovery of most, if not all, psychotropic drugs in current use reveals a repeated story of accident and serendipity (Ayd & Blackwell, 1970). Indeed, those few drugs which were developed with some sort of rationale have almost all been of little practical value but I shall draw a discreet veil over these failures. Many of the drugs in clinical use were discovered in the course of the search for other compounds such as antihistamines or hypotensive agents. Often, when a new psychotropic compound was discovered, the pharmacologist in the laboratory had to develop techniques to characterise the spectrum of action of these drugs de novo. Chlorpromazine, for example, has a profile of action so different from the previous psychotropic drugs such as paraldehyde and the barbiturates that even now it is impossible to see how it could have been developed and discovered in a logical, rational manner. Only recently has it become probable that the mechanism of the major tranquillising action of drugs like chlorpromazine is related to their interference with dopamine turnover.

The emphasis in research has also been on basic biochemical mechanisms presumed to underlie abnormal mental states. Such systems, for example catecholamines in the brain, are certainly altered by many psychotropic drugs but the relevance of these changes to clinical effects remains unproven. The constantly recurring basic problem is that there are no adequate animal models for any common psychiatric condition. Consequently, hypotheses regarding the modes of action of psychotropic drugs have to be tested in man with all the problems and limitations which this implies.

PHARMACOKINETICS

Even in the applied clinical sphere there have been difficulties which have often been glossed over and certainly infrequently examined in pharmacological terms. Despite substantial advances in the treatment of anxiety, depression and acute schizophrenia, and despite the euphoric, mutually congratulatory tone which too often typified meetings of psychopharmacologists, a group of sceptics remained who pointed out that an appreciable proportion of patients did not respond to the new pharmacological treatments. For example, about a fifth of patients admitted to hospital with depression show an inadequate response to antidepressive medication (Medical Research Council, 1965). This failure to respond was regarded by some as an arcane mystery which reinforced their view that psychiatric patients formed a heterogeneous group. The circularity of this argument hardly needs emphasising but the defeatism which it can produce must not be underestimated.

All along, the pharmacological factors governing drug response in patients have received surprisingly little attention. For example, the number of studies using classical pharmacological concepts such as dose-effect curves and bioassays is nugatory. The problems of absorption, distribution and metabolism were also neglected in comparison with the study of psychiatric, psychological and social factors. Nevertheless, some psychopharmacologists have refused to lose sight of the basic fact that these innovatory treatments were **drugs** and therefore could be presumed to be subject to the same processes as any other drugs, namely, absorption, distribution, metabolism and excretion. One major problem until very recently has been the difficulty of estimating many psychotropic drugs in body fluids. In the past few years a more pharmacological approach to psychotropic drugs has been apparent pari passu with the development of techniques for the measurement of plasma levels of many psychotropic drugs. The refinement of techniques such as gas-liquid chromatography has been a great impetus. Furthermore, the emphasis of official bodies such as the Committee on Safety of Medicines in this country and the Food and Drugs Administration in the USA on the pharmacokinetics of new psychotropic drugs has accelerated this trend (Martin, 1971). Until the last few years it was possible for a psychotropic drug to be marketed with no evidence that it was present in the body or having any effects other than the verbal reports of a few patients regarding their symptoms and mood.

Much work has been carried out, especially in Scandinavia, on the pharmacokinetics of the tricyclic antidepressives. Nortriptyline has been mainly used as it is the easiest to measure in plasma. Desmethylimipramine, amitriptyline and imipramine have also been investigated. The plasma half-life of nortriptyline following single oral doses (1 mg/kg) averaged 27 hours and that of desipramine was 18 hours (Alexanderson, 1972). Those for the parent dimethyl compounds, amitriptyline and imipramine, are at least as long. These long half-lives explain why many clinicians have adopted the practice of giving such drugs in a once daily dosage schedule (International Drug Therapy Newsletter, 1972). Amitriptyline is the favourite drug for this type of approach, 100 - 150 mg being given in a single dose at night. The unwanted effects such as hypotension and dry mouth are circumvented and the drowsiness effect is put to good use, the drug acting as a hypnotic. Patients are probably more likely to remember to take their medication and to persist with it when it is prescribed once daily rather than thrice daily.

After about a week of taking a tricyclic antidepressive drug, plasma levels reach a 'steady-state', the amount of drug metabolised and eliminated over 24 hours equalling the amount ingested. Much interest has centred around the relationship between the steady-state levels in patients and their clinical response to tricyclics, it being a reasonable assumption that rational advances in drug therapy would result from evaluation of pharmacological factors of this kind. However, different studies have produced different results.

The bulk of studies from Scandinavia support the idea of an inverted U-shaped curve between clinical response and plasma tricyclic levels (Figure 1). It is entirely reasonable that little clinical effect would be seen

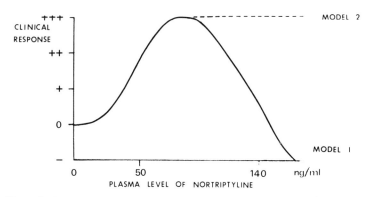

Figure 1. Diagrammatic representation of the two types of postulated relationship between clinical response and plasma level of nortriptyline in depressed patients

in patients with low plasma levels (less than 50 ng/ml). At high plasma levels unwanted effects would be expected to be sufficiently frequent and intense to interfere with treatment. Further, it is claimed that high levels of nortriptyline (over 140 ng/ml) are associated with lack of clinical response, the optimum levels lying between 50 and 140 ng/ml (Asberg et al, 1971). However, the data on which this claim was originally based, while suggestive, is not really significant when the correct statistics for the significance of a curvilinear relationship are applied.

Work in this country has not supported this data as high rectilinear rank-order correlations have been claimed between plasma levels of amitriptyline and nortriptyline and improvement on the Hamilton Depression Scale (Braithwaite et al, 1972). The correlations reported (mainly between 0.80 and 0.88) are high, at least as high as the test-retest or inter-rater reliabilities for the Hamilton Scale itself and this suggests that these correlations may partly have arisen by chance. The data of this study have been reanalysed by Gruvstad (1973) in an attempt to demonstrate that the curvilinear relationship of the earlier study was similarly present, so that this question is still an open one.

Yet another study, carried out in Australia, showed no relationship between plasma level and clinical response, nor any difference in clinical response in two groups of patients maintained at high and low drug levels respectively (Burrows et al, 1972).

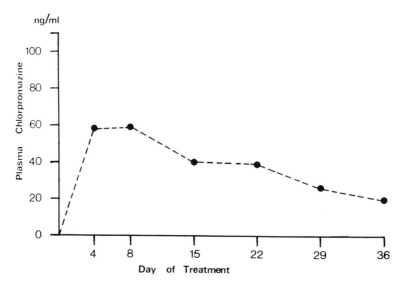

Figure 2. Mean plasma chlorpromazine levels in 10 acutely disturbed patients treated with chlorpromazine elixir, 100 mg 8 hourly orally, for at least five weeks. Measurements taken immediately prior to 8 am dose

Although steady-state levels are attained with tricyclic antidepressives, we have been unable to find such a stable situation with the chemically similar phenothiazine, chlorpromazine (Sakalis et al, 1972). Ten patients, previously drug-free for at least 4 weeks, were treated with chlorpromazine, 100 mg 8-hourly orally for 5-6 weeks. Plasma chlorpromazine levels were measured on the 4th, 8th, 15th, 22nd, 29th and last day of treatment, at 0, 2, 4 and 6 hours after the morning dose. The mean values for the 0 hour points are shown in Figure 2. There was an initial rise in level but thereafter the levels declined and no 'steady-state' was reached. We suggested that chlorpromazine accelerates its own metabolism by an induction effect on liver and/or gut hydroxylating enzymes but that the metabolite produced is itself psychotropically active so that there is no falling off in clinical effect (unlike the situation with barbiturates). In a further study, using the plasma half-life of the drug antipyrine as an index of liver hydroxylating 'power', our preliminary results suggest that an increase in this ability does occur consistently during the course of a month's treatment with chlorpromazine.

The finding of this induction effect of chlorpromazine has led us to mount some current experiments on drug interactions. Phenobarbitone is a well-known inducer and interactions with chlorpromazine are to be expected (Remmer, 1972). What is less well known is that orphenadrine ('Disipal'), an anti-Parkinsonian agent commonly given with chlorpromazine, is also an inducer of liver enzymes (Conney et al, 1960). It is tempting to speculate that orphenadrine works, at least in part, by inducing liver enzymes and thereby lowering the plasma concentration of chlorpromazine to less toxic levels. However, this would be a premature assumption because: (a) the accelerated metabolism of chlorpromazine may result in pharmacologically active compounds, and (b) drugs may compete for liver enzymes and reciprocally raise plasma levels (see Figure 3). The latter mechanism has been described for tricyclic antidepressives and phenothiazine tranquillisers. Combined administration of a representative of each class produces elevated plasma levels of both, presumably because partial blocking of the liver metabolising enzymes outweighs any induction effects (Gram & Overø, 1972). Thus, interactions between drugs must always be investigated empirically in man under realistic conditions of clinical use.

One final aspect of this young but growing area concerns the injectable tranquillisers. The first of these was fluphenazine formulated as the enanthate or decanoate in sesame oil. Injected intramuscularly as a 'depot' every 2 to 3 weeks, it has enabled patients who were uncontrolled and ill on oral medication to be maintained in a fairly stable state in the community. Placebo injections are ineffective so that non-specific factors such as increased social support or continuing detailed evaluation cannot be important (Hirsch et al, 1973). It has been shown that over 80 per cent of ingested

LIVER ENZYMES

INDUCTION	COMPETITION	NET RESULT ON PLASMA LEVELS
O [+] [+ +]	O [+] [+ +]	O
+ +	O	↓↓
+ [O]	+ + [+]	↑
O	+ +	↑↑
+ + [+]	+ [O]	↓

Figure 3. Interactions of drugs on liver enzymes. The net effect on plasma levels depends on the relative predominance of induction or competition

chlorpromazine is metabolised to inactive metabolites such as the sulphoxide as it passes through the gut-wall. By giving a phenothiazine intramuscularly, not only is one certain that the drug has been taken but the rate of breakdown is much less as there is no 'first-pass' breakdown in the liver. Studies are at present in progress to confirm whether patients who do well with depot injections but poorly on oral phenothiazine have low plasma drug levels while on the latter, presumably due to rapid metabolism.

The study of the pharmacokinetics of the important psychotropic drugs such as chlorpromazine and nortriptyline has already shown that these treatments discovered by chance and introduced empirically are subject to the same pharmacological principles as any other medication. The use of such an approach may well solve some of the outstanding problems in clinical psychopharmacology.

LITHIUM

I shall now turn to lithium, which has the longest and the most involved story of all of the modern generation of psychotropically active agents. Even now, the situation is confused and the need for continuing controlled evaluation of this cation's actions in mania and depression has not lessened.

In the 19th century lithium was used as a treatment for gout, the rationale being that lithium urate was the most soluble of the urates and therefore lithium might be expected to dissolve gouty deposits. However, the levels attained in practice were far too low for the lithium to exert any uricosuric effect. A second use for lithium at this time was as the bromide in the treatment of epilepsy.

Both these uses of lithium lapsed and the substance was little used until the 1940's when it was introduced as a sodium-substitute in the diet of cardiac and hypertensive patients. Its toxicity, including three deaths, was quickly recognised and it was withdrawn after a great deal of alarm had been produced in physicians and patients in the USA.

The discovery of the psychotropic actions of the lithium ion was made serendipitously in 1948 by the Australian psychiatrist John Cade (1970). He had hypothesized that mania was attributable to an excess of a hypothetical toxic substance, that this substance was excreted in the urine and should be demonstrable on injection into animals such as guinea pigs. In the course of this work, Cade became interested in the interactions between uric acid and the toxic effects of urea and he injected lithium urate, the most soluble salt. He noted that 'the animals, although fully conscious, became extremely lethargic and unresponsive to stimuli for one to two hours before once again becoming normally timed and active' (Cade, 1970). This was due to the lithium ion as lithium carbonate also produced this effect.

Because of his interest in mania, Cade tried lithium in 10 manic patients and noted dramatic improvement in all. Little notice was taken when these results were published but, gradually, mainly because of the persistent efforts of the Danish psychiatrist, Mogens Schou, lithium became established as a treatment for mania. The slowness of the acceptance of lithium for this purpose is of interest and reflects a large number of factors such as the availability of other effective drugs such as chlorpromazine, the memory of the debacle when lithium was used in the 1940's, the lack of commercial incentive as lithium, per se, is not patentable, and a suspicion among many psychopharmacologists that lithium must act in some blunderbuss fashion akin to bromide in epilepsy. Nevertheless, a few small-scale controlled trials were carried out which indicated that lithium was effective in combating manic symptoms (eg. Schou et al, 1954; Maggs, 1963; Wharton & Fieve, 1966; Bunney et al, 1968).

Mania is an uncommon condition as evidenced by the relatively small numbers in these trials, and lithium would have continued to play a minor role in psychiatry if it had not been for the claims of Baastrup and Schou (1967) that lithium was effective in the prophylaxis not only of recurrent attacks of mania but also of recurrent attacks of depression. This was so whether the patient suffered from manic-depressive episodes (so-called 'bipolar' illnesses) or from depressive episodes only ('unipolar' illnesses). As recurrent affective disorders represent a common disorder and as the establishment of prophylactic, as opposed to curative, drug effects is a complex scientific problem, this claim needed very careful evaluation. Unfortunately, the data supporting this claim, and several other trials in

149

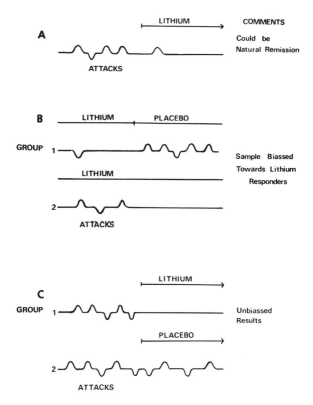

EXPERIMENTAL DESIGNS

Figure 4. Experimental designs to assess prophylactic properties of lithium. See text for further details

this area, stemmed from the unacceptable design of comparing episode frequency while on lithium with that in a similar period before treatment commenced (see Figure 4A). As the natural history of affective disorders is not usefully predictable, such a design will inevitably bias the results in favour of lithium.

The criticisms were partly met by taking a group of patients maintained on lithium and dividing it into two sub-groups, one continued on lithium and the other switched, under double-blind procedures, to placebo (Baastrup et al, 1970). The relapse rate in the placebo group was high suggesting that patients successfully maintained on lithium are still deriving benefit from it after one or more years (Figure 4B).

The most scientifically acceptable design is to take patients with recurrent affective disorders and to randomly allocate them to lithium therapy or placebo (Figure 4C). This was done in a group of 65 patients studied for periods up to 112 weeks by Coppen and his colleagues (1971). The patients were carefully assessed by a psychiatrist and by a psychiatric social worker. The results showed the great superiority of lithium: no patient on lithium needed ECT whereas 43 per cent of those on placebo received one or more courses. Similarly, 86 per cent of lithium-treated patients were rated as showing little or no affective pathology during the course of the trial whereas only 8 per cent of the placebo group fell in these categories. Lithium seemed as effective in patients with unipolar illnesses as in those with bipolar illnesses.

These results would indicate the undoubted usefulness of lithium in the prophylaxis of recurrent affective disorders. However, the results of Coppen's trial are much better than any other published trial including the original report of Baastrup and Schou. This might be due to careful selection of patients, to routine lithium plasma level monitoring and dosage adjustment or to chance. A large-scale multi-centre American trial is almost concluded and one hopes its results will be equally conclusive.

One should note that the term 'prophylaxis' is not really appropriate. It seems that affective episodes, both manic and depressive, still occur but are muted and sub-clinical. 'Symptom-Suppressant' would be a less ambiguous label.

Meanwhile, the use of lithium in the treatment of mania has been challenged. A large-scale American study has recently been published which compared lithium to chlorpromazine in a total of 255 manic and hypomanic patients (Prien et al, 1972). Patients were classified as highly active or mildly active according to the amount of motor activity and treatments were compared in terms of early terminations, symptom change and toxicity. In highly active patients, chlorpromazine was clearly superior to lithium in acting more quickly, producing significantly fewer dropouts, and having a lower incidence of severe unwanted effects. In mildly active patients, differences were less clearcut: both drugs controlled the symptoms but lithium left the patients feeling less sluggish and fatigued and produced fewer unwanted effects. Many psychiatrists prefer haloperidol to chlorpromazine for the treatment of mania so that the comparison of lithium to haloperidol would be interesting. Nevertheless, it may still be, as Schou (1968) contends, that the combination of lithium with a major tranquilliser is the most effective therapy.

A similar comparison was evaluated in excited schizo-affective patients (Prien et al, 1973). Again, chlorpromazine was superior to lithium especially in the more ill patients.

The present position, in my opinion, is that lithium is not the treatment of choice on its own in controlling manic or excited schizo-affective patients, being both less effective and slower in onset of effect, especially in the more ill patients. In the prophylaxis of recurrent mania or depressive episodes, lithium, on current evidence, seems to be a useful therapy. Nevertheless, after nearly 25 years the place of lithium in psychiatry is not entirely clear.

There is a link between the previous section on pharmacokinetics and plasma levels and the practical use of lithium. Lithium is the first drug in psychiatry for which the monitoring of plasma levels is not only advisable but essential. The level should be maintained between about 0.8 and 1.4 meq/l, levels above this being commonly associated with toxic effects. Levels below this seem to be related to absence of or incomplete therapeutic response. It might well be that the tardy but undoubted success of lithium is partly due to the care with which optimum blood levels are routinely maintained.

AMINE PRECURSORS

The next topic I shall outline is one of the most exciting and important in drug therapy in psychiatry, namely, the use of amine precursors in the treatment of depressed patients (Carroll, 1971). Current biological theories of brain mechanisms in depression have in common their postulation of a key role for a brain monoamine deficiency underlying the disorder. There is no concensus concerning the particular monoamine of greatest importance in this respect, dopamine, noradrenaline, serotonin (5-hydroxytryptamine) and tryptamine, all being suggested. The relationships between these amines is complex with mutual influences on the various metabolic pathways. Similarly, the experimental and clinical evidence is confusing, the latter being derived from observations often of a necessarily unsystematic nature. Nevertheless, the theory that depression is related to a deficit of an amine such as noradrenaline or serotonin in the brain has provided an impetus for the empirical testing of amine precursors in clinical treatment.

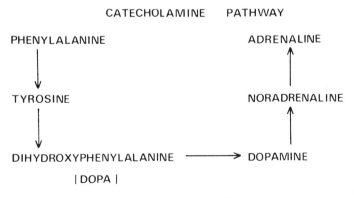

Figure 5. Catecholamine pathway

L-DOPA (see Figure 5)

The early studies of the effects of dopa in patients with depression were equivocal for the same reason as those in patients with Parkinsonism – the doses used can be seen with hindsight to have been far too low. Even so, in some studies using up to 50 mg L-dopa intravenously, it seemed that **retarded** depressive patients showed some transient improvement in the akinesia, if not in the mood (Ingvarsson, 1965; Matussek et al, 1970; Persson & Roos, 1967).

More recently, a controlled trial has been carried out in which depressed patients were given either a large dose (3 - 12.5 g/day) of L-dopa or a smaller dose (0.3 - 1.5 g/day) combined with an inhibitor of peripheral dopa decarboxylase (Goodwin et al, 1970). Of 16 patients, only 4, all retarded depressives, improved; 7 other retarded and 5 agitated patients failed to respond. In 3 of the 4 responders, relapse followed the substitution of a placebo. In all 5 patients with a previous history of mania, the L-dopa induced manic behaviour and in those who failed to show an antidepressive response, anger was noted. Psychotic features such as delusions and bizarre behaviour were often increased as well (Bunney et al, 1970), suggesting that L-dopa has a non-specific activating effect raising general arousal: this manifests itself as increased psychotic behaviour, mania or anger depending on the previous disposition of the patient. There is thus little support for the hypothesis that depression is associated with a diminution in brain catecholamines.

TRYPTOPHAN

Two precursors of serotonin are available which are able to cross the blood-brain barrier, namely, tryptophan, the naturally occurring amino acid, and 5-hydroxytryptophan (Figure 6).

The first trial of tryptophan was reported in 1963 when the amino acid was used in conjunction with the monoamine oxidase inhibitor, tranylcypromine (Parnate – Coppen et al, 1963). Tryptophan (10 - 17 g of D-L isomer) or placebo was added during the second of a four week period of treatment with tranylcypromine. The Hamilton Depression Rating scale scores fell more rapidly in weeks 2, 3 and 4 in the tryptophan-addition group than in the placebo-addition group. The conclusion was drawn that tryptophan potentiated the MAOI and that this effect persisted after withdrawal of the amino acid supplements. Other studies have supported the claim that tryptophan potentiates MAOI's (Pare, 1963; Glassman & Platman, 1969).

Further claims have been made that tryptophan on its own is an effective antidepressive agent culminating in the marketing of a proprietary preparation

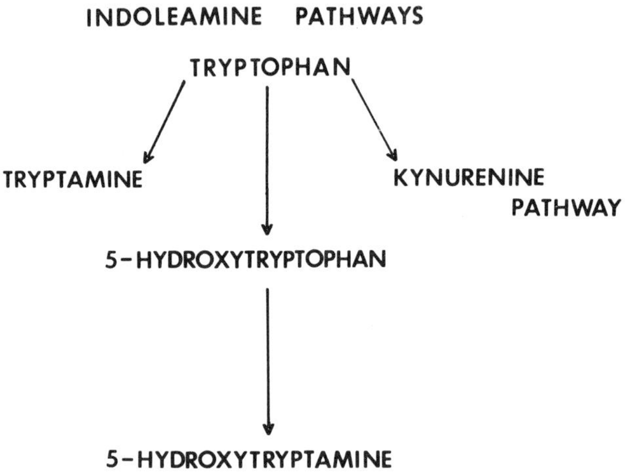

INDOLEAMINE PATHWAYS

TRYPTOPHAN

TRYPTAMINE   KYNURENINE
                                         PATHWAY

5-HYDROXYTRYPTOPHAN

5-HYDROXYTRYPTAMINE

Figure 6. Indoleamine pathways

Optimax, which consists of tryptophan plus pyridoxine and ascorbic acid, the vitamins being believed to facilitate the conversion to serotonin. This claim is based on the results of a trial comparing the effects of D-L-tryptophan (5-6 g/day) with and without MAOI's with the effects of ECT in a previously studied group (Coppen et al, 1967). Not only is this an unsatisfactory method of control but reliance was placed on self-rating scales which are suspect in a condition such as depression in which loss of insight often occurs. The various treatments appeared more or less equally effective and the authors implied that tryptophan was a potential alternative to ECT.

The deficiencies in this trial were such that replication is urgently called for especially as a more carefully conducted trial in Australia suggested that tryptophan had little or no activity (Carroll et al, 1970). Of 12 patients given L-tryptophan 7 g/day plus 170 mg of pyridoxine, only one improved in 3 weeks; of 12 treated with ECT, all improved.

A further mystery concerns the acute effects of L-tryptophan in normals. It is generally held that a few grams of the amino acid given orally have a soporific and hypnotic effect and that this might be exploited to provide a 'natural' sleeping tablet. In my laboratory Dr M Greenwood has infused up to 8 g L-trytophan over a period of 2 hours. The free (unbound) tryptophan in the plasma rose as much as 30-fold and yet the psychotropic effects detected were minimal. Recently, Oswald and his colleagues in Edinburgh reported their inability to note any change in time to onset or character of sleep following 7.5 g given to patients (Březinová et al, 1972).

5-hydroxytryptophan. As seen in Figure 6, tryptophan is hydroxylated to 5-hydroxytryptophan which is the immediate precursor of serotonin. As tryptophan is primarily metabolised through pathways other than the serotonin pathway, while 5-hydroxytryptophan is not, it would appear preferable to administer the latter. Clinical trials have been carried out and the preliminary results are as equivocal as those with L-tryptophan. Certainly, the rate and degree of response are less than 100 per cent.

To summarise, the biochemistry of both dopamine and serotonin precursors are very complex, so complex, in fact, that even if such precursors are found to be powerful antidepressive agents the interpretation of the mode of action will be difficult. For example, after large doses of tryptophan and especially 5-hydroxytryptophan, serotonin levels are raised in many areas of the brain, including some which are not usually serotoninergic. Also, administration of one precursor such as L-dopa may interfere with others like tryptophan by competing for brain uptake mechanisms and for decarboxylase enzymes and by acting as a false transmitter. Metabolites of biogenic amines may influence the effects of the amines themselves; for example, several of the metabolites of tryptophan in the kynurenine pathway (see Figure 6) competitively interfere with the uptake of tryptophan into the brain. For these and many other reasons it would be premature to assume that the demonstration of the antidepressive properties of an amine precursor would quickly lead to the elucidation of biochemical mechanisms in depressior Nevertheless, such a treatment would represent a very welcome addition to our armamentarium.

TRH

With respect to depression, mention should be made of the intriguing results following the injection of thyrotrophin-releasing hormone (TRH) (Prange et al, 1972; Kastin et al, 1972). In the first of these studies using a double-blind controlled cross-over design, the effects of a single TRH injection (600 μg) were compared with placebo in ten euthyroid depressed women. TRH caused a marked amelioration in depressive symptoms, maximal about 30 hours after the injection with a return of the symptoms over the next 5 days. There was no significant change in serum tri-iodothyronine (T_3) or free-thyroxine index during the day of the injection, and serum-TSH levels, although rising in response to the TRH, did so to a lesser extent than in normal subjects. The mechanism for this effect is obscure but may represent a direct action on the brain, perhaps on the hypothalamus. This area of the brain is believed to be underactive in patients with severe depression. As Papavisiliou et al (1972) have recently reported psychotropic actions of the pineal hormone melatonin in patients with Parkinson's disease it seems possible that brain hormones may play a significant role in the future in the treatment of behavioural disorders.

Turning now to the treatment of anxiety, we have been witnessing the inexorable procession of newly introduced benzodiazepines. However, I want to deal with a much more interesting topic, namely, the role of beta-adrenergic blocking agents in the treatment of anxiety. Let us go back to examine some of the basic theoretical issues. William James (1884) postulated 'that the bodily changes follow directly the perception of the exciting fact and that our feeling of the same changes as they occur is the emotion. Every one of the bodily changes, whatsoever it be, is felt acutely or obscurely the moment it occurs'. The following year, Lange put forward essentially the same ideas except that he limited the bodily changes to those of the cardiovascular system. The hypothesis has never been disproved because it is not susceptible to direct disproof as it is a philosophical viewpoint rather than a scientific hypothesis.

One indirect approach is to induce bodily changes by means of drugs acting peripherally, adrenaline being the most popular for this purpose, and then to evaluate the emotional responses produced. As with most drug studies of emotional states the results have been ambiguous. After receiving injections of adrenaline, many subjects report subjective changes of a rather indefinable, vague and inchoate nature without any genuine emotional colouring. These have been deemed 'as if' emotions. Other subjects or the same subjects on other occasions have experienced apparently genuine anxiety attacks but these could have been panic responses to the experimental situation and not directly attributable to the adrenaline.

The alternative experimental approach is to block physiological activity using pharmacological means and then to ascertain whether emotional blunting has occurred. Agents such as curare and atropine have been used but interest has centred recently on the effects of beta-blocking agents. Unfortunately, there is some evidence that many beta-blocking agents also have central effects which would make the interpretation of any emotional changes very difficult. Thus, evidence for a central action has been reported in animal studies (Leszkovszky & Tardos, 1965; Bainbridge & Greenwood, 1971) and in human subjects (Gillam & Prichard, 1965; Hinshelwood, 1969). In all these cases, however, the dosage was much greater than that used in therapeutic practice. The initial report that propranolol was therapeutically effective in anxious patients suggested that the autonomic symptoms were primarily ameliorated (Granville-Grossman & Turner, 1966); this is in favour of a peripheral mode of action in anxiety. Further evidence is the absence of therapeutic effects with D-propranolol which has the same properties as the L-isomer with the exception of beta-blockade (Bonn & Turner, 1971).

Dr Tyrer and I have attempted to detect central effects in normal subjects after single doses of beta-blocking agents (Lader & Tyrer, 1972). A wide range of central effects was measured using a small on-line laboratory computer and included the electroencephalogram, electroencephalic evoked response, and a range of psychological tests such as reaction time and key-tapping. Peripheral measures included the pulse rate, palmar sweat gland activity and finger tremor. Subjective mood scales were also used.

There was a significant drop in pulse rate over time for both agents as compared with placebo showing that adequate peripheral blockade had occurred. However, none of the other physiological or behavioural measures showed significant drug effects. For example, we have previously found one of the most sensitive measures of central drug effects to be the percentage of fast wave activity in the electroencephalogram. No drug effects on this variable were apparent. However, three of the subjective scales showed significant drug effects: the beta-blockers produced drowsiness, muzziness and caused the subjects to feel less tranquil. These effects showed the expected time effect course.

When one attempts to interpret the results the same sort of difficulties still intrude as those in interpreting results with infusion of adrenaline and indeed with the original formulation of the James-Lange hypothesis. Firstly,

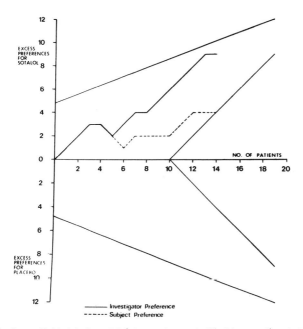

Figure 7. Sequential trial of sotalol (a beta-adrenergic blocking agent) and placebo in the treatment of patients with anxiety states (by kind permission of the editor and publishers of 'Clinical Pharmacology and Therapeutics')

157

the results could have been due to chance. Secondly, the beta-blocking agents could have had direct central effects although the measures which we used have been found in other studies to be very sensitive and one would have expected to have found more objective evidence of direct central effects. Thirdly, the subjective effects could be mediated indirectly because of the definite cardiovascular changes. Fourthly, the subjective effects could have been secondary to the perception of the peripheral physiological effects.

However, a second interest was in the use of these compounds therapeutically. Previous trials had reported only psychiatrists' rating of anxiety as indicators of drug effect (eg. Granville-Grossman & Turner, 1966; Bonn et al, 1972). We carried out a sequential trial of sotalol against placebo using a double-blind crossover design (Tyrer & Lader, 1973). If the psychiatrist's rating was taken as the criterion then the active drug showed every indication of being superior to placebo. However, if the patient's self-rating was used then the superiority of the drug could not be established (see Figure 7). Examination of individual symptoms suggested that the expected lessening of such symptoms as palpitations and gastric upset and tremor was, in fact, occurring but the patients still felt anxious. It appeared, therefore, that it is easy for a psychiatrist to mistake the peripheral symptoms of anxiety for anxiety itself but that the patient has no doubt as to the distinction between these two aspects of his condition and regards himself as unimproved if the central feelings persist. Our conclusions were that any reinforcement of anxiety by means of peripheral mechanisms was not important in the majority of patients and that such compounds as the beta-blocking agents would only be of use as adjuvants to treatment with centrally acting anxiolytic agents.

CONCLUSIONS

To conclude, I shall again stress that the undoubted advances in the area of drug treatment in psychiatry are based on the accidental discoveries of experienced physicians in psychological medicine working in the clinic with ill patients. No animal models of high predictive value have been developed so that further major advances must come by yet more serendipity. Nevertheless, the full realisation of the potential of the drugs already available has not yet been achieved and it is in this area that clinical psychopharmacology will play its most useful role.

REFERENCES

Alexanderson, B. (1972) European Journal of Clinical Pharmacology, **5**, 1
Asberg, M., Crönholm, B., Sjöqvist, F. and Tuck, D. (1971) British Medical Journal, **3**, 331
Ayd, F. J. and Blackwell, B. (1970) (Eds.) 'Discoveries in Biological Psychiatry', Lippincott, Philadelphia

Baastrup, P. C. and Schou, M. (1967) Archives of General Psychiatry, **16**, 162
Baastrup, P. C., Paulsen, J. C., Schou, M., Thompsen, K. and Amdisen, A. (1970) Lancet, **ii**, 326
Bainbridge, J. G. and Greenwood, D. T. (1971) Neuropharmacology, **10**, 453
Bonn, J. A. and Turner, P. (1971) Lancet, **i**, 1355
Bonn, J. A., Turner, P. and Hicks, D. C. (1972) Lancet, **i**, 814
Braithwaite, R. A., Goulding, R., Theano, G., Bailey, J. and Coppen, A. (1972) Lancet, **i**, 1297
Brézinova, V., Loudon, J. and Oswald, I. (1972) Lancet, **ii**, 1086
Bunney, W. E., Goodwin, F. K., Davis, J. M. and Fawcett, J. A. (1968) American Journal of Psychiatry, **125**, 499
Bunney, W. E., Murphy, D. L., Brodie, H. K. H. and Goodwin, F. K. (1970) Lancet, **i**, 352
Burrows, G., Turecek, S. and Davies, B. (1972) Psychopharmacologia, suppl. **26**, 80
Cade, J. F. J. (1970) In 'Discoveries in Biological Psychiatry'. (Eds.) F. J. Ayd and B. Blackwell, Lippincott, Philadelphia
Carroll, B. J. (1971) Clinical Pharmacology and Therapeutics, **12**, 743
Carroll, B. J., Mowbray, R. M. and Davies, B. M. (1970) Lancet, **i**, 967
Conney, A. H., Davison, C., Gastel, R. and Barns, J. J. (1960) Journal of Pharmacology and Experimental Therapeutics, **130**, 1
Coppen, A., Shaw, D. M. and Farrell, J. P. (1963) Lancet, **i**, 79
Coppen, A., Shaw, D. M., Herzberg, B. and Maggs, R. (1967) Lancet, **ii**, 1178
Coppen, A., Noguera, R., Bailey, J., Burns, B. H., Swani, M. S., Hare, E. H., Gardner, R. and Maggs, R. (1971) Lancet, **ii**, 275
Gillam, P. M. S. and Prichard, B. N. C. (1965) British Medical Journal, **2**, 337
Glassman, A. H. and Platman, S. R. (1969) Journal of Psychiatric Research, **7**, 83
Goodwin, F. K., Brodie, H. K. H., Murphy, D. L. and Bunney, W. E. (1970) Biological Psychiatry, **2**, 341
Gram, L. F. and Overø, K. F. (1972) British Medical Journal, **2**, 463
Granville-Grossman, K. L. and Turner, P. (1966) Lancet, **i**, 788
Gruvstad, M. (1973) Lancet, **i**, 95
Hinshelwood, R. D. (1969) British Medical Journal, **2**, 445
Hirsch, S. R., Gaind, R., Rohde, P. D., Stevens, B. C. and Wing, J. K. (1973) British Medical Journal, in press
Ingvarsson, V. C. G. (1965) Arzneimittel-Forschung, **15**, 849
International Drug Therapy Newsletter (1972) Nov-Dec issue Baltimore
James, W. (1884) Mind, **19**, 188
Kastin, A. J., Ehrensing, R. H., Schalch, D. S. and Anderson, M. S. (1972) Lancet, **ii**, 740
Lader, M. H. and Tyrer, P. J. (1972) British Journal of Pharmacology, **45**, 557
Leszkovszky, G. and Tardos, L. (1965) Journal of Pharmacology and Pharmaceutics, **17**, 518
Maggs, R. (1963) British Journal of Psychiatry, **109**, 56
Martin, E. W. (1971) 'Hazards of Medication'. Lippincott, Philadelphia
Matussek, N., Benkert, O., Schneider, K., Otten, H. and Pohlmeier, H. (1970) Arzneimittel-Forschung, **20**, 934
Medical Research Council (1965) British Medical Journal, **1**, 881
Papavasiliou, P. S., Cotzias, G. C., Duby, S. E., Steck, A. J., Bell, M. and Lawrence, W. H. (1972) Journal of the American Medical Association, **221**, 88
Pare, C. M. B. (1963) Lancet, **ii**, 527
Persson, T. and Roos, B. E. (1967) Lancet, **ii**, 987
Prange, A. J., Wilson, I. C., Lara, P. P., Alltop, L. B. and Breese, G. R. (1972) Lancet, **ii**, 99
Prien, R. F., Caffey, E. M. and Klett, C. J. (1972) Archives of General Psychiatry, **26**, 146

Prien, R. F., Caffey, E. M. and Klett, C. J. (1973) Archives of General
   Psychiatry, in press
Remmer, H. (1972) European Journal of Clinical Pharmacology, 5, 116
Sakalis, G., Curry, S. H., Mould, G. P. and Lader, M. H. (1972) Clinical
   Pharmacology and Therapeutics, 13, 931
Schou, M. (1968) Journal of Psychiatric Research, 6, 67
Schou, M., Juel-Nielsen, N., Strömgren, E. and Voldby, H. (1954) Journal
   of Neurology and Psychiatry, 17, 250
Tyrer, P. and Lader, M. (1973) Clinical Pharmacology and Therapeutics,
   in press
Wharton, R. N. and Fieve, R. R. (1966) American Journal of Psychiatry,
   123, 706

Physiological and Pharmacological Problems Related to Migraine

ELEANOR ZAIMIS

The field of migraine is still full of uncertainties and disagreements. I shall therefore refer first to the facts which are known and accepted and then discuss the areas where little is known and speculation flourishes.

In classical migraine, the attacks may be mild or completely incapacitating and are preceded or accompanied by transient focal neurological phenomena, such as visual, sensory or speech disturbances. The headache is usually unilateral, and may be associated with nausea and vomiting. At some stage, the pain assumes a throbbing quality, accentuated by coughing, sneezing or head movement.

VASCULAR CHANGES

There is almost complete agreement that the early phase of the attack (prodromal) must be due to vasoconstriction within the internal carotid system and the second phase (headache) to vasodilatation within the external carotid system and possibly other arteries. However, the existing evidence is based on very few quantitative measurements (Table I). Furthermore, some of the concepts regarding cerebral circulation are in the process of changing. For example, for many years the part played by cerebral vasomotor nerves was dismissed as negligible. But recent evidence leaves no doubt that cerebral blood vessels have a rich nerve supply and that there are both vasoconstrictor and vasodilator pathways. Moreover, physiological studies demonstrating that these nerves have a significant function are beginning to accumulate. Purves (1972), in his excellent monograph on "The Physiology of the Cerebral Circulation", points out that on the available evidence, vasomotor nerves could be important in at least three ways. Firstly, vasomotor activity could interact with and act as a fine control for other factors which are known to affect vascular smooth muscle — eg carbon dioxide, oxygen and hydrogen ions in plasma or extracellular fluid. In addition, James et al (1969) have shown that the neural contribution becomes progressively more important as

Table I. Vascular Changes

EARLY PHASE OF THE ATTACK (prodromal)

Vasoconstriction, within the internal carotid system

Dukes and Vieth (1966)	- angiography
O'Brien (1967)	- ^{133}Xe - inhalation
Skinhøj and Paulson (1969)	- ^{133}Xe - internal carotid artery

SECOND PHASE (headache)

Vasodilatation, within the external carotid system, and possibly other arteries

Tunis and Wolff (1952)	- recording of the pulsations of the superficial cranial arteries
Skinhøj and Paulson (1969)	- ^{133}Xe - internal carotid artery

---

arterial pressure or blood gas tensions depart from the physiological range. A second way in which vasomotor nerves could be involved is in determining the rate at which cerebral vascular responses occur. Purves indicates that the response of cerebral vascular smooth muscle may consist of two principal components, a fast component which is reflexly determined and which may be initiated by stimulation of peripheral arterial baroreceptors and chemoreceptors, and a slow component which represents either the intrinsic response of vascular smooth muscle or its response to an altered chemical environment. The third function of vasomotor activity in the cerebral blood vessels might be to integrate the response of the cerebral vascular bed with those of other peripheral beds. Studies on these lines coupled with electrophysiological and biochemical studies should one day solve the question — at present unanswered — of whether migraine results primarily from a neural or a vascular disorder.

PRECIPITATING FACTORS

There is also good agreement about the factors which may precipitate a migraine attack. These include dietary and physical factors, fasting, hypnotics, hormonal influences, psychological mechanisms and vasoactive substances. Amongst the foods considered to be migraine precipitants in some patients are chocolate, milk and milk products, alcohol and fish. The similarity between such foods and those reported to give rise to headaches and hypertensive incidents in patients treated with monoamine oxidase inhibitors was noted by Hanington (1967). Since Asatoor et al (1963) had found that tyramine was the only pressor amine consistently present in significant amounts in several types of fermented cheese, Hanington gave tyramine to patients who had a clear dietary history and found that this monoamine did indeed precipitate attacks of migraine. Later, Hanington, Horn and Wilkinson (1969) reported that tyramine appeared to have a graded effect, producing severe headaches frequently in those with a history of migraine, but only mild headaches infrequently in those with no history of headache. More recently, a defect in the ability of migrainous subjects to conjugate tyramine was discovered (Youdim et al, 1971). However, it is unlikely that a defect in tyramine metabolism is the only factor involved in dietary migraine, since chocolate, the food most commonly implicated as a precipitating factor, contains very little tyramine.

Although the pharmacology of tyramine has been extensively discussed during the last few years, marked differences still exist between both the results obtained and the interpretations given to them. Many authors have put forward the hypothesis that the pharmacological effects of tyramine are indirect and depend on the release of noradrenaline from tissue stores. Studies of tyramine in our own department, however, strongly suggest a direct action on the effector cells themselves (Zaimis, 1972). Moreover, comparisons of the pharmacological actions of various sympathomimetic amines in man produced results which are difficult to reconcile with the view that the action of tyramine is entirely the result of noradrenaline liberation from tissue stores (Mueller & Horwitz, 1962; Cohn, 1965; Pilkington et al, 1966. For further details, see Zaimis, 1964 and 1968). It will be a pity, therefore, if the direct action of tyramine is ignored and theories related to the pathogenesis of migraine are built on the uncertain basis that the only action of this amine is to release a number of vasoactive substances from various tissues. One such recent example involves the prostaglandins. Because prostaglandins are known to be associated with the experimental production of headache (Carlson, 1967), Sandler (1972) suggested that in migraine, pharmacologically active substances, such as tyramine, gaining access to portal venous blood, may provoke the secondary release from the lungs of a prostaglandin or other active substance into the systemic circulation. However, attempts to detect them either in venous blood, or indeed in cerebrospinal fluid during a migraine attack, have so far failed.

There is little doubt that hormones play a significant role although by no means all migraine attacks are hormonally dependent or triggered. The same is true for physical factors: exposure to excess heat, cold, flashes of bright light etc are well known precipitating factors. Many people with migraine know that alcohol or hypnotics may induce migraine, usually the following morning. Unusually heavy or long sleep on weekends or holidays is also a recognised cause for migraine (Friedman, 1969). Indeed, Gans (1951) reported that reducing the amount of sleep in his patients was followed by a reduction in the frequency and severity of the attacks. Blau (1971) has recently suggested that attacks of migraine precipitated by these factors may be related to the depth or length of sleep, "when carbon dioxide accumulation or relative anoxia can affect the intracranial circulation". It is an interesting point, worth testing.

Precipitating factors should always be investigated as their removal can be the most successful method of treatment.

DRUGS IN THE TREATMENT OF MIGRAINE

A further area of agreement concerns the usefulness of certain drugs in the treatment of migraine. For example, ergotamine, analgesics such as aspirin and paracetamol and antiemetics such as cyclizine or prochlorperazine, are generally considered the most effective drugs in treating the attack itself (Wilkinson, 1971). Other drugs such as methysergide and clonidine have proved quite successful in reducing the frequency and intensity of the attacks.

The antiemetics and the non-narcotic analgesics control the manifestations associated with a migraine attack. On the other hand, ergotamine, methysergide and clonidine have been introduced for a more specific reason — to reverse or prevent the abnormal vascular conditions.

Ergotamine

Ergotamine has a number of pharmacological actions but its therapeutic effect during an attack of migraine is generally considered to be due to its vasoconstrictor action. For example, Friedman (1972) has found a good correlation between the vasoconstriction of the cranial arteries and the reduction in headache intensity. Moreover, Brooke and Robinson (1970), have shown that ergotamine in man has an important constrictor effect on veins, even in the lower clinical dose-ranges. These authors also suggest that ergotamine's powerful venoconstriction may be the cause of the harmful cardiovascular side-effects (such as angina and pulmonary oedema) that are sometimes observed in patients with pre-existing heart disease.

More recently, doubts have been expressed as to the mechanism of action of ergotamine. For example, Lance et al (1969) suggest that vasoconstriction takes place because ergotamine mimics the constrictor effects of 5-HT. On the other hand, Berde (1972) and Salzmann and Kalberer (1973) have put forward the hypothesis that ergotamine is useful in migraine because it inhibits the re-uptake of noradrenaline and 5-HT by the specific stores.

Methysergide

Although it is an ergot derivative, methysergide has weak vasoconstrictor and oxytocic activity. However, Cerletti and Doepfner (1958) found that the drug inhibits the vasoconstrictor effects of 5-HT as well as its other actions on a variety of non-vascular smooth muscles. Because of these results and because the suggestion was made that the blood levels of 5-HT may be increased during a migraine attack, methysergide was introduced by Sicuteri in 1959, for the prophylactic treatment of migraine, and, indeed, methysergide has since proved its value (for details see Curran et al, 1967; Friedman, 1972). But, as with ergotamine, scientists differ in their opinions about the mechanism of action of methysergide. For example, Curran et al (1965) conclude that the beneficial effect of methysergide in the prophylaxis of migraine may depend "on it simulating the action of 5-HT". Similarly, Caroll and Hilton (1973) believe that methysergide is not a competitive inhibitor of 5-HT but that it exerts a 5-HT 'mimicking' effect on receptor sites throughout the body. Thus, according to them it constitutes a type of replacement therapy, with methysergide molecules standing in for 5-HT whenever reductions in the latter occur. On the other hand, Dalessio et al (1961) and Saxena (1972) suggest that a methysergide-induced increase in the sensitivity of the vessels to the action of circulating vasoconstrictor substances (especially noradrenaline and adrenaline) might explain its therapeutic value.

Clonidine

Clonidine, an imidazoline derivative, synthesised by Stähle et al in 1962, was introduced first in the treatment of moderately severe or severe hypertension and later on in the prophylactic treatment of migraine.

Clonidine is a powerful drug and, according to the dose and the route of administration, can produce a wide range of effects. For example, when the drug is administered to animals parenterally in large doses, or in smaller doses locally (into the cisterna magna, the lateral cerebral ventricle or the vertebral artery), a variety of central nervous system effects can be produced. Because of this, the assumption that the pharmacological effects of clonidine result from a central action underlies a great many statements made during the past few years (Kobinger & Walland, 1967; Sattler & Van Zwieten, 1967; Kobinger & Hoefke, 1968; Schmitt et al, 1968). Some of the central effects are specific: disturbances of thermoregulation (Maskrey et al, 1970); chemical changes in the brain and the spinal cord, evoked by stimulation of central noradrenaline receptors (Anden et al, 1970), and behavioural changes (Laverty & Taylor, 1969). Others are the result of a generalised depression of the central nervous system; these include severe sedation, depression of the vasomotor centre (bringing about a reduction of the sympathetic outflow) and inhibition of reflex pressor responses to carotid occlusion. Maskrey et al (1970) found that in the sheep and the goat an intraventricular injection of 3 μg of clonidine caused disturbances of thermoregulation without there being evidence of other central nervous changes such as sedation, which was seen only when 50 μg were injected into the lateral cerebral ventricle. Such doses of clonidine, however, if transferred to man would be completely outside the therapeutic range. In hypertensive patients, the daily oral dose is rarely larger than 0.5 mg while in the prophylactic treatment of migraine, it is no more than 0.15 to 0.2 mg a day. Our own conclusion is that in both man and animals, clonidine, in doses below 10 μg/kg, acts mainly by a direct effect on vascular smooth muscle. It is only when larger doses are given that the central nervous system effects become significantly involved. This conclusion is based on the following experimental results and clinical observations.

The drug, administered chronically to cats, reduces both the magnitude and the duration of vasoconstrictor and vasodilator responses elicited either by the electrical stimulation of the lumbar sympathetic chain, or by the close-arterial administration of vasoconstrictor and vasodilator drugs (Zaimis, 1970; Larbi,1970). It appears, therefore, that under the influence of clonidine, a change occurs in the smooth muscle which makes the vessels less capable of responding to, or of sustaining, either vasoconstriction or vasodilatation.

One of the most important aspects of the action of clonidine in man is that it does not interfere with vasomotor reflexes. The drug lowers recumbent blood pressure as effectively as it lowers the standing pressure and there have been no instances of serious orthostatic hypotension; the response to the Valsalva manoeuvre is not modified; and there is normal cardiovascular adaptation to exercise (Barnett & Cantor,1968; Muir et al,1969; Raftos,1969; Macdougall et al,1970). Obviously, under clinical conditions, the nervous control of the vessels is very little or not at all affected. Sedation is present in some but not all patients and then only when the dose exceeds 0.5 mg per day. Moreover, there is no correlation between the duration of hypotension and that of sedation, and in long-term treatment sedation appears to become less troublesome. Finally, the hypotensive response is clearly not dose-dependent but the incidence of side-effects increases with increased doses.

The fact that clonidine was found to affect both vasoconstrictor and vasodilator responses in animals, led to the suggestions that the drug should be given a trial in the prophylactic treatment of migraine (Zaimis & Hanington, 1969). The clinical results obtained so far are encouraging (Wilkinson,1969; Shafar et al,1972) and support the view that the drug has a direct vascular effect.

Further support of a direct action of clonidine on vascular smooth muscle comes from more recent findings. Because of the beneficial effects of clonidine in migraine, Clayden (1972) has made a preliminary evaluation of clonidine in the treatment of menopausal flushing. Eleven unselected patients were treated over a period of six weeks with doses varying from 25 to 75 μg twice

166

daily. Nine of them showed definite benefit. The side effects were minimal, and gave no cause for concern.

Clayden's findings are supported by the results of a recent study of ours in man. Ian James and I compared the effect of clonidine and two other hypotensive drugs, guanethidine and methyldopa, on the vasodilation induced by reactive hyperaemia. In healthy volunteers, forearm blood flow was measured by means of radioactive xenon, before and after the administration of the three hypotensive drugs. Each drug treatment lasted for seven days and all drugs were administered orally. In the clonidine-treated subjects, the reactive hyperaemia was significantly reduced; in contrast, it was considerably increased in the guanethidine and methyldopa-treated subjects. As in Clayden's cases, therefore, the response of the vessels, after clonidine, to the locally-released vasodilator substances was reduced.

WORKING HYPOTHESES RELATED TO THE PATHOGENESIS OF MIGRAINE

In the last twenty years many hypotheses concerning the pathogenesis of migraine have been put forward. Many of these are very attractive but only when experimental evidence becomes available shall we know which of these provides the true explanation.

Because the headache in migraine is thought to result from vasodilatation, Chapman et al (1960) and Karlsberg et al (1962) put forward the hypothesis that the pain is due to the combined effects of vasodilatation and the accumulation in the walls of the arteries and in the perivascular tissue of substances that lower the threshold to pain. A similar but somewhat more elaborate proposal was that made by Ostfeld (1960). According to him, "during the attack, a substance or substances are released that have the capacity to induce arteriolar vasodilatation and oedema and to bring about reversible tissue damage. The substance may be released locally by nerves, or may be a blood constituent that accumulates in the local oedema fluid entering through the more permeable scalp capillaries. Once damaged, local cells could in turn manufacture and release other noxious agents to maintain the process and make the pain of arterial dilatation more intense."

Many vasoactive substances, such as acetylcholine, noradrenaline, histamine, substance P, bradykinin and adenosine triphosphate have been discussed as probable headache substances (for details and references, see Ostfeld, 1960; Sicuteri, 1967) but the prime target of most research and discussion has been 5-HT.

Because locally applied 5-HT is a powerful pain-producing substance (Armstrong et al, 1952), Sicuteri (1959) introduced methysergide, a 5-HT antagonist, in the prophylactic treatment of migraine. The therapeutic efficacy of the drug was confirmed and this encouraged the speculation that the blood levels of 5-HT are increased during a migraine attack. Indeed, Sicuteri et al (1961) reported the presence in the urine of large amounts of 5-hydroxy-indoleacetic acid (5-HIAA), a 5-HT metabolite. However, further investigations have shown wide differences in 5-HIAA levels during migraine attacks. For example, Curran et al (1965) found that the urinary excretion of 5-HIAA was increased in 16 out of 31 patients while Curzon et al (1966) were able to correlate augmented 5-HIAA excretion with migraine headache in only 2 out of 9 patients. Variable results have also been obtained with plasma 5-HT levels. Since 1965 Lance and his group (for references see Anthony et al, 1969) have repeatedly reported that "plasma 5-HT drops sharply at the onset of a migraine attack and remains low while headache persists". This, they thought, was specific and not simply a reaction to headache, vomiting or stress. Because 5-HT has a vasoconstrictor action on scalp vessels, they suggested that "the sudden drop in plasma 5-HT, which may prove to be caused by a variety of 5-HT releasing agents, probably plays a part in the unrestrained extracranial vasodilatation of migraine headache, in patients who have an hereditary instability of extracranial vascular control." Reduced 5-HT blood levels during attacks of migraine were also found by Hilton and Cumings (1972). On the other hand, Kimball et al (1960) found the plasma level of 5-HT unaltered during a migraine attack and, more recently, Sandler and his colleagues (personal communication) concluded that there is no consistent pattern in the changes of the blood 5-HT levels or the MAO activity in platelets.

One has to ask why there is so much disagreement between the results of various investigators. Curran et al (1965) believe that the disagreement exists because the normal diurnal and individual variation of plasma 5-HT is so great that random sampling is meaningless. They insist that the results become meaningful only when a baseline has been established for each patient by frequent estimations. Dr Denis Sharman has drawn my attention to another possibility. In most investigations 5-HT blood levels are measured by means of a rapid spectrophotofluorimetric method (Ashcroft et al, 1964). With human blood under normal circumstances, the fluorescence as recorded by this method can be taken as a measure of 5-HT, as this is the only 5-OR indolyl compound normally detectable. However, other 5-OR indolyl compounds can give rise to a similar fluorescence (Sharman, 1960) and in pathological conditions such substances (as 5-HT precursors or metabolites) may be present in the blood in sufficiently high concentrations to contribute to the values for 5-OR indolyl concentrations given by the method.

Thus, over the last few years, a new theory has slowly emerged according to which, normal 5-HT turnover is necessary to prevent pain sensation. It is the reduction, therefore, and not the increase in 5-HT levels that induces the headache in migraine.

Fenclonine (p-chlorophenylalanine) a potent depletor of brain and peripheral 5-HT in both animals and man (Cremata & Koe, 1966) has played an important role in the growth of this theory. In 1967, Tenen demonstrated that in rats, the drug increases the animal's sensitivity to pain. Using a venoconstriction test in man, Sicuteri (1973) found that after fenclonine, the sensitivity of the veins to 5-HT but not to noradrenaline increased. Moreover, in migraine sufferers, the administration of fenclonine was followed by deep and superficial hyperalgesia and spontaneous pain in the limbs, trunk, neck and scalp (Sicuteri, 1971). Finally, the previous administration of either 5-hydroxytryptophan or tryptophan reduced the effects of fenclonine in both animals and man (Tenen, 1967; Sicuteri, 1973). Because of all these results and because the 'pain syndrome' does not appear after fenclonine in normal subjects, Sicuteri suggested that "a brain deficiency of 5-HT and consequently a state of central supersensitivity to the amine may be the basic condition in headache".

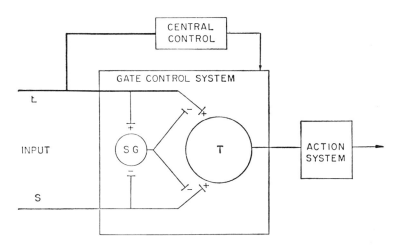

Figure 1. Schematic diagram of the gate control theory of pain mechanisms: (L) the large-diameter fibres; (S) the small-diameter fibres. The fibres project to the substantia gelatinosa (SG) and first central transmission (T) cells. The inhibitory effect exerted by SG on the afferent fibre terminals is increased by activity in L fibres and decreased by activity in S fibres. The central control trigger is represented by a line running from the large-fibre system to the central control mechanisms; these mechanisms, in turn, project back to the gate control system. The T cells project to the entry cells of the action system. + = excitation; − = inhibition (see text). (Melzack & Wall, 1965). Reproduced by kind permission of the Editor of 'Science'

All pain information is known to travel to the spinal cord via small-diameter fibres while stimulation of the larger-diameter fibres is never painful (Shealy, 1966). Moreover, it has been demonstrated that activity in the large fibre inhibits at the first spinal synapse, and subsequently activity in the small-diameter fibres, an activity considered essential to pain conduction. Melzack and Wall (1965) suggested that this mechanism normally acts as a gate to balance pain and non-pain input (Figure 1). Since the dorsal columns contain almost pure and concentrated large-diameter fibres, it was suggested that they offered the best sites for selective stimulation of these large fibres. And indeed Shealy et al (1967) demonstrated a significant increase in pain threshold during dorsal column stimulation. This technique has subsequently been applied to patients with chronic intractable pain (Shealy, 1970). Sicuteri (1973) suggests that 5-HT may be the biochemical mediator at this gate.

There is no doubt that workers in the field are trying hard to understand the problems of the pathogenesis of migraine but, as they themselves admit, experimental evidence for each of the existing theories is still scanty.   A closely-knit multidisciplinary approach may prove of value in future research.

REFERENCES

Andén, N. E., Corrodi, H., Fuxe, K., Hökfelt, B., Hökfelt, T., Rydin, C. and Svensson, T. (1970) Life Sciences, **9**, 513

Anthony, M., Hinterberger, H. and Lance, J. W. (1969) Research and Clinical Study of Headache, **2**, 29

Armstrong, D., Dry, R. M. L., Keele, C. A. and Markham, J. W. (1952) Journal of Physiology, **117**, 70

Asatoor, A. M., Levi, A. J. and Milne, M. D. (1963) Lancet, ii, 733

Ashcroft, G. W., Crawford, T. B. B., Binns, J. K. and MacDougall, J. E. (1964) Clinica Chimica Acta, **9**, 364

Barnett, A. J. and Cantor, S. (1968) Medical Journal of Australia, **1**, 87

Berde, B. (1972) Headache, **11**, 139

Blau, J. N. (1971) British Medical Journal, **2**, 751

Brooke, O. G. and Robinson, B. F. (1970) British Medical Journal, **1**, 139

Carlson, L. A. (1967) in 'Prostaglandins'. Nobel Symposium 2, page 123. (June 1966). (Ed) S. Bergström and B. Samuelsson. Almqvist and Wiksell. New York

Caroll, J. D. and Hilton, B. P. (1973) in 'Background to Migraine'. 5th Migraine Symposium. Heinemann, London (in press). Page 122

Cerletti, A. and Doepfner, W. (1958) Helvetica physiologica et pharmacologica acta, **16**, 55

Chapman, L. F., Ramos, A. D., Grodell, H., Silverman, G. and Wolff, H. G. (1960) Transactions of the American Neurological Association, **85**, 200

Clayden, J. R. (1972) Lancet, ii, 1361

Cohn, J. N. (1965) Circulation Research, **16**, 174

Cremata, V. Y. and Koe, B. K. (1966) Clinical Pharmacology and Therapeutics, **1**, 768

Curran, D. A., Hinterberger, H. and Lance, J. W. (1965) Brain, **88**, 997

Curran, D. A., Hinterberger, H. and Lance, J. W. (1967) Research and Clinical Study of Headache, **1**, 74

Curzon, G., Theaker, P. and Phillips, B. (1966) Journal of Neurology, Neurosurgery and Psychiatry, **29**, 85

Dalessio, D. J., Camp, W. A., Goodell, H. and Wolff, H. G. (1961) Archives of Neurology, **4**, 235

Dukes, H. T. and Vieth, R. G. (1966) Neurology (Minn.), **14**, 636

Friedman, A. P. (1969) in 'Background to Migraine'. 3rd Migraine Symposium. (Ed) A. L. Cochrane. Heinemann, London. Page 165

Friedman, A. P. (1972) International Encyclopaedia of Pharmacology and Therapeutics, Section 33, Volume 1. (Section Ed) A. Capi. Pergamon Press, Oxford

Gans, M. (1951) Journal of Nervous and Mental Disease, **113**, 405

Hanington, E. (1967) British Medical Journal, **1**, 550

Hanington, E., Horn, M. and Wilkinson, M. (1969) in 'Background to Migraine'. 3rd Migraine Symposium. (Ed) A. L. Cochrane. Heinemann, London

Hilton, B. P. and Cumings, J. N. (1972) Journal of Neurology, Neurosurgery and Psychiatry, **35**, 505

James, I. M., Millar, R. A. and Purves, M. J. (1969) Circulation Research, **25**, 77

Karlsberg, P., Adams, J. E. and Elliot, H. W. (1962) Surgical Forum, **13**, 425

Kimball, R. W., Friedman, A. P. and Vallejo, E. (1960) Neurology, **10**, 107

Kobinger, W. and Hoefke, W. (1968) in 'Hochdruck Therapie'. (Ed) L. Heilmeyer, H. J. Hothmill and E. F. Pfeiffer. Thieme, Stuttgart. Page 4

Kobinger, W. and Walland, A. (1967) European Journal of Pharmacology, **2**, 155

Lance, J. W., Anthony, M. and Hinterberger, H. (1969) 'Background to Migraine'. 34d Migraine Symposium. (Ed) A. L. Cochrane. Heinemann, London. Page 155

Larbi, E. B. (1970) On the Pharmacology of Clonidine. PhD Thesis, University of London

Laverty, R. and Taylor, K. M. (1969) British Journal of Pharmacology, **35**, 253

Maskrey, M., Vogt, M. and Bligh, J. (1970) European Journal of Pharmacology, **12**, 297

Melzack, R. and Wall, T. D. (1965) Science, **150**, 971

Mueller, P. S. and Horwitz, D. (1962) Journal of Lipid Research, **3**, 251

Muir, A. L., Burton, J. L. and Lawrie, D. M. (1969) Lancet, **ii**, 181

Macdougall, A. I., Addis, G. J., Mackay, N., Dymock, I. W., Turpie, A. G. G., Ballingall, D. L. K., Maclennan, W. J., Whiting, B. and Macarthur, J. G. (1970) British Medical Journal, **3**, 440

O'Brien, M. D. (1967) Lancet, **i**, 1036

Ostfeld, A. M. (1960) Journal of the American Medical Association, **174**, 1188

Pilkington, T. R. E., Lowe, R. D. Foster, R., Robinson, B. F. and Antonis, A. (1966) Journal of Lipid Research, **7**, 73

Purves, M. J. (1972) 'The Physiology of the Cerebral Circulation'. Monograph of the Physiological Society. Cambridge University Press, Cambridge

Raftos, J. (1969) Medical Journal of Australia, **2**, 684

Salzmann, R. and Kalberer, F. (1973) 'Background to Migraine'. 5th Migraine Symposium. Heinemann, London (in press)

Sandler, M. (1972) Lancet, **i**, 618

Sattler, R. W. and Van Zwieten, P. A. (1967) European Journal of Pharmacology, **2**, 9

Saxena, P. R. (1972) Headache, **12**, 44

Schmitt, H., Schmitt, Mme H., Boissier, J. R., Giudicelli, J. F. and Fichelle, J. (1968) European Journal of Pharmacology, **2**, 340

Shafar, J., Tallett, E. R. and Knowlson, P. A. (1972) Lancet, **i**, 403

Sharman, D. F. (1960) PhD Thesis, University of Edinburgh

Shealy, C. N. (1966) Headache, **6**, 101

Shealy, C. N. (1970) Journal of Neurosurgery, **32**, 560

Shealy, C. N., Tastitz, N., Mortimer, J. T. and Becker, D. P. (1967) Anesthesia and Analgesia - Current Researches, **46**, 299

Sicuteri, F. (1959) International Archives of Allergy and Applied Immunology, **15**, 300

Sicuteri, F. (1967) Research and Clinical Study of Headache, **1**, 6

Sicuteri, F. (1971) Pharmacological Research Communications, **3**, 401

Sicuteri, F. (1973) 'Background to Migraine'. 5th Migraine Symposium. Heinemann, London (in press). Page 45

Sicuteri, F., Testi, A. and Anselmi, B. (1961) International Archives of Allergy and Applied Immunology, **19**, 55

Skinhøj, E. and Paulson, O. B. (1969) British Medical Journal, **3**, 569

Stähle, H., Hauptmann, K. H. and Zeile, K. (1962) From the laboratories of C. H. Boehringer, Sohn, Ingelheim, Rhein

Tenen, S. S. (1967) Psychopharmacologia (Berlin), **10**, 204

Tunis, M. M. and Woolf, H. G. (1962) American Journal of Medical Science,

224, 565
Wilkinson, M. (1969) Hemacrania, **1**, 6
Wilkinson, M. (1971) British Medical Journal, **2**, 754
Youdim, M. B. H. , Carter, S. B. , Sandler, M. , Hanington, E. and
Wilkinson, M. (1971) Nature, **230**, 127
Zaimis, E. (1964) Annual Review of Pharmacology, **4**, 365
Zaimis, E. (1968) Anesthesiology, **29**, 732
Zaimis, E. (1970) in 'Catapres in Hypertension'. (Ed) M. E. Conolly.
Butterworth, London
Zaimis, E. (1972) in 'Nerve Growth Factor and its Antiserum'.
(Ed) E. Zaimis. Athlone Press, London
Zaimis, E. and Hanington, E. (1969) Lancet, **ii**, 298

Carcinoid Syndrome

P ISAAC

Disease states which produce paroxysmal symptoms attract the interest not only of the clinician but also that of the pharmacologist, who by tradition has concerned himself with the agents responsible for producing the symptoms. The carcinoid syndrome with its classically paroxysmal symptomatology provides a good example of how this shared interest can lead to a wider understanding of the biochemical basis of the disease and also provide useful suggestions for its treatment.

This syndrome is produced by tumours of the enterochromaffin system – a scattered series of cells derived from neuroectodermal stem cells which migrated into the primitive alimentary tract during embryological development (Weichert, 1970). Carcinoid tumours can occur anywhere in this system but are especially common in the small intestine and appendix (Table I – Sanders & Axtell, 1964).

Table I. The anatomical distribution of carcinoid tumours in the gastrointestinal tract (from Sanders & Axtell, 1964)

Site	Number	% with Metastases
Stomach	86	28
Duodenum	64	23
Jejunum and Ileum	841	33
Appendix	1173	2.9
Meckel's diverticulum	30	17
Caecum	40	71
Colon	28	52
Rectum	302	28
Gall Bladder	5	0
Abdominal Metastases (no primary found)	10*	10

* 8 of these patients had the carcinoid syndrome

173

With the exception of the somewhat rare bronchial and ovarian carcinoids which drain directly into the systemic circulation, metastatic spread to the liver appears to be necessary for the production of the diverse symptoms that constitute the carcinoid syndrome.

5-HYDROXYTRYPTAMINE

Histologically, carcinoid tumours are composed of clusters of small polygonal cells which contain granules that are capable of binding, and in some instances reducing silver salts. This argentaffinity appears to depend on the presence of high intracellular concentrations of 5-hydroxytryptamine (5HT – Pentilla & Lempinen, 1968). Tumour cells take up tryptophan from the plasma. This aminoacid is then converted by tryptophan hydroxylase to 5-hydroxytryptophan (5HTP) which is then decarboxylated to 5HT (Grahame-Smith, 1967 – Figure 1).

Although the actual amount of 5HT present in the tumour depends on rates of synthesis and metabolism, the extent of intracellular storage or release

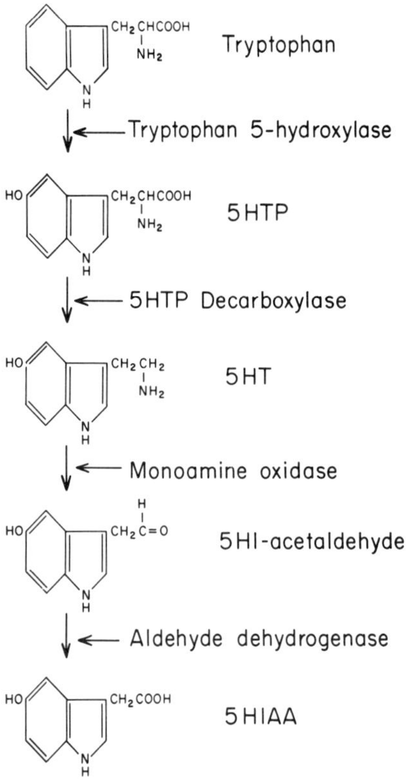

Figure 1. The synthesis and metabolism of 5-hydroxytryptamine

into the circulation, most small bowel carcinoids contain 100 - 1,000 $\mu g/G$ (Gowenlock & Platt, 1962).

What happens to the 5HT that is released from carcinoid tissue is not clear. The majority is probably taken up by the lungs (Davis, 1968) and much of the 5HT remaining in the circulation appears to be bound to platelets, which in some way give up their 5HT to tissue binding sites where it is converted by monoamine oxidase to 5-hydroxyindole acetaldehyde (5HIA) and eventually to 5-hydroxyindole acetic acid (5HIAA - Page et al, 1955). The result is that although whole blood 5HT levels are markedly raised, the plasma level of free 5HT - which is probably what is important for the production of symptoms - is only slightly elevated (Robertson et al, 1962). The increased 5HT turnover frequently leads to low plasma tryptophan levels, and, in practically all cases, greatly increased urinary 5HIAA excretion - the actual amounts of metabolite produced depending to a certain extent on the availability of tryptophan for 5HT synthesis. Although certain drugs such as chlorpromazine may interfere with the estimation of urinary 5HIAA there are very few instances of the syndrome reported with apparently normal 5HIAA excretion (Sandler & Snow, 1958); on the other hand bananas which contain large quantities of 5HT, increase 5HIAA excretion and may give false positive results.

It was at one time widely accepted that paroxysmal release of 5HT into the circulation was the cause of carcinoid flushing attacks. In support of this theory was the demonstration that intravenous injection of 5HT (0.3 - 1.8 mg) could produce flushing, both in normal subjects and in patients with the carcinoid syndrome (Page & McCubbin, 1953). However, Robertson and his colleague[(1962) pointed out that this 5HT-induced flushing was not impressive and was of a rather cyanotic nature. It was also accompanied by facial tingling and overbreathing, and sometimes, severe headaches and moderate hypertension - features that are not usually associated with spontaneous carcinoid flushing, but are pharmacological effects of 5HT. They also measured free plasma 5HT levels during noradrenaline-provoked flushing in their carcinoid patients and showed that flushing attacks were not usually accompanied by a rise in 5HT levels. There was one exception in which there was a paroxysmal rise in plasma free 5HT concentration during flushing - which was cyanotic in colour and accompanied by marked hyperventilation. It was concluded from these studies that although 5HT may occasionally be involved in flushing, another agent was also involved.

KALLIKREIN

In the search for this other agent some interesting earlier work came to light. This showed that certain catecholamines which provoke flushing attacks in carcinoid patients were also capable of stimulating kinin secretion

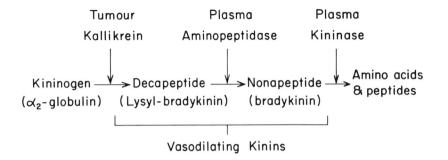

Figure 2. Synthesis and metabolism of bradykinin

in salivary glands (Hilton & Lewis, 1956). The **kinins** are polypeptides formed by the action of a proteolytic enzyme (kallikrein) on an α_2-globulin (kininogen) – (Figure 2). They are extremely potent vasodilators and intravenous injection of bradykinin in carcinoid patients produced a transient flushing and tachycardia which was quite similar to that seen in spontaneous attacks (Oates et al, 1964). The same authors showed that kallikrein was present in carcinoid tissue and was capable of converting human kininogen to bradykinin (Melmon et al, 1965). They also demonstrated that bradykinin levels in hepatic venous blood draining liver metastases increased considerably during flushing attacks and it has since been shown that arterial bradykinin levels are increased during spontaneous flushing and flushing provoked by pharmacological agents (Adamson et al, 1969).

FLUSH PROVOCATION

During these studies it was noticed that the time taken to produce the raised kinin levels and concomitant flushing varied consistently from one provoking agent to another (Figure 3). Intravenous bradykinin produced flushing within 40 seconds, the flush lasting for about a minute.

Noradrenaline intravenously produced its usual physiological effects of pallor and hyperventilation rapidly, but then, after about 75 seconds a flush began which was accompanied by raised blood bradykinin levels which fell again as the flush subsided. This led to the suggestion that whereas the injected bradykinin acts directly on the arterioles to produce vasodilatation and flushing, noradrenaline first has to circulate to, and stimulate, receptors in the carcinoid tissue. As a result of this, kallikrein is released from the tumour and acts on plasma kininogen to produce bradykinin which then circulates to produce the flush. In support of this sequence of events is the finding that phentolamine and phenoxybenzamine – α-adrenergic blocking agents, can prevent noradrenaline-provoked increases in plasma bradykinin

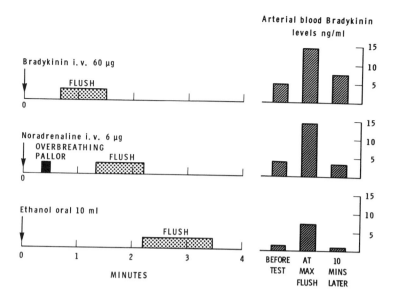

Figure 3. Carcinoid flush provocation

levels, presumably by blocking the tumour catecholamine receptors, and
also concomitantly prevent flushing. These α-adrenergic blocking agents do
not, however, inhibit the flush produced by intravenous bradykinin. In some
patients oral and intravenous **alcohol** produce flushes which take $2\frac{1}{2}$ - 3
minutes to develop and are again accompanied by raised plasma bradykinin
levels. In addition, alcohol induced flushing can sometimes be prevented by
α-adrenergic blocking agents. These findings have led to the proposal that
alcohol acts by releasing an endogenous catecholamine which, like intravenous noradrenaline, triggers the release of kallikrein from carcinoid
tissue. Flush provocation by intravenous noradrenaline 1 - 10 μg and oral
ethanol 10 cc in 15 cc orange juice, is an extremely valuable diagnostic tool
(Adamson et al, 1969).

FLUSH VARIATION

From these studies it would seem that bradykinin is an important factor in
the production of flushing but there are objections to it being the only factor
involved. Not all patients who flush have elevated plasma bradykinin levels,
and on closer examination, the flush produced by intravenous bradykinin is
not a perfect reproduction of a spontaneous flush. The bradykinin flush is
much pinker and lacks the usual patchy distribution. Tachycardia and hypotension are also more marked. It may be that in many patients 5HT acts

177

synergistically with bradykinin to produce the characteristic features of carcinoid flushing.

In other patients, particularly those with gastric carcinoids the flushing is a vivid red and has an unusual 'geographical' distribution. These patients have been shown to excrete large quantities of **histamine** in their urine and the histamine content of a gastric carcinoid tumour has been shown to be very high (Campbell et al, 1963). This suggests that some carcinoid tumours are composed of cells that not only produce 5HT and kallikrein but also make histamine. It also illustrates how predominance of a particular tumour product can lead to variations in the clinical picture (Grahame-Smith, 1968). The flushing associated with bronchial carcinoids sometimes lasts for several hours and is often accompanied by facial oedema and profuse lacrimation and perhaps one should be looking for yet another tumour product to account for this further variation. In this respect it may be relevant that Sandler and Snow (1958) have discovered that some bronchial carcinoids contain prosta-glandins.

Diarrhoea is another common symptom and is often accompanied by cramping abdominal pains and explosive defaecation. Although diarrhoea sometimes occurs during flushing attacks, these two major symptoms occur independently so often that one must conclude that they are probably **not** caused by the same agent. Whereas flushing may be due to kallikrein release it appears more likely that 5HT is responsible for the gastrointestinal symptoms. 5HT is present in normal gut mucosa and is also synthesized and stored in nerve endings of the myenteric plexus. Its overall effects are to increase small bowel activity while inhibiting the motility of the colon – effects which could well account for the observed symptoms (Misiewicz et al, 1966). Furthermore, drugs such as para-chlorophenylalanine and methysergide which interfere with 5HT synthesis and activity are often effective in relieving these symptoms.

In spite of this evidence, there are some difficulties in accepting the role of 5HT in the production of these symptoms. First, attacks of diarrhoea and pain tend to be paroxysmal yet paroxysmal elevations of free plasma 5HT levels are rare. Secondly, both bradykinin and prostaglandings have their own effects on gut motility and these might well contribute towards the clinical picture.

Fibrosis is one of the most striking features of the carcinoid syndrome and may affect the peritoneum, pleura and pericardium, and also, in a characteristic fashion, the heart itself. The cardiac lesions consist of sub-endothelial deposits of fibrous tissue on the luminal surface of the internal elastic lamina. The right side of the heart is mainly affected, especially the arterial aspect of the pulmonary valve cusps, and the ventricular aspect of the tricuspid valve. Plaques of fibrous tissue also tend to occur on the papillary muscles and chordae tendinae. Constriction and rigidity of the valves usually lead to pulmonary stenosis and tricuspid regurgitation. In those rare instances where left sided heart lesions have been reported, there has either been a right to left shunt at atrial level (McKusick, 1956) or a bronchial carcinoid draining into the pulmonary veins has been present (Roberts & Sjoerdsma, 1964). This distribution suggests that the agent responsible for producing the fibrosis (not yet identified but possibly 5HT) is effectively removed from the blood during circulation through the lungs.

Respiratory symptoms have frequently been reported (Mattingly & Sjoerdsma, 1956). The **hyperventilation** that often occurs during flushing attacks has been ascribed to 5HT, and intravenous injections of this agent are very effective in producing this symptom. As noted earlier, plasma 5HT levels were transiently increased in the patient who had marked overbreathing during cyanotic flushing (Robertson et al, 1962). Many patients who have pre-existing chronic bronchitis or emphysema notice a worsening in airways obstruction during flushing attacks. There are other patients without pre-vious chest disease who develop asthma-like symptoms during a flush. This **bronchoconstriction** can usually be relieved by Salbutamol or Isoprenaline. There are isolated reports of relief with phenoxybenzamine and also with methysergide. This 5HT antagonist when used intravenously also appears to be effective in overcoming the bronchoconstriction sometimes encountered in carcinoid patients during surgery and general anaesthesia (Mengel, 1965).

TREATMENT

Because the tumour and its metastases are slow-growing most patients with the carcinoid syndrome face several years of distressing symptoms. In carefully selected patients surgical removal of the primary tumour and its hepatic metastases affords dramatic relief and greatly reduces urinary 5HIAA excretion (Zeegen et al, 1969). Where possible it is the treatment of choice. Unfortunately, because of the widespread nature of the hepatic secondaries most patients are unsuitable for this form of therapy (Stephen & Grahame-Smith, 1972). In these patients pharmacological intervention is the mainstay of management. Reference to Figure 4 shows that there are several stages at which drugs may potentially interfere with the tumour products thought to be responsible for the major symptoms of the carcinoid syndrome.

α-methyl dopa interferes with the synthesis of 5HT by inhibiting the decarboxylation of 5HTP. It has been most helpful in those patients with cyanotic flushing.

179

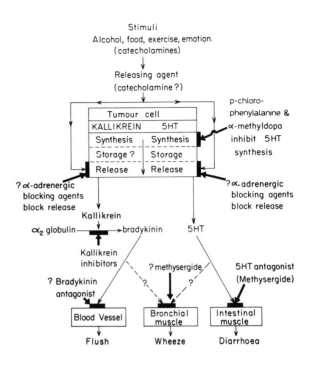

Figure 4. Clinical pharmacology of the Carcinoid Syndrome

Para-chlorophenylalanine inhibits tryptophan hydroxylation and effectively decreases 5HT synthesis and 5HIAA excretion. It usually has little effect on flushing but does sometimes relieve the diarrhoea and occasionally dramatically improves the patient's appetite and sense of well-being.

Methysergide is a potent 5HT antagonist and is at present the drug of choice in the treatment of severe carcinoid diarrhoea. However, its potentially dangerous side-effects such as retroperitoneal fibrosis and vascular spasm should be weighed against its beneficial effects.

As yet, very little has been achieved in the attempt to interrupt kallikrein production or activity. Rather surprisingly, **trasylol** which will inhibit carcinoid kallikrein in vitro (Melmon et al, 1965) failed to prevent flushing even when 170,000 units were infused into one patient over a 20 hour period (Grahame-Smith et al, 1965).

As mentioned earlier, release of 5HT and kallikrein from the tumour can be reduced by α-adrenergic blocking agents. Long term treatment with **phenoxybenzamine** (10 - 20 mg t.d.s.) can sometimes decrease both the frequency and severity of flushing attacks. Finally, **corticosteroids** have been tried. They appear to be ineffective in patients with gastrointestinal carcinoids but, inexplicably, prednisone in a dose of 20 mg daily can often produce significant improvement in the severe flushing and diarrhoea associated with bronchial carcinoid tumours.

I have tried to indicate that although progress has undoubtedly been made in understanding the pharmacological nature of the symptoms of the carcinoid syndrome there are still several features which demand further explanation. Another agent besides kallikrein will probably be found to be involved in flushing and yet another along with 5HT in the production of gastrointestinal symptoms. There are even fewer clues as to how the heart disease is produced. In conclusion, and perhaps most importantly, we should ask ourselves what is the carcinoid syndrome trying to tell us about the normal function of the enterochromaffin system?

REFERENCES

Adamson, A. R., Grahame-Smith, D. G., Peart, W. S. and Starr, M. (1969) Lancet, ii, 2, 293

Campbell, A. C. P., Gowenlock, A. H., Platt, D. S. and Snow, P. J. D. (1963) Gut, 4, 61

Davis, V. E. (1968) Advances in Pharmacology, 6B, 143

Gowenlock, A. H. and Platt, D. S. (1962) In 'The clinical chemistry of monoamines'. (Eds.) H. Varley and A. H. Gowenlock, Eisever, New York. Vol. 2, page 140

Grahame-Smith, D. G., Peart, W. S. and Ferriman, D. G. (1965) Proceedings of the Royal Society of Medicine, 58, 701

Grahame-Smith, D. G. (1967) Clinical Science, 33, 147

Grahame-Smith, D. G. (1968) American Journal of Cardiology, 21, 376

Hilton, S. M. and Lewis, G. P. (1956) Journal of Physiology, 174, 400

McKusick, V. A. (1956) Bulletin of the Institute of the History of Medicine, Johns Hopkins University, 98, 13

Mattingly, T. W. and Sjoerdsma, A. (1956) Modern Concepts of Cardiovascular Disease, 25, 7

Melmon, K. L., Lovenberg, W., Sjoerdsma, A. (1965) Clinica chimica acta, 12, 292

Mengel, C. E. (1965) Annals of Internal Medicine, 62, 587

Misiewicz, J. J., Waller, S. L. and Eisner, M. (1966) Gut, 7, 208

Oates, J. A., Melmon, K. L., Sjoerdsma, A., Gillespie, L. and Mason, D. T. (1964) Lancet, i, 514

Page, I. H. and McCubbin, J. W. (1953) Circulation Research, 1, 354

Page, I. H., Corcoran, A. C., Udenfriend, S., Sjoerdsma, A. and Weissbach, H. (1955) Lancet, i, 198

Pentilla, A. and Lempinen, M. (1968) Gastroenterology, 54, 375

Roberts, W. C. and Sjoerdsma, A. (1964) American Journal of Medicine, 36, 5

Robertson, J. I. S., Peart, W. S. and Andrews, T. M. (1962) Quarterly Journal of Medicine, 31, 103

Sanders, R. J. and Axtell, H. K. (1964) Surgery, Gynecology and Obstetrics with International Abstracts of Surgery, 199, 369

Sandler, M. and Snow, P. J. D. (1958) Lancet, i, 137

Stephen, J. L. and Grahame-Smith, D. G. (1972) Proceedings of the Royal Society of Medicine, 65, 444

Weichert, R. F. (1970) American Journal of Medicine, 49, 232

Zeegen, R., Rothwell-Jackson, R. and Sandler, M. (1969) Gut, 10, 617

Prostaglandins in Disease

ALAN BENNETT

The title 'Prostaglandins in Disease' embraces several entirely separate aspects. For example, there are diseases in which prostaglandins (PGs) may be used in treatment, diseases in which PG formation and release may contribute to the pathology, and diseases which might be due to drugs which interfere with PG synthesis. In order to understand these relationships, it is necessary to know what PGs are and how their metabolism or actions can be affected by drugs.

The PGs are 20-carbon fatty acids which are produced from straight chain C-20 essential fatty acids by the formation of a 5-membered ring from C-8 to C-12 (Figure 1). The substituents on this ring, and the position of ring C=C bonds which may be present, determine the type of PG (E, F, A, B or C) and its biological actions. The precursor fatty acid determines the number of double bonds in the side-chains. Dihomo-γ-linolenic acid gives rise to one C=C bond (as in PGE_1 and $PGF_{1\alpha}$ both of which can be formed from the same substrate depending on the co-factors present); arachidonic

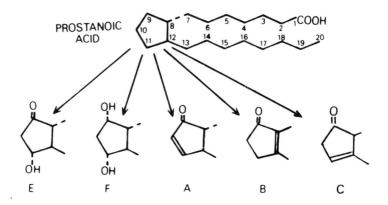

Figure 1. All the prostaglandins are derivatives of prostanoic acid. The substituents on the five-membered ring determine the name given to the prostaglandins (PGE, F, A, B or C). PGC has been discovered only recently (Jones, 1972)

182

acid, two C=C bonds (as in PGE_2 etc); eicosapentaenoic acid, three C=C bonds (as in PGE_3 etc). The subscripts used with the PGF compounds refer to the configuration of the -OH at C-8 which may be α (naturally occurring) or β. Biological activity is dependent on various factors including the ring substituents which determine the qualitative type of action, the presence of an -OH at C-15, and the number of C=C bonds in the side chains which usually alters the effects of the PGs quantitatively, but seldom qualitatively.

PGs are formed from their precursors by enzymes often referred to collectively as 'PG synthetase'. Recently Vane (1971, 1972) showed that aspirin and similarly acting anti-inflammatory drugs inhibit the synthesis of PGs (but not their actions), and this seems to be important therapeutically. The PG synthetase systems may differ at different sites. Whereas aspirin and paracetamol inhibit PG synthetase in rabbit and dog brain, only aspirin has a marked effect on synthesis by dog spleen in concentrations reached in the plasma with therapeutic doses in man (Flower & Vane, 1972). This seems to explain why both aspirin and paracetamol are antipyretic but only aspirin is anti-inflammatory (see later), and it might now be possible on this basis to produce drugs with higher degrees of selectivity. Another group of drugs of potentially great therapeutic importance are the PG antagonists (eg. the dibenzoxazepine derivative SC-19220 and polyphloretin phosphate – Sanner, 1969; Eakins et al, 1970; Bennett & Posner, 1971; Eakins & Sanner, 1972). These compete with PGs (mainly Es and Fs have been tested) at most, but not all, of their sites of action. Antagonists of action are mainly of theoretical interest at present since only polyphloretin phosphate is known to be safe to give to man, and there has been little attempt to use it in human disease conditions. The ability to block some receptors and not others may be of importance in drug selectivity.

PGs are rapidly inactivated in the body by various routes. For example, 95% of PGE and F compounds are inactivated by one passage through the pulmonary circulation (Ferreira & Vane, 1967). Two important pathways which have been identified are PG-15 dehydrogenase and delta 13 reductase. The dehydrogenation is prevented in analogues in which $-CH_3$ replaces the -H at C-15 (see later). An effective inhibitor of PG-15 dehydrogenase itself (ie analogous to the inhibition of acetylcholine hydrolysis by anticholinesterases) has yet to be found, but it might be of great value in conditions helped by PG administration.

DISEASES WHICH MIGHT BE TREATED WITH PGS

The logical situations for treating diseases with PGs are those in which the cause is due to a deficiency of PG production. In most cases, however, no such link has been clearly established, and the situations discussed are either in the experimental stage or are still hypothetical.

Asthma

PGE compounds relax the isolated bronchiolar smooth muscle of man and laboratory animals, whereas PGF compounds cause contraction (Main, 1964; Sweatman & Collier, 1968). Aerosols of PGE_1 and E_2 have been used in asthmatic patients to produce bronchodilatation and are many times more potent than isoprenaline (Cuthbert, 1969; Herxheimer & Roetscher, 1971). The problem so far is that the PGs are irritant and tend to cause coughing, and it is not yet known whether this can be improved by pharmaceutical formulation or whether a PG analogue would be more suitable. Aerosols of PGE compounds would seem to be desirable therapeutically because they are rapidly inactivated in the lungs, at least when infused intravenously. Their use in asthma has been based so far only on the inhibition of bronchial muscle, and the subject has been reviewed fully by Smith (1972). However, PGs can stimulate fluid secretion in the gut, and it will be important to see if such an effect occurs in the lung.

It has been postulated that bronchoconstriction in asthma might be due partly to disordered synthesis of PGs (Horton, 1969). Both PGE_2 and $PGF_{2\alpha}$ occur in human lung, and both are formed from the same precursor depending on the co-factors present. If formation of $PGF_{2\alpha}$ were to occur at the expense of PGE_2, bronchoconstriction would be expected. A somewhat analogous approach has been used in considering the occasional severe bronchoconstriction caused in a few asthmatics by aspirin and indomethacin. Perhaps there is inhibition of PGE_2 synthesis which normally maintains bronchodilatation.

Peptic Ulcers

PGE_1 or A_1 infused i.v. into human subjects reduces basal- and pentagastrin-stimulated gastric acid secretion (Classen et al, 1970, 1971; Wada & Ishizawa, 1970; Wilson et al, 1970). The mechanism by which this reduction occurs is not clear, however, since both PGs are highly vaso-active and might merely alter mucosal blood flow rather than affect the acid-secreting mechanism directly. Karim et al (1973) have studied analogues of PGE_2 which have the C-15 -OH group protected by a C-15 methyl group (15-methyl (S) PGE_2 methyl ester and 15-methyl (R) PGE_2 methyl ester) (the S and R show the configuration at C-15). These act orally in low doses to inhibit basal and pentagastrin-stimulated secretion for a period of a few hours. The R analogue is preferable because it lacks unwanted effects, although the dose required (0.2mg) is more than with the S-analogue. The drug appears to have a local action, rather than acting after absorption into the systemic circulation, since the same dose injected i.v. has no effect on secretion. The mechanism of action is unclear since substantially higher amounts of

PGE_1 or PGE_2 given orally do not inhibit secretion (Horton et al, 1968; Karim et al, 1973); perhaps this is due to rapid inactivation within the mucosa. It cannot be assumed that the PG analogue acts on receptors normally activated by PGE_2, since studies with the PG synthesis inhibitor indomethacin suggest that the PGE_2-like substance occurring in human gastric mucosa (Bennett et al, 1967) is unlikely to play an inhibitory role in gastric acid secretion (Bennett et al, 1972; 1973). But regardless of its mode of action the drug may be of value in the treatment of duodenal ulceration.

It is interesting that the anti-inflammatory drugs such as aspirin, indomethacin and phenylbutazone have in common the fact that they are acidic, they inhibit PG synthesis, and they cause gastric bleeding. Numerous reasons have been advanced to explain this (eg. see Salter, 1968), and it is tempting to speculate that inhibition of PG synthesis may be involved. PG release might maintain vasodilatation (see below under 'Hypertension'), and aspirin-like drugs might produce vasoconstriction and ischaemia. In support of this view, aspirin and indomethacin reduce gastric mucosal blood flow in the dog (A Bennett, B P Curwain and P Holton, unpublished).

Hypertension

PGE and PGA compounds are potent vasodilators, and the view has been expressed that they might circulate as peripheral vasodilators, that they might be produced and act locally in small blood vessels, or that they might regulate distribution of blood flow in the kidney (Lee, 1967). A role for PGA compounds as circulating antihypertensive agents is possible, because they (unlike PGE and PGF compounds) are not inactivated on passage through the lungs (Horton & Jones, 1969; McGiff et al, 1969). However, studies with the kidney, the organ from which the PG might originate, indicate that in the rabbit, renal levels of PGE_2 are much greater than of PGA_2 (Daniels et al, 1967). There is circumstantial evidence that PGs maintain vasodilatation locally in peripheral blood vessels, since the PG synthesis inhibitor indomethacin causes cerebral and conjunctival vasoconstriction (Sicuteri et al, 1965; Vecchio & Fontana, 1965). PG release appears to maintain tone in certain gastrointestinal muscles (Ferreira et al, 1972), and there is also some evidence that PGE release maintains relaxation of the circular muscle of guinea-pig colon (unpublished). The evidence for a role within the kidney is stronger, since PGE_2 is released from the dog kidney during ischaemia (McGiff et al, 1970; Aiken & Vane, 1971).

In several studies with hypertensive patients, PGA_1 has been infused i.v. at rates of $0.22/\mu g/kg/min$ (Lee et al, 1969) and above (see review by Karim & Somers, 1972). This produces a fall in systolic and diastolic pressures, tachycardia which appears to be reflex, and an increase in cardiac output. PG infusions are clearly unsuitable for the routine treatment of hypertension, but it remains to be seen whether orally acting analogues can be produced, or whether drugs can be used to inhibit the breakdown of PGs released into the bloodstream.

Thrombosis

Platelet adhesion and aggregation play a vital role in the initial phases of thrombus formation, and they might also be important factors in atherosclerosis (Robinson & LeBeau, 1967). It is therefore of particular interest that low concentrations of PGE_1 inhibit aggregation of human platelets in vitro in response to ADP and a variety of other agents (Kloeze, 1969). However, PGE_1 or PGE_2 infused i.v. in vivo (E_1 0.2μg/kg/min for 15 min – Elkeles et al, 1969; E_2 5μg/kg/min for several hours – Karim & Filshie, 1972) did not affect platelet aggregation. Perhaps this was due to rapid inactivation. PG ω-homo E_1 is more potent than PGE_1, but PGE_2 and other types of PG are less effective in vitro, and PGE_2 actually stimulates aggregation of pig and rat platelets (Kloeze, 1969). Further details of this subject are given in an excellent review by Mody (1972). It remains to be seen whether a stable analogue will be of value in the treatment and prevention of thrombosis and possibly of atherosclerosis.

Peripheral vascular disease

The potent vasodilator effect of PGE_1 has been used recently in peripheral atherosclerotic vascular disease by Carlson and Eriksson (1973). They infused PGE_1 1ng/kg/min into the femoral artery for about 10 minutes every hour for 24-72 hours, and found that the pain disappeared completely after the first infusion in 3 out of 4 patients, without any side effects. Subsequently there was a considerable improvement in rest pain in all cases and in no instance was amputation necessary. The action of PGE_1 may have been due to a relaxant effect on the vascular muscle, but the authors point out that an effect on metabolism or platelet aggregation might also be involved. In addition, it is possible that PGs cause muscle relaxation by inhibition of noradrenaline release; such a mechanism has been demonstrated in the cat spleen (Hedqvist, 1969).

DISEASES IN WHICH PGs APPEAR TO CONTRIBUTE
TO THE PATHOLOGY

Fever

The fever produced by pyrogen may involve PG, since PGE_1 injected into the third ventricle in cats is the most potent pyretic substance so far tested, and the amount of PG-like activity in the CSF is increased three-fold by pyrogen (Milton & Wendlandt, 1970, 1971; Feldberg & Saxena, 1971, 1972; Feldberg & Gupta, 1972). Paracetamol, which inhibits PG synthesis by the brain, reduces pyrogen-induced fever but not PGE_1-induced fever. The evidence in man that PGs may be involved in fever are that PGE_2 infused i.v. in obstetric patients may cause pyrexia (Hendricks et al, 1971), and that antipyretic drugs such as aspirin are inhibitors of PG synthesis.

Inflammation

There is strong evidence that PGs contribute to the inflammation at a variety of sites in the body. PG-like activity has been found, together with other substances, in the inflammatory exudate induced in cats by carrageenin (Willis, 1969), and in various inflamed human tissues (skin – Greaves et al, 1971; eye – Eakins et al, 1972a). Small amounts of injected PGE_1 and E_2 produce changes seen in inflammation such as vasodilatation and increased vascular permeability (Kaley & Weiner, 1971). Although an acute inflammatory reaction to thermal injury or the injection of turpentine can occur in the absence of polymorphonuclear leucocytes (Willoughby & Giroud, 1969), it seems likely that PG can also be released from white blood cells. This seems to be so with the PGE_1 appearing in the aqueous humour of the rabbit eye during experimental immunogenic uveitis: polymorphonuclear leucocytes which enter the inflamed eye contain PGE_1-like material whereas material resembling PGE_2 and $PGF_{2\alpha}$ occur in the ocular tissue (see Eakins et al, 1972b). It remains to be seen whether PG release from white cells occurs generally in inflammation, along with the many other factors which are involved.

Inhibition of PG synthesis appears to be an important factor in the mode of action of non-steroidal anti-inflammatory drugs (Vane, 1972). Whether the steroidal anti-inflammatory drugs act similarly is in doubt since the concentrations of hydrocortisone or fluocinolone ($100\mu g/ml$ – Greaves & McDonald-Gibson, 1972) which reduce PG synthesis by homogenates of rat skin are approximately 100 times higher than plasma levels reached with clinical dosages. Inhibition of PG synthetase could be involved with locally applied steroids, but another of several possibilities is that steroids 'stabilise' membranes and so may prevent essential steps in the synthesis of PGs. Or perhaps steroids prevent white cells entering the inflamed site and so reduce the amount of released PG.

Pain

PGE_1 and E_2 are potent pain-inducing substances in the mouse, as shown by the abdominal constrictions which occur when PGs are injected intraperitoneally (Collier & Schneider, 1972). Subdermal infusions of PGE_1 or E_2 alone in man may cause some pain. Ferreira (1972) showed that PGE_1 (30 ng/min) infused subdermally greatly increased the pain caused by bradykinin and/or histamine infused simultaneously. Inhibition of PG synthesis might therefore explain the analgesic action of aspirin-like drugs. Ferreira also pointed out, however, that lipoperoxides which act similarly to PGE_1 may be involved, and since their formation is not antagonised by inhibitors of PG synthesis some types of pain might be resistant to aspirin. Fuller details of the relationship of PGs to fever, inflammation and pain are presented in an excellent review by Vane (1972).

Cholera and other diarrhoeal states

The stimulant effect of cholera enterotoxin on fluid and electrolyte secretion into the intestinal lumen is mimicked qualitatively by PGE compounds, and in both cases stimulation of adenyl cyclase appears to be involved (Kimberg et al, 1971). The possibility that cholera toxin acts at least in part by releasing PG (Bennett, 1971) is supported by experiments in the rat and cat in which aspirin and indomethacin inhibit cholera-induced intestinal secretion (Jacoby & Marshall, 1972; Finck & Katz, 1972). The action of these drugs in the human disease has yet to be evaluated, and it is not yet known whether other gastrointestinal infections act through a similar pathway. However, there is some evidence for an involvement of PGs in the diarrhoea following X-irradiation of the bowel. The diarrhoea improved within 24 hours in 9 out of the 10 patients treated so far, when aspirin 600-900 mg was given four times daily; conventional forms of treatment (codeine etc) had been ineffective (A T Mennie, personal communication). One can speculate that the X-ray treatment causes tissue damage and leads to PG release which affects intestinal secretion and motility.

Since diarrhoea frequently accompanies the i.v. infusion of $PGF_{2\alpha}$ and sometimes of PGE_2 into obstetric patients (Karim & Filshie, 1970), it may be that secretion of $PGF_{2\alpha}$ - and E_2-like material into the blood from certain tumours contributes to the diarrhoea (eg. medullary carcinoma of the thyroid, Williams et al, 1968). However it is important to remember that tumours secrete more than one substance, and that since PGE and F compounds are rapidly metabolised in the lungs and other vascular beds, little would be expected to reach the gut.

Bone resorption by dental cysts

Bone resorption by dental cysts has been shown to be due to material released from the cyst wall (Harris & Goldhaber, 1973). PGE compounds are potent bone-resorbing agents (Klein & Raisz, 1970), and material resembling PGE_2 is formed during incubation of the outer part of the cyst capsule (ie. the part which comes into contact with the jaw bone – Harris et al, 1973). The production of PG-like material in tissue culture is inhibited by indomethacin, but it remains to be seen whether inhibitors of PG synthesis have any place in the treatment of this condition.

Obesity

The release of free fatty acids and glycerol from human adipose tissue in response to noradrenaline is inhibited in vitro by PGE_1 (Carlson & Hallberg, 1968; Micheli et al, 1969). This raises the question of a possible involvement of PGs in obesity, and Haessler and Crawford (1966) found a lipid inhibitor of lipolysis in the adipose tissue of rats which became obese following hypothalamic lesions. Furthermore, PG antagonists and low concentrations of indomethacin enhance lipolysis in rat isolated fat cells (Illiano & Cuatrecasas, 1971). However, since there are no reports that aspirin-like drugs are weight-reducing agents in man, it would seem that PGs are not normally involved in obesity, or that the drugs used do not (adequately) prevent PG synthesis in adipose tissue.

The preceding discussion covers several of the aspects of PGs in disease. There are of course many others where the link between PGs and disease may be even more tenuous than some of the examples given. There are also disorders – rather than diseases – such as male infertility and constipation where PGs might be used medically, and there are menstrual and obstetric problems. No doubt the list will grow at an impressive rate. Fortunately, there are several drugs available which antagonise the synthesis or many of the actions of PGs. In addition to their therapeutic value, these drugs can be used as tools to evaluate the involvement of PGs in various processes.

REFERENCES

Aiken, J. W. and Vane, J. R. (1971) The Pharmacologist, **15**, 564
Bennett, A. (1971) Nature, **231**, 536
Bennett, A., Murray, J. G. and Wyllie, J. H. (1967) British Journal of Pharmacology and Chemotherapy, **32**, 339
Bennett, A. and Posner, J. (1971) British Journal of Pharmacology, **42**, 584
Bennett, A., Stamford, I. F. and Unger, W. G. (1972) Journal of Physiology, **226**, 96P
Bennett, A., Stamford, I. F. and Unger, W. G. (1973) Journal of Physiology, in press
Carlson, L. A. and Eriksson, I. (1973) Lancet, i, 155
Carlson, L. A. and Hallberg, D. (1968) Journal of Laboratory and Clinical Medicine, **71**, 368
Classen, M., Koch, H., Birkhardt, J., Topf, G. and Demling, L. (1971) Digestion, **4**, 333
Classen, M., Koch, H., Deyhle, P., Weidenhiller, S. and Demling, L. (1970) Klinische Wochenschrift, **48**, 876
Collier, H. O. J. and Schneider, C. (1972) Nature New Biology, **236**, 141
Cuthbert, M. F. (1969) British Medical Journal, **4**, 723
Daniels, E. G., Hinman, J. W., Leach, B. E. and Muirhead, E. E. (1967) Nature, **215**, 1298
Eakins, K. E., Karim, S. M. M. and Miller, J. D. (1970) British Journal of Pharmacology, **39**, 556
Eakins, K. E. and Sanner, J. H. (1972) In 'The prostaglandins: progress in research'. (Ed.) S. M. M. Karim, Medical and Technical Publishing Co. Ltd., Oxford. page 263

Eakins, K. E., Whitelocke, R. A. F., Bennett, A. and Martenet, A. C. (1972a) British Medical Journal, **3**, 452
Eakins, K. E., Whitelocke, R. A. F., Perkins, E. S., Bennett, A. and Unger, W. G. (1972b) Nature New Biology, **239**, 248
Elkeles, R. S., Hampton, J. R., Harrison, M. J. G. and Mitchell, J. R. A. (1969) Lancet, **ii**, 111
Feldberg, W. and Gupta, K. P. (1972) Journal of Physiology, **222**, 126P
Feldberg, W. and Saxena, P. N. (1971) Journal of Physiology, **217**, 547
Feldberg, W. and Saxena, P. N. (1972) Journal of Physiology, **219**, 739
Ferreira, S. H. (1972) Nature New Biology, **240**, 200
Ferreira, S. H., Herman, A. and Vane, J. R. (1972) British Journal of Pharmacology, **44**, 328P
Ferreira, S. H. and Vane, J. R. (1967) Nature, **216**, 868
Finck, A. D. and Katz, R. L. (1972) Nature, **238**, 274
Flower, R. J. and Vane, J. R. (1972) Nature, **240**, 410
Greaves, M. W. and McDonald-Gibson, W. (1972) British Medical Journal, **2**, 83
Greaves, M. W., Søndergaard, J. and McDonald-Gibson, W. (1971) British Medical Journal, **2**, 258
Haessler, H. A. and Crawford, J. D. (1966) Science, **154**, 909
Harris, M. and Goldhaber, P. (1973) British Journal of Oral Surgery, in press
Harris, M., Jenkins, M. V., Bennett, A. and Wills, M. R. (1973) in press
Hedqvist, P. (1969) Acta Physiologica Scandinavica, **75**, 511
Hendricks, C. H., Brenner, W. E., Ekbladh, L., Brotamek, V. and Fishburne, J. I. (1971) American Journal of Obstetrics and Gynecology, **3**, 564
Herxheimer, H., and Roetscher, I. (1971) European Journal of Clinical Pharmacology, **3**, 123
Horton, E. W. (1969) Physiological Review, **49**, 122
Horton, E. W. and Jones, R. L. (1969) British Journal of Pharmacology, **37**, 705
Horton, E. W., Main, I. H. M., Thompson, C. F. and Wright, P. (1968) Gut, **9**, 655
Illiano, G. and Cuatrecasas, P. (1971) Nature New Biology, **234**, 72
Jacoby, H. I. and Marshall, C. H. (1972) Nature, **235**, 163
Jones, R. L. (1972) British Journal of Pharmacology, **45**, 144P
Kaley, G. and Weiner, R. (1971) Annals of the New York Academy of Sciences **180**, 338
Karim, S. M. M., Carter, D. C., Bhana, D. and Ganesan, P. A. (1973) British Medical Journal, **1**, 143
Karim, S. M. M. and Filshie, G. M. (1970) Lancet, **i**, 157
Karim, S. M. M. and Filshie, G. M. (1972) Journal of Obstetrics and Gynaecology of the British Commonwealth, **79**, 1
Karim, S. M. M. and Somers, K. (1972) In 'The prostaglandins: progress in research'. (Ed.) S. M. M. Karim, Medical and Technical Publishing Co. Ltd., Oxford. page 165
Kimberg, D. V., Field, M., Johnson, J., Henderson, A. and Gershon, E. (1971) Journal of Clinical Investigation, **50**, 1218
Klein, D. C. and Raisz, L. G. (1970) Endocrinology, **86**, 1436
Kloeze, J. (1969) Biochimica et Biophysica Acta, **187**, 285
Lee, J. B. (1967) New England Journal of Medicine, **277**, 1073
Lee, J. B., McGiff, J. C., Kannegiessier, H., Mudd, J. G., Aykent, Y. and Frawley, T. F. (1969) Clinical Research, **17**, 456
Main, I. H. M. (1964) British Journal of Pharmacology and Chemotherapy, **22**, 511
McGiff, J. C., Crowshaw, K., Terragno, N. A. and Lonigro, A. J. (1970) Circulation Research, **27**, Suppl. 1, 121
McGiff, J. G., Terragno, N. A., Ng, K. K. F. and Lee, J. B. (1969) Federation Proceedings, **28**, 286
Micheli, H., Carlson, L. A. and Hallberg, D. (1969) Acta Chirurgica Scandinavica, **135**, 663

Milton, A. and Wendlandt, S. (1970) Journal of Physiology, **207**, 76P
Milton, A. S. and Wendlandt, S. (1971) Journal of Physiology, **218**, 325
Mody, N. J. (1972) In 'The prostaglandins: progress in research'. (Ed.) S. M. M. Karim, Medical and Technical Publishing Co. Ltd., Oxford, page 239
Robinson, R. W. and LeBeau, R. J. (1967) American Journal of Medical Science, **253**, 76
Salter, R. H. (1968) American Journal of Digestive Diseases, **13**, 38
Sanner, J. H. (1969) Archives internationales de pharmacodynamie et de therapie, **180**, 46
Sicuteri, F., Michelacci, S. and Anselmi, B. (1965) Clinical Pharmacology and Therapeutics, **6**, 336
Smith, P. A. (1972) In 'The prostaglandins: progress in research'. (Ed.) S. M. M. Karim, Medical and Technical Publishing Co. Ltd., Oxford. page 223
Sweatman, W. J. F. and Collier, H. O. J. (1968) Nature, **217**, 69
Vane, J. R. (1971) Nature New Biology, **231**, 232
Vane, J. R. (1972) In 'Inflammation: Mechanisms and Control'. (Ed.) I. H. Lepow and P. A. Ward, Academic Press Inc., New York. page 261
Vecchio, C. and Fontana, S. (1965) In 'Recenti Acquisizioni nella Terapia Antireumatica non Steroidea'. Atti del Simposia Internazionale, Milan. Edizioni Minerva Medica, page 166
Wada, T. and Ishizawa, M. (1970) Japanese Journal of Clinical Medicine, **28**, 2465
Williams, E. D., Karim, S. M. M. and Sandler, M. (1968) Lancet, **i**, 22
Willis, A. L. (1969) In 'Prostaglandins, peptides and amines'. (Ed.) P. Mantegazza and E. W. Horton, Academic Press, London. page 31
Willoughby, D. A. and Giroud, J. P. (1969) Journal of Pathology, **98**, 53
Wilson, D. E., Phillips, C. and Levine, R. A. (1971) Gastroenterology, **61**, 201

Clonidine (Catapres) in Hypertension

M E CONOLLY

Serendipity, which means the making of a happy discovery quite by chance, well describes the accidental discovery of the hypotensive properties of the imidazoline derivative clonidine ('Catapres', St 155, 2-(2,6-dichlorophenyl-amino)-2-imidazoline hydrochloride).

As a group, the imidazolines, some of which are shown in Figure 1, have

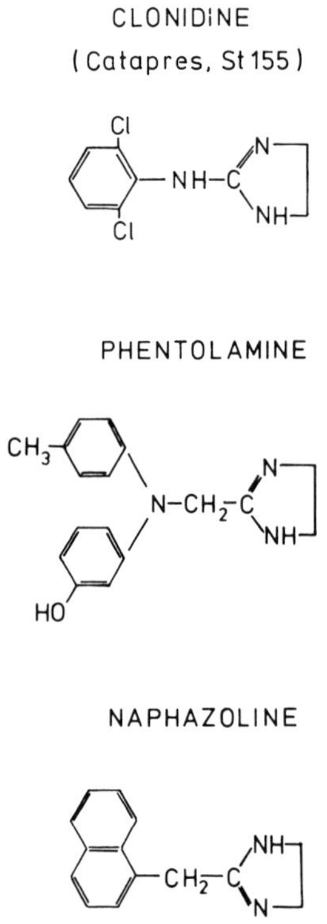

Figure 1. Some imidazoline derivatives in clinical use

a wide range of pharmacological activities. Phentolamine is well known as an α adrenoceptor blocking agent, and tolazoline, which has similar properties, has been used as a peripheral vasodilator. In contrast, the analogue naphazoline is an α stimulant and is used as such to produce nasal decongestion. Clonidine was synthesized and tested with this use in mind, and it caused considerable surprise when it was found that the nasal instillation of a few drops caused marked sedation and a considerable fall in blood pressure (Graubner & Wolf, 1966).

Extensive studies since that time (Ehringer, 1966; Nayler et al, 1968; Constantine & McShane, 1968; Barnett & Cantor, 1968; McRaven et al, 1971; Onesti et al, 1971) have shown that in man and animals it is a highly effective blood-pressure lowering agent. A striking feature of clonidine is that it achieves this effect when given in only microgram doses.

In this paper, animal studies will be considered only in so far as they contribute to our understanding of the mechanism of action of clonidine, since in considering the nature of the changes it produces, there is now an ample body of human data.

ANIMAL STUDIES

In all species examined, rapid injections of clonidine produce an initial rise in blood pressure. This has been shown to be due to a direct α adrenoceptor agonist effect, and is abolished by α blocking agents (Nayler et al, 1968). This phase is followed by a prolonged fall in arterial pressure. Both the initial pressor and subsequent depressor phase are accompanied by a bradycardia. As the heart rate falls, there is also a variable reduction in stroke volume and force of myocardial contraction, although clonidine is without direct effect on the heart (Constantine & McShane, 1968). A fall in cardiac output occurs, which is caused by the cardiac changes mentioned above and also by a fall in venous return, itself a result of systemic venodilation (Nayler et al, 1968) which causes pooling of blood peripherally. Peripheral resistance is at first increased by the direct α stimulant effect, but later falls to normal or low levels, which, in the face of a reduced cardiac output, indicates a reduction in vasomotor activity.

Clonidine is known to cross the blood-brain barrier (Rehbinder, 1970) and it now seems clear that the principal changes are caused by the central action of this drug on medullary vasomotor centres, which decreases sympathetic activity while increasing vagal tone. Thus Schmitt (1970) has shown that intravenous injection of clonidine produces a period of hypotension characterised by a decrease in activity recorded in splanchnic and cardiac sympathetic nerves. Transection of the brain stem at the mid-collicular level did not alter the response to clonidine, whereas disruption of the sympathetic outflow tracts by section of the upper cervical cord produced a fall in blood

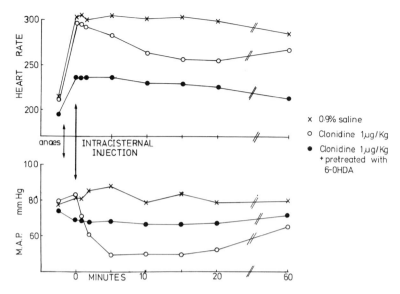

Figure 2. Prevention of the effects of intracisternal injection of clonidine by
pretreatment with intracisternal 6-hydroxydopamine (6 OHD) ten days earlier

pressure which was not further lowered by clonidine. Indeed, owing to its α
agonist action, a sustained rise in pressure was observed.

Further support for a predominantly central effect has been obtained by
showing that blood pressure can be lowered by giving very small doses of
clonidine either into the vertebral artery (Constantine & McShane, 1968), the
cerebral ventricle (Sherman et al, 1968) or the cisterna magna (Kobinger,
1967). Onesti et al (1971) have shown that 1 μg/kg clonidine intracisternally
reduces blood pressure and also causes a fall in renal vein renin in a manner
very similar to that of 30 times the dose of clonidine given intravenously.
More recently it has been shown (Dollery & Reid, 1973) that biochemical partial ablation of brain stem and spinal adrenergic neurones with 6 hydroxy
dopamine will also reduce the hypotension and bradycardia produced by clonidine (Figure 2).

It has been suggested (Bolme & Fuxe, 1971) that clonidine may mediate
its central effects by stimulating central α receptors, and they have shown
that centrally acting α receptor blocking drugs will prevent clonidine from
lowering blood pressure.

In addition to its centrally mediated effects, clonidine has a number of
direct peripheral effects, and although their importance relative to the central
actions is not known, it is possible that they contribute significantly to the
final lowering of blood pressure achieved. Zaimis (1970) has shown that
prolonged treatment with clonidine reduces the response of vascular smooth
muscle to both α and β adrenergic stimulants. Shaw et al (1971) have also

shown a peripheral vasodilator action in animals with complete autonomic block.

Clonidine has also been shown to have an inhibitory effect on the release of noradrenaline from postganglionic sympathetic nerve terminals and of acetyl choline from postganglionic parasympathetic fibres (Werner et al, 1972) when present in concentrations which might reasonably be expected to occur when normal therapeutic doses are given.

CLINICAL PHARMACOLOGY

Studies in man, unlike those in animals, are limited by the need to use less traumatic and, where possible, non-invasive techniques. Nevertheless, the human data which have been gathered serve to indicate those features of the drug's pharmacology which determine the usefulness of clonidine as a hypotensive agent. In particular, whereas the adrenergic neurone blocking drugs lower the blood pressure at the cost of abolishing circulatory regulating mechanisms, often leading to profound orthostatic and exercise induced hypotension, clonidine has the important advantage of leaving the homeostatic mechanisms intact (Barnett & Cantor, 1968).

ACUTE INTRAVENOUS ADMINISTRATION

Intravenous injection of clonidine produces a brief rise in blood pressure followed by a prolonged hypotensive phase. Both phases may be accompanied by a reduction of heart rate if the dose of clonidine is sufficiently large. Representative studies are those of McRaven et al (1971). They studied eight hypertensive patients in the supine position, giving them two injections of $150\mu g$ each over $2\frac{1}{2}$ minutes, 30 minutes apart. The first dose produced a brief pressor effect in 5 subjects, the average increase being 26/16 mm Hg. Blood pressure returned to baseline within $2\frac{1}{2}$ minutes and after that in all 8 subjects a 17% fall in mean pressure from 135 to 110 mm Hg occurred. The second $150\mu g$ dose reduced the mean pressure further to 99 mm Hg. The cardiac index was reduced by both doses, to 84% and 76% of control values respectively, there being a reduction in stroke volume, but not in heart rate until the full $300\mu g$ had been given (81 to 76 beats/min). Since both cardiac output and arterial blood pressure fell, no change in total systemic vascular resistance was observed.

ACUTE ORAL ADMINISTRATION

Onesti et al (1971) studied 7 hypertensive patients, both supine and tilted to 45° after oral administration of $300-750\mu g$ clonidine. There was no initial pressor phase, but lowering of the arterial blood pressure was observed from 30 minutes after dosing. The maximal effect was observed at 2 to 4 hours, and some effect persisted for 6 to 10 hours.

With the patients studied supine, mean arterial pressure fell by 17%, from 155 to 128 mm Hg as the cardiac output fell by 21%, there being a 10% reduction in heart rate and a 15% reduction in stroke volume. Calculated peripheral resistance was unchanged.

When the same subjects were studied at a 45° tilt, mean arterial pressure fell by 33%, from 151 to 101 mm Hg. The cardiac output fell 15% and heart rate by 14%. In this position, as opposed to the supine studies, there was an apparent 21% reduction in peripheral resistance because of an inability to vasoconstrict in response to the tilted position, the absolute value of the 'tilted' total peripheral resistance after clonidine being identical with control values observed in the supine position.

The ability to produce haemodynamic changes in response to being tilted after dosing was also modified in that a 21% orthostatic fall in pressure occurred after clonidine (mean pressure falling from 128 to 101 mm Hg). This was largely accounted for by a failure to increase peripheral resistance in a normal manner.

Renal haemodynamic changes were documented in the same subjects. Strikingly, despite a 17% fall in mean arterial pressure in supine studies, and a 33% fall in the 45° tilt studies, because of a concomitant fall in renal vascular resistance, renal blood flow and glomerular filtration rate were unchanged. Peripheral vein renin levels studied in four patients were reduced after clonidine by 60% in the supine position, and the increase normally seen on tilting was abolished.

Hökfelt et al (1970) have studied the effect on plasma renin, urinary aldosterone secretion rate and urinary catecholamines in more detail, in patients with essential and renovascular hypertension and also in one patient with a phaeochromocytoma. Clonidine administration ranged from a single injection of 150μg to chronic oral therapy with 1200μg/day. In all cases except that of the phaeochromocytoma there was a reduction in blood pressure, heart rate, plasma renin activity, urinary catecholamine levels and aldosterone secretion rate. The reduction in catecholamine excretion was a dose related phenomenon, but the changes in renin and aldosterone were not necessarily always dependent on changes in noradrenaline excretion, since it was found that if sodium deprivation was introduced during clonidine administration, plasma renin activity and aldosterone secretion rate rose in the face of suppressed catecholamine excretion.

Muir et al (1969) studied the response at rest and on exercise in the supine and the erect position in 8 hypertensive patients given 150μg clonidine intravenously. As in other studies, the initial injection of clonidine given at rest produced a biphasic change in blood pressure with a maximum average fall in mean blood pressure of 17%. Cardiac output and peripheral resistance fell by 9% each. The calculated cardio-pulmonary blood volume fell in each case, suggesting a redistribution of the blood volume. The overshoot response to the Valsalva manoeuvre was not altered by clonidine.

The response to exercise was of great interest in that although baseline values of blood pressure, heart rate and peripheral resistance after clonidine were all lower than the control values, the changes in response to exercise were all qualitatively unchanged by clonidine in both the supine and erect positions.

CLINICAL EVALUATION

Numerous clinical trials of the effectiveness of clonidine have now been reported, in which the drug has been used alone or with a diuretic (Smet et al, 1969; Onesti et al, 1971; Mathew & Parker, 1971). In other trials, clonidine has been directly compared with established antihypertensive drugs such as guanethidine (Hoobler & Sagastume, 1970) or methyldopa (Amery et al, 1970; Putzeys & Hoobler, 1972; Mroczek et al, 1972; Conolly et al, 1972). Unfortunately, the majority of published trials have used the drug in combination with a diuretic. Also some trials have employed clonidine only in fixed, arbitrary and often inadequate doses. Both these practices make it difficult to form a clear idea of its potency as a blood pressure lowering agent. However, the picture which has emerged is of a drug which closely matches methyldopa in terms of ability to lower blood pressure without producing orthostatic hypotension; the side effects of the two drugs are similar although those caused by clonidine may be more troublesome and more persistent. Two recent trials will be reviewed.

The first by Mroczek et al (1972) was a double-blind comparison of clonidine and methyldopa in 41 negro patients, both drugs being given in combination with a constant dose of chlorthalidone. The dose of the two drugs was

Table I. A comparison of methyldopa-chlorthalidone and clonidine-chlorthalidone

Treatment	Control	Chlorthalidone	Methyldopa	Clonidine
Average sitting blood pressure (mm Hg)	$176/116$	$163/107$	$145/96$	$143/92$
Average standing blood pressure	$175/102$	$161/106$	$144/96$	$144/90$
Average daily dose	-	90mg	1000mg	660μg
Number (out of 41) made normotensive (sitting BP)	0	1	15	19

titrated against the blood pressure, until control was achieved or side effects prevented any further increase.

The dose of clonidine used was 150 to 1800μg/day (mean 660μg/day) and of methyldopa was 150 to 2500mg/day (mean 1000mg/day). The results reported in terms of the sitting and standing mean blood pressures are summarized in Table I. The principal side effects noted were sedation, which was more common with clonidine treatment (13:9), and dry mouth (7 patients on each drug). Dizziness occurred more often with methyldopa (10:4). However, only 3 patients were lost from the trial because of side effects, and in general side effects were found to diminish with time. Repeated examination of blood count, carbohydrate metabolism and renal and hepatic function revealed no changes while on either drug.

Table II. A comparison of clonidine and methyldopa

Position	Presenting BP	Control achieved with	
		Clonidine	Methyldopa
(lying)	$196/123$	$148/94$	$146/93$
(sitting)	$201/121$	$162/97$	$156/95$
(standing)	$196/109$	$160/91$	$151/88$
Average daily dose	-	1330μg	4150mg

The second trial (Conolly et al, 1972) was a titrated-dose cross-over comparison of clonidine and methyldopa, without the use of diuretics. The dose used was increased until pressure control was achieved or side effects became intolerable. Both drugs produced a very comparable control of blood pressure (Table II), the average doses used being 1330μg clonidine/day (range 375-4200μg/day) or 4150mg methyldopa/day (range 750-10,000mg). Side effects were more prominent in this trial because of the larger doses used; the major side effects encountered in the 13 patients who completed the trial are shown in Table III. In general it was found that sedation lessened with time, whereas dry mouth did not. Six patients were withdrawn from the trial because of side effects, 4 due to clonidine and 2 due to methyldopa.

Neither drug produced serious toxicity, although 9 of the 13 patients developed a positive direct Coomb's test while on methyldopa (Carstairs et al, 1966). Regular examination of retinal appearance and function in patients

Table III. Side effects of clonidine and methyldopa

Symptom	Clonidine	Methyldopa
Dry mouth	12	8
Sedation	8	7
Depression	1	1

receiving clonidine revealed no changes. One patient became pregnant while on clonidine. The pregnancy was terminated for reasons not related to her hypertension. The foetus was examined and found to be normal. Normal foetal development in patients taking clonidine has been noted elsewhere (Mathew & Parker, 1971).

It has been noted previously that drugs such as the tricyclic antidepressant drugs interfere with the hypotensive action of adrenergic neurone blocking drugs (Mitchell et al, 1967) by blocking their uptake into the nerve endings.

During the course of this trial, loss of pressure control was seen in a patient taking clonidine when imipramine was added to his treatment, and this phenomenon has now been documented more fully (Briant et al, 1973). Details of a patient taking desmethylimipramine (DMI) are shown in Figure 3. Loss of pressure control takes some days to reach maximum, and is readily

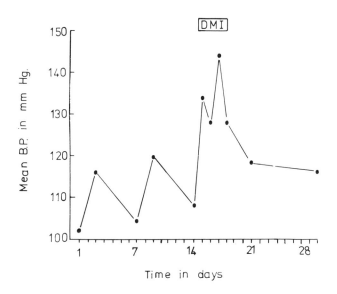

Figure 3. Interaction between clonidine and desmethyl imipramine (DMI)

199

reversed by withdrawing the antidepressant.

During the course of this trial we encountered several cases in which abrupt withdrawal of clonidine precipitated a severe hypertensive crisis, associated with high circulating and urinary catecholamines, exactly comparable to that described elsewhere (Hökfelt et al, 1970). Data from one patient are shown in Table IV.

Table IV. Biochemical and clinical features of
clonidine-withdrawal hypertensive crisis

Biochemical data	Observed		Normal
Plasma:			
Adrenaline	69ng/l		< 60
Noradrenaline	614ng/l		150-200
Free fatty acid	790μEq/l		470-620
Urine:			
Adrenaline	18.4μg/G Creatinine		2-6
Noradrenaline	121 μg/G Creatinine		15-26
Clinical data			
Blood pressure	190/160	200/170	180/160
Heart rate	120	148	152

Patients must be warned of the possibility of this dangerous complication; they must guard against running out of or forgetting tablets and attendant physicians must take care to avoid too rapid withdrawal of clonidine if a change of therapy is needed. If for any reason oral therapy cannot be maintained (eg surgery with general anaesthesia), clonidine may be continued by intramuscular injection. Anaesthetists should be aware of this problem.

CONCLUSION

Clonidine appears to be a useful alternative drug in the treatment of arterial hypertension and exerts its effects, at least in part, via central mechanisms. If used alone, side effects may be troublesome, especially early in therapy. However, concomitant use of a diuretic enables a lower dose to be used. Pressure control is free from orthostatic and exercise induced hypotension. Abrupt withdrawal may precipitate a severe hypertensive crisis.

ACKNOWLEDGMENTS

The author is grateful to Doctors R H Briant, C T Dollery and J L Reid for permission to use some of their unpublished data.

Figure 2 is reproduced from a paper by C T Dollery and J L Reid by kind permission of the Editor of the British Journal of Pharmacology.

REFERENCES

Amery, A., Verstraete, M., Bossaert, H. and Verstreken, G. (1970) British Medical Journal, **4**, 392

Barnett, A. J. and Cantor, S. (1968) Medical Journal of Australia, **1**, 87

Bolme, P. and Fuxe, K. (1971) European Journal of Pharmacology, **13**, 168

Briant, R. H., Reid, J. L. and Dollery, C. T. (1973) British Medical Journal (in press)

Carstairs, K. C., Breckenridge, A., Dollery, C. T. and Worlledge, S.M. (1966) Lancet, **ii**, 133

Conolly, M. E., Briant, R. H., George, C. F. and Dollery, C. T. (1972) European Journal of Clinical Pharmacology, **4**, 222

Constantine, J. W. and McShane, W. K. (1968) European Journal of Pharmacology, **4**, 109

Dollery, C. T. and Reid, J. L. (1973) British Journal of Pharmacology, **47**, 206

Ehringer, H. (1966) Arzneimittel-Forschung (Drug Research), **16**, 1165

Graubner, W. and Wolf, M. (1966) Arzneimittel-Forschung (Drug Research), **16**, 1055

Hökfelt, B., Hedeland, H. and Dymling, J. F. (1970) European Journal of Pharmacology, **10**, 389

Hoobler, S. W. and Sagastume, E. (1970) 'Catapres in Hypertension'. (Ed) M. E. Conolly. Butterworth, London

Kobinger, W. (1967) Naunyn-Schmiedebergs Archiv für Pharmakologie und experimentelle Pathologie, **258**, 48

Mathew. J. Y. and Parker, M. L. (1971) Medical Journal of Australia, **2**, 1120

McRaven, D. R., Kroetz, F. W., Kioschos, J. M. and Kirkendall, W. M. (1971) American Heart Journal, **81**, 482

Mitchell, J. R., Arias, L. and Oates, J. A. (1967) Journal of the American Medical Association, **202**, 149

Mroczek, W. J., Leibel, B. A. and Finnerty, F. A. (1972) American Journal of Cardiology, **29**, 712

Muir, A. L., Burton, J. L. and Lawrie, D. M. (1969) Lancet, **ii**, 181

Nayler, W. G., Price, J. M., Swann, J. B., McInnes, I., Race, D. and Lowe, T. E. (1968) Journal of Pharmacology and Experimental Therapeutics, **164**, 45

Onesti, G., Schwartz, A. B., Kim, K. E., Paz-Martinez, V. and Swartz, C. (1971) Circulation Research, **28** (Suppl.2), 53

Putzeys, M. R. and Hoobler, S. W. (1972) American Heart Journal, **83**, 464

Rehbinder, D. (1970) 'Catapres in Hypertension'. (Ed) M. E. Conolly. Butterworth, London

Schmitt, H. (1970) 'Catapres in Hypertension'. (Ed) M. E. Conolly. Butterworth, London

Shaw, J., Hunyor, S. N. and Korner, P. I. (1971) European Journal of Pharmacology, **14**, 101

Sherman, G. F., Grega, G. I., Woods, R. J. and Buckley, J. R. (1968) European Journal of Pharmacology, **2**, 326

Smet, G., Hoobler, S. W., Shafeek, S. and Julius, S. (1969) American Heart Journal, **77**, 473

Werner, U., Starke, K. and Schumann, H. J. (1972) Archives internationales de pharmacodynamie et de thérapie, **195**, 282

Zaimis, E. (1970) 'Catapres in Hypertension'. (Ed) M. E. Conolly. Butterworth, London

Paget's Disease and Calcitonin Therapy
N J Y WOODHOUSE

INTRODUCTION

A considerable reawakening of interest in Paget's disease has occurred in the last few years. This has been almost entirely due to the therapeutic success of calcitonin which can produce healing of the disease process.

Paget's disease is more common than is generally recognised and although usually occurring in middle age or later, it rarely presents in early life. It is most often diagnosed in people of West European stock, is sometimes familial and affects men more frequently than women. The cause of Paget's disease is unknown but the underlying abnormality seems to be a purposeless proliferation of osteoclasts which invade normal bone, this being followed by a compensatory increase in new bone formation. The turnover of the abnormal bone tissue is accelerated, bone resorption and formation occurring at rates in excess of the normal skeleton with the formation of woven, non-lamellar bone. This leads to a rise in serum alkaline and acid phosphatase levels and in urine hydroxyproline excretion. The bone formed is structurally abnormal and is consequently liable to deformity and fracture, and may in addition be very painful.

The effect of calcitonin is dramatic and is associated with a reversal of these abnormalities: bone turnover is reduced, normal lamellar bone is again formed and radiological healing of the disease with remodelling of bone occurs.

PAGET'S DISEASE
Incidence

The true incidence of Paget's disease was not realised until Schmorl (1932) and later Collins (1956) reported values of 3.0% and 3.7% from necropsy studies in patients over 40 years of age. Hobson and Pemberton (1955) reported an incidence of 4.9% in 162 older subjects, which compares well with Collins' results when age corrected. From population statistics and using Collins' figures, the estimated number of affected individuals in England and

Table I. Estimated incidence of the number of patients with
Paget's disease in England and Wales

Age group	Population	Incidence of disease	Estimated number of affected people
40 - 54	9,065,800	1.8%	163,184
55 - 69	8,206,800	3.6%	295,445
70 - 84	3,600,100	5.0%	180,005
85+	393,600	9.1%	35,818
Total	21,266,300	3.7%	786,853

Calculation based on Collins' 1956 necropsy data and Registrar General's
Quarterly report, September 1970

Wales lies somewhere between 700,000 - 800,000 (Table I). Many are probably asymptomatic, but if, as Collins suggests, 5% have symptoms, then
40,000 people in this country alone may require treatment.

Natural History

The original clinical observations made by Sir James Paget (1877) which
extended over many years, and the serial serum alkaline phosphatase levels
reported by Woodard (1959) indicate that the disease is slowly progressive.
Radiological observations also support this view, but there may be considerable individual variation with the disease advancing rapidly in months in a
small number of patients. On occasion the disease burns out, but evidence
of spontaneous radiological bone healing has not been reported to date.

Complications

1. **Deformity** which may produce mechanical disability, damage to surrounding joints and compression of neurological tissue.

2. **Structural weakness** which in addition to promoting deformity renders the
bone more liable to fractures. These usually occur in the lower limb, but
when vertebrae collapse, cord compression and paralysis can occur.

3. **Bone pain** is of two types, that due to the Pagetic tissue alone, or to the
secondary arthritis. Both are often seen together. The former is variously
described as stabbing, burning or tingling and may be worse at night.

4. **Hypercalcaemia** occurs when bone resorption exceeds bone formation,
and the capacity of the kidney to excrete the calcium load is exceeded. This
is most likely during immobilisation.

5. **Congestive cardiac failure.** A considerable increase in bone blood flow

and cardiac output occurs in patients with extensive and active disease, and when myocardial reserve is impaired, high output failure will occur.

6. Sarcoma. This complication is fortunately rare and probably occurs in less than 0.1% of affected individuals.

CALCITONIN IN PAGET'S DISEASE

Introduction

Calcitonin is a single chain polypeptide hormone of 32 amino acids and is secreted by the parafollicular or 'C' cells. In mammals these are found mainly in the thyroid gland, but in non-mammals form a separate structure called the ultimobranchial body (Copp et al, 1967; MacIntyre, 1969). The secretion rate of calcitonin is controlled by the level of serum calcium and is increased by hypercalcaemia and reduced by hypocalcaemia. Calcitonin inhibits osteoclastic bone resorption and may be important in the regulation of the normal bone remodelling process.

When the rate of bone resorption is greater than in normal adult man, eg in experimental animals or patients with Paget's disease, the acute administration of calcitonin inhibits bone resorption and causes a fall in serum calcium and phosphate levels and urinary hydroxyproline excretion. These observations, together with the reported relief of bone pain in Paget's disease (Bijvoet & Jansen, 1967), first prompted the long term use of this hormone in man (Woodhouse et al, 1970).

Three different calcitonin species — porcine, human and salmon — have now been synthesised and are currently being used in clinical studies. In man the calcium-lowering ability of these hormones is different: weight-for-weight, an intravenous injection of salmon calcitonin is ten times more potent than human and one hundred times more potent than porcine calcitonin (Galante et al, 1973). Although each hormone has 32 amino acids, the amino acid composition of porcine and salmon calcitonin differs from that of human calcitonin.

Antibody formation against the non-human hormones can occur and may limit their clinical usefulness in some cases (Singer et al, 1972).

Treatment

Several groups have now published their results of long-term (3-36 months) treatment using porcine (Shai et al, 1971), human (Woodhouse et al, 1971) and salmon calcitonin (Singer et al, 1970). In general the clinical and biochemical response has been similar and is summarised below.

Patients claimed relief of bone pain and this was associated with a reduction in skin temperature over affected peripheral bones. A sharp fall in hydroxyproline excretion occurred at the onset of treatment and then excretion subsequently declined more slowly towards normal. Serum alkaline phosphatase levels fell in parallel with the hydroxyproline, but without the acute initial fall. Additional evidence for a declining bone turnover rate included a progressive fall in the number of osteoclasts and a reduction in calcium-47 uptake by bone. Calcium balance improved immediately and this effect still persisted at four months. In some patients, with initially mild to moderate disease activity, normal alkaline phosphatase and hydroxyproline levels were achieved. Serum immunoreactive parathyroid hormone levels remained within the normal range after many months of treatment.

The therapeutic potential of calcitonin, suggested by these observations, was boosted further when histological studies revealed that progressively more normal lamellar bone was being laid down during treatment (Woodhouse et al, 1971; Bordier et al, 1973). More recently, radiological studies have

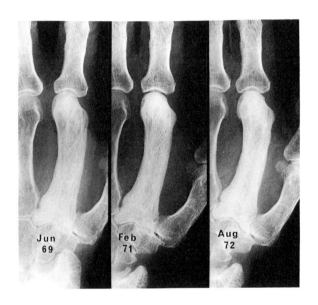

Figure 1. Index metacarpal of a patient with Paget's disease before (June, 1969) and during human calcitonin therapy. On treatment, a more normal cortical and trabecular bone pattern was restored and the external diameter of the bone was reduced. (Reproduced by kind permission of the Editor of the Lancet, 11, 992)

clearly revealed that remodelling of the diseased bone occurs (Figure 1) with healing of the disease (Woodhouse et al, 1972a). These two observations are of considerable practical and theoretical importance. As bone remodels during treatment, and its shape returns towards normal, it seems likely that long-term calcitonin administration will eventually result in complete healing of the disease. In practice, however, this could take as long as the disease took to develop. Treatment should, therefore, be started early in those patients liable to develop complications. These findings also suggest that a major physiological role of calcitonin is to control the normal process of bone remodelling.

The Hydroxyproline 'Plateau'

In some patients, instead of gradually declining towards normal values, urinary hydroxyproline excretion levels off or remains unchanged — the so-called 'plateau' effect. This type of response occurred in a patient with juvenile Paget's disease receiving human calcitonin (Woodhouse et al, 1972b) and in an adult patient receiving salmon calcitonin (Rapoport, 1973). In the plateau phase, however, a striking radiological improvement was observed in both patients. It seems likely, therefore, that this effect reflects the continuous healing process necessary for bone remodelling to occur. In patients with extensive disease, hydroxyproline levels could remain elevated for years during the healing phase.

Relapse on Treatment

A relapse is defined as a rise in serum alkaline phosphatase and urinary hydroxyproline levels towards control values in spite of continuing calcitonin therapy with a biologically active compound. This occurs in a high proportion of patients given porcine calcitonin and may reflect inadequate dosage. The development of high titre antibodies against the non-human calcitonins may also produce a relapse, but this has so far been reported in only one case. Antibodies to human calcitonin have not been found in over 30 patients undergoing treatment.

Withdrawal of treatment is also associated with a rise in serum alkaline phosphatase and urinary hydroxyproline levels.

Dose of Calcitonin

The optimal therapeutic dose of calcitonin is unknown, and so far patients on long-term treatment have been given arbitrary amounts based on acute responses to the hormone. Most studies have employed approximately 100 MRC Units per patient per day, but it must be remembered that this unit is derived from a rat bio-assay. As mentioned previously, salmon calcitonin is ten times more potent than human and one hundred times more potent than porcine calcitonin in man, whereas in the rat assay human and porcine are equipotent and salmon calcitonin forty times more potent than either. Equivalent doses for a patient with Paget's disease in MRC units would therefore be: salmon — 10 MRC units, human — 100 MRC units, and porcine — 1000 MRC units. For clinical use, it seems preferable to use the weights of synthetic hormones rather than MRC units. Experience with human calcitonin indicates that a dose of 0.5mg to 1.0mg (1.0mg = 100 MRC units) per day is effective, but lower doses have been inadequately studied, and may prove equally effective.

Side Effects of Treatment

Injections of the synthetic calcitonins are painless and local reactions are rare. Sometimes there is mild flushing of the face lasting 30-120 minutes, and this may be associated with mild nausea.

In over 40 patients receiving human calcitonin, treatment has been withdrawn in two — one with osteoporosis, the other with Paget's disease. These patients felt unwell for several hours following the injections, and complained of nausea, shivering and a sensation of cold in the arms, legs and pharynx.

SUMMARY

Calcitonin will produce relief of bone pain and a reduction in bone turnover in patients with Paget's disease. During treatment normal lamellar bone is formed and radiological healing of bone is seen to occur. This hormone is the treatment of choice for Paget's disease, and its early use should prevent the development of complications.

ACKNOWLEDGMENTS

I should like to express my thanks to Professor Iain MacIntyre, Dr Graham Joplin and Dr Frank Doyle for their constant advice and encouragement during my studies, and to my many colleagues from Ciba-Geigy for supplies of human calcitonin.

REFERENCES

Bijvoet, O. L. M. and Jansen, A. P. (1967) Lancet, ii, 471
Bordier, Ph., Woodhouse, N. J. Y., Joplin, G. F . and MacIntyre, I. (1973) Journal of Bone and Joint Surgery B (in press)
Collins, D. H . (1956) Lancet, ii, 51
Copp, D. H., Cockcroft, D. W. and Kueh, Y. (1967) Canadian Journal of Physiology, 45, 1095
Galante, L., Joplin, G. F., MacIntyre, I. and Woodhouse, N. J. Y . (1973) Clinical Science (in press)
Hobson, W. and Pemberton, J. (1955) 'The Health of the Elderly at Home'. Butterworth, London. Page 137
MacIntyre, I. (1969) in 'Fifth Symposium on Advanced Medicine'. (Ed) R. Williams. Pitman Medical, London. Page 91
Paget, J. (1877) Medico-chirurgical Transactions, 60, 37
Rapoport, A. (1973) personal communication
Schmorl, G. (1932) Virchows Archiv für pathologische Anatomie und Physiologie und für klinische Medizin, 283, 694
Shai, F., Baker, R. K. and Wallach, S. (1971) Journal of Clinical Investigation, 50, 1927
Singer, F. R., Neer, R. M., Parsons, J. A., Krane, S. M. and Potts, J. T. Jnr. (1970) Journal of Clinical Investigation, 49, 89a
Singer, F. R., Aldred, J. P., Neer, R. M., Krane, S. M., Potts, J. T. Jnr. and Bloch, K. J. (1972) Journal of Clinical Investigation, 51, 2331
Woodard, H. Q. (1959) Cancer, 12, 1226
Woodhouse, N. J. Y., Reiner, M., Kalu, D. N., Galante, L., Joplin, G. F.

and MacIntyre, I. (1970) in 'Proceedings of the Calcitonin 1969
Symposium'. (Ed) S. Taylor. Heinemann Medical, London. Page 504
Woodhouse, N. J. Y., Reiner, M., Bordier, Ph., Kalu, D. N., Fisher, M.,
Foster, G. V., Joplin, G. F. and MacIntyre, I. (1971) Lancet, i, 1139
Woodhouse, N. J. Y., Joplin, G. F., MacIntyre, I. and Doyle, F. H.
(1972a) Lancet, ii, 992
Woodhouse, N. J. Y., Sigurdsson, G., Joplin, G. F. and MacIntyre, I.
(1972b) British Medical Journal, 4, 267

Current Status of Digoxin Therapy

D G GRAHAME-SMITH

Several important advances have occurred in the general area of therapy with cardiac glycosides during recent years. These advances concern particularly:

1. Further understanding of their mode of action in the therapy of cardiac failure.
2. Appreciation of the factors which determine the amount of a cardiac glycoside which after administration exerts its pharmacological effects (ie the pharmacokinetics of cardiac glycosides).
3. Increasing knowledge of the manifestations, incidence, causes, mechanisms, treatment and prognosis of digitalis toxicity.

MODE OF ACTION

To understand why cardiac glycosides are beneficial in cardiac failure, the action of these drugs upon the myocardium must be examined. Cardiac glycosides increase the force and speed of contraction of myocardial muscle in normal hearts, non-failing but diseased hearts, and in the failing heart, ie they have a positive inotropic effect (for review see Mason et al, 1969). Several different methods have been used to demonstrate this effect. Mason and Braunwald (1963) showed that ouabain greatly increased the peak rate of rise of intraventricular pressure (dp/dt) during isovolumic contraction of the right ventricle in normal subjects, increased dp/dt of the left ventricle in patients with uncomplicated atrial septal defects, and also intensified the ventricular dp/dt during atrial systole, suggesting a positive inotropic effect upon the atrial myocardium. Acetylstrophanthidin increased the force of isometric myocardial tension in patients with congenital cardiac defects with stressed but non-failing hearts as measured with the Walton-Brodie strain gauge arch in surgery (Braunwald et al, 1961). Sonnenblick et al (1966) sutured small radio-opaque markers to the external surface of the ventricles at the time of surgery for the correction of valvular defects. Subsequent to the operation the changes in ventricular dimensions were assessed by a cineradiographic technique and intraventricular pressure was measured at a constant length point in each contraction. After ouabain the velocity of movement of the markers was about doubled while intraventricular pressure at a constant length was only minimally increased.

Now the total cardiovascular situation in regard to the normal heart, and the non-failing but diseased heart, differs from that with the failing heart in that with the latter there is a lowered cardiac output, lowered stroke volume and elevated ventricular end-diastolic pressure and volume. These changes are accompanied by systemic arteriolar and venous constriction produced by increased sympathetic nervous activity which serve to support (however inadequately) the circulation, by which is really meant tissue perfusion and the supply of oxygen to tissues.

When cardiac output is **not** lowered, although cardiac glycosides augment myocardial contractability this is not translated into increased cardiac output and total blood flow because cardiac glycosides also cause direct arteriolar constriction and perhaps venoconstriction. However, in cardiac failure the cardiac glycosides produce an increased cardiac output through their inotropic effect, the increased reflex sympathetic tone relaxes, and there is overall arteriolar and venous dilatation which masks the mild direct vasoconstrictor effects which these drugs otherwise have. The total effect of the cardiac glycosides to improve the function of the heart as a pump for the circulation of the blood is therefore only really seen when heart failure is clinically evident. It is possible that cardiac glycosides might be beneficial in improving the contractility of the diseased heart in patients without clinical evidence of congestive heart failure. Kahler et al (1962) showed that digoxin reduced the post-exercise oxygen debt in patients with cardiac disease without heart failure. Williams and Braunwald (1965) found that the mortality from heart failure and the degree of ventricular hypertrophy resulting from experimental aortic constriction in animals was reduced by chronic digitalisation. Theory would suggest that the inotropic effect of cardiac glycosides on the non-failing but diseased heart might allow the circulation to be adequately maintained without excessive sympathetic nervous activity and ventricular dilatation and hypertrophy. Obviously only long term clinical studies will solve this problem.

What has been outlined above refers specifically to the inotropic activity of cardiac glycosides, though of course these drugs improve the function of the heart as a pump when used to control supraventricular tachyarrhythmias.

SUBCELLULAR MECHANISMS OF ACTION

Here we leave the realm of complex cardiac dynamics which are difficult to measure precisely, and enter the equally complex realm of the biochemistry and biophysics of myocardial muscular contraction and relaxation. It is not known exactly how cardiac glycosides produce their inotropic effect upon the myocardial muscle cell. However, if the present body of knowledge is on the right track the focal point seems to be an effect upon the processes by which excitation of the membrane of the myocardial muscle cell are linked to contraction of the muscle (for an extensive review see Lee & Klaus, 1971). Certain possibilities seemed to have been ruled out. Cardiac glycosides do not appear to affect the contractile proteins directly. None of the well defined enzymes involved in energy production such as glycolysis and oxidation are apparently consistently affected by the drugs. Mitochondrial oxidative phosphorylation and myocardial energy-rich phosphate are likewise affected. It is probable that cardiac glycosides do not induce their inotropic affect by a primary action on energy production by metabolic processes.

When the muscle membrane is excited and an action potential occurs, sodium and calcium ions enter the cell, followed by potassium efflux. The concentration of free calcium ions in the cytoplasm near the myofibrils increases and when this concentration reaches a critical level it appears that in the presence of intracellular membrane ATPase and ATP, contraction of actomyosin is initiated leading of course to shortening of the muscle cell. Interest at present concerns the influence of cardiac glycosides on the critical level of free calcium within the myocardial cell. There is evidence that these drugs increase this level, though there is controversy about how this effect is produced. There are two main theories. First, the correlation between the effect of cardiac glycosides in inhibiting membrane bound $(Na^+ + K^+)$-activated ATPases and their inotropic effect is impressive, though not conclusive (Okita, 1972). This enzyme is part of a membrane transport system involved in the regulation of $Na^+ + K^+$ ion flux across cell membranes. When this enzyme is inhibited by cardiac glycosides the active transport of Na^+ ions outwards and of K^+ ions inwards is blocked, intracellular Na^+ concentrations increase and intracellular K^+ ion concentrations decrease. It is suggested that the increase in Na^+ ion concentrations in some way releases Ca^{++} ions from intracellular binding sites and increases the free Ca^+ ion concentration in the area of the myofibrils. Second, another proposition is that cardiac glycosides directly affect Ca^{++} binding by cell and intracellular membranes and that it is by this mechanism that free Ca^{++} ion concentrations are increased.

FACTORS DETERMINING THE OVERALL THERAPEUTIC EFFECT OF CARDIAC GLYCOSIDES

PHARMACOKINETICS OF DIGOXIN

Because digoxin is the most commonly used cardiac glycoside in the UK, the details of the clinical pharmacology will refer mainly to this glycoside.

Digoxin is lipid soluble and is rapidly absorbed when it is fully available for absorption. Recently there have been reports of differences between brands and batches of digoxin tablets in terms of the bioavailability of their contained digoxin (Lindenbaum et al, 1971; Shaw et al, 1972; Lancet, 1972). Such differences can cause quite marked variability in the therapeutic potency of oral digoxin preparations and are very likely due to differences in the pharmaceutical preparation of tablets. Efforts to define the physical properties of digoxin tablets and to correlate these with bioavailability in man and improve the standardisation of digoxin tablets are currently being made.

In man some 85% of administered digoxin is absorbed, probably from the stomach and certainly from both the proximal and distal small bowel by a non-saturable transport process (Greenberger & Caldwell, 1972). After absorption digoxin passes to the liver in portal venous blood. Very little metabolism of digoxin occurs in the liver or the rest of the body, about 85% (80% urine, 5% stool) appearing in the excreta as unchanged digoxin (see Doherty, 1972). The metabolites which do result from liver metabolism are due to the removal of one or two sugar (digitoxose) molecules from the digoxin molecule. These metabolic products are either secreted in the bile to appear in the stool or pass through the liver into the systemic circulation and appear in the urine. Liver metabolism and biliary secretion is of little overall importance to the therapeutic or toxic effects of digoxin. The unchanged (85%) digoxin undergoes distribution or renal excretion.

Distribution

Digoxin is about 20% bound to plasma protein in contrast to digitoxin which is about 90% bound, and is distributed to all tissues including the brain. Doherty et al (1967) studied the tissue distribution of tritiated digoxin in patients who came to autopsy. The concentration in the kidney was very high and that in the heart was appreciable, though in terms of the total reservoir of the drug, skeletal muscle contained a considerable amount. In these studies, myocardial/plasma ratios of about 30:1 were found. There is some controversy about how reliably a plasma concentration will predict the myocardial concentration and thus how predictable is the myocardial/ plasma concentration ratio. Binnion et al (1969) found a mean atrial digoxin concentration of 219 $m_{\mu}g/G$ tissue in atrial appendages removed during mitral valvotomy in digitalised patients but the values varied from 34 $m\mu g/G$ to 648 $m\mu g/G$. If we assume a therapeutic plasma concentration of about 1 ng/ml there is certainly a very high myocardial/plasma ratio. However, after an oral dose of digoxin 0. 5mg (Figure 1) the plasma level rises quickly, fall rapidly initially and then much more slowly to an equilibrium 'plateau'. The half-life of plasma digoxin calculated from the slope of the equilibrium

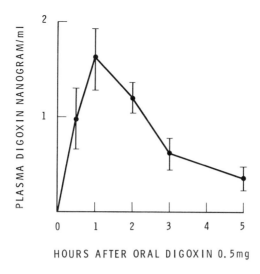

Figure 1. Plasma level/time curve after oral digoxin

'plateau' is about 33 hours (Doherty, 1968). Consideration of the plasma
level after dosage reveals that the myocardial/plasma ratio must be altering
much of the time after a dose of digoxin, in addition it seems likely that the
initial fast fall in plasma digoxin levels represents the phase of distribution
of the drug and myocardial levels might be more influenced by this phase
than by the 'plateau' phase. The total pharmacokinetic situation is thus very
complex and a great deal more work is necessary to understand the relationship between the time course of the plasma level and the myocardial concentration after dosage of cardiac glycosides.

Excretion

Glomerular filtration is the major mechanism for the renal excretion of
digoxin in man and bears a direct relationship therefore to creatinine clearance (Marcus, 1972). Renal functional impairment resulting in decreased
glomerular filtration and a fall in creatinine clearance results in a decreased
digoxin turnover time, increased plasma concentration and a greater tendency
to intoxication. Mathematical methods are available relating body surface
area, creatinine clearance, and plasma levels to predict future digoxin
dosage (Jelliffe, 1968).

OTHER FACTORS INFLUENCING DIGITALIS THERAPY

Plasma potassium concentration

Hyperkalaemia protects against digitalis induced arrhythmias (see Marcus,

213

1972). An important factor here is the effect of raised extracellular potassium in inhibiting digoxin binding to tissues. Marcus (1972) has shown that the production of hyperkalaemia in dogs lowers the myocardial concentration of digoxin, raises the plasma digoxin level and lowers the myocardial/plasma ratio after the administration of tritiated digoxin. However, the greater sensitivity of the heart to digitalis in hypokalaemia is not accounted for by a greater myocardial uptake of digoxin and it appears that there is a true hypersensitivity of the heart in the presence of hypokalaemia (Marcus, 1972). The hyperkalaemia of renal failure and the hypokalaemia associated with the use of thiazide diuretics, frusemide and ethacrynic acid are common situations requiring review of digitalis requirements.

Thyroid function

Doherty and Perkins (1966) have shown that in hyperthyroidism the half-life of serum digoxin is shortened and that in hypothyroidism it is prolonged. Thus patients with hyperthyroidism tend to be resistant to digoxin and those with hypothyroidism more sensitive, and thyroid status demands appropriate dosage adjustment. This is particularly important when continuing digitalisation in patients returning with treatment to euthyroidism from either a hypothyroid or hyperthyroid state.

THE MEASUREMENT OF PLASMA DIGOXIN CONCENTRATIONS

During the past 4 years several methods have been developed for the accurate assay of plasma digoxin concentrations.

1. Radioimmunoassay

Butler and Chen (1967) immunised rabbits with a digoxin-bovine serum albumin conjugate and raised antibodies specific for the digoxigenin moiety of digoxin. Smith et al (1969) utilised these antibodies to assay digoxin. Briefly, the patient's serum is incubated with tritiated digoxin and digoxin antibodies. The amount of tritiated digoxin binding to the antibody depends upon the amount of non-radioactive digoxin present in the serum. Unbound tritiated digoxin is removed by charcoal absorption and the antibody-bound tritiated digoxin measured by liquid scintillation counting.

2. Red-cell rubidium ^{86} (Rb^{86}) uptake inhibition assay

Cardiac glycosides inhibit (Rb^{86}) uptake by human red cells. Lowenstein and Corrill (1966) demonstrated that it was feasible to assay plasma digoxin using this principle and the method was developed for routine use by Grahame-Smith and Everest (1969), Binnion et al (1969) and Bertler and Redfors (1970). The assay requires extraction of digoxin from plasma and by comparison with digoxin standards, the measurement of the ability of the extract to inhibit the

uptake of Rb^{86} by human red cells, in vitro. Other assay methods, not yet
fully assessed, are based upon the inhibition of Na-K activated ATPase
activity by cardiac glycosides (Burnett & Conklin, 1968) or upon the competition of non-radioactive digoxin with isotopically labelled digoxin for the
binding sites on an Na-K activated ATPase (Brooker & Appelman, 1968).

Until all the factors relating the time-course of plasma digoxin levels to
myocardial levels after a dose of digoxin are known, absolutely rational use
of plasma digoxin concentrations in guiding therapy will not be possible.
Nevertheless a knowledge of the plasma digoxin concentration can be useful
in two situations, first when there appears to be an inadequate therapeutic
response to what should be adequate doses of digoxin, as may occur in malabsorption states (Heizer et al, 1971) and, second, as a help in the diagnosis
of digoxin toxicity.

DIGITALIS TOXICITY

Digitalis toxicity is a considerable problem. Various studies have shown the
incidence of digitalis toxicity amongst hospitalised patients to be from 7%
to 20% and in one study digoxin toxicity accounted for one-third of all drug
reactions monitored (Hurwitz & Wade, 1969). Mortality amongst intoxicated
patients is more than twice as high as amongst non-toxic patients (Beller et
al, 1971) although this may not be due solely to intoxication but rather to the
severity of the disease for which the drugs are being administered and also
the effect of the disease on renal function and digoxin excretion.

Criteria used to diagnose digitalis toxicity are non-cardiac and cardiac.
The non-cardiac criteria are well known (Chung, 1969) but in one study
where only cardiac criteria were accepted in the diagnosis of digitalis
toxicity, only anorexia rated a significant positive correlation with toxic
arrhythmias (Beller et al, 1971) and many patients with digitalis-induced
cardiac arrhythmias may lack gastrointestinal and other symptoms.

There has been increasing knowledge of the arrhythmias caused by
digitalis over the last few years (Fisch & Knoebel, 1970). Ectopic ventricular
rhythms are most common and include ventricular ectopic beats, ventricular
bigeminy and ventricular tachycardia. Atrioventricular (A V) nodal arrhythmias are frequent and include non-paroxysmal A V junctional exit block. Other
arrhythmias encountered are A V dissociation, atrial tachycardia with A V
block and sinoatrial arrhythmias. Arrhythmias and conduction disturbances
in the presence of atrial fibrillation are particularly difficult to recognise.
The largest prospective study of this problem so far came from Boston
(Beller et al, 1971). Of 931 consecutive patients admitted to a single medical
service 135 were taking a cardiac glycoside. On the basis of electrocardio-
graphic arrhythmias 23% were considered toxic and 6% possibly toxic. The
toxic group had more advanced heart disease, atrial fibrillation and chronic

pulmonary disease and renal failure. In this study the toxic groups did not differ from the non-toxic in the type of preparation, age, sex, prevalence of other medication or concentration of serum potassium. The mean serum digoxin concentration was 2.3 ng/ml in toxic patients and in non-toxic patients 1 ng/ml. There was, however, considerable overlap and a diagnosis of digitalis toxicity cannot be made on the serum level alone. However, when using the serum level certain general points can be made: If an adult patient has been digitalised with digoxin and is on maintenance therapy, and presents with symptoms and signs suggestive of digoxin toxicity and the plasma potassium is not less than 3.5 mEq/L then: (1) If the plasma digoxin concentration is 1 ng or less the patient's problem is unlikely to be due to digoxin therapy. (2) If the plasma digoxin concentration lies between 1 ng/ml and 2.5 ng/ml then digoxin toxicity may be the cause. Digoxin therapy should be temporarily stopped and restarted at a lower dose. Certainly increasing the dose would be contra-indicated. If emergency therapeutic measures were indicated then if there were no other factors to consider one could assume digoxin toxicity and institute appropriate measures. (3) If the plasma concentration is greater than 3 ng/ml then digoxin toxicity is extremely likely. The overlap of plasma digoxin in non-toxic and toxic groups of patients emphasises the extremely small margin between therapeutic and toxic doses.

Wotman et al (1971) have found that the saliva of patients with digitalis toxicity contains higher potassium and calcium concentrations than that of non-toxic patients and suggest that the $[K^+] \times [Ca^{++}]$ product might be helpful in the diagnosis of digitalis toxicity.

In a very interesting article Lown and his colleagues (1972) consider other aids to the diagnosis of digitalis toxicity. Carotid sinus pressure will induce vagal slowing of the heart and may temporarily precipitate arrhythmias due to digitalis toxicity. Acetylstrophanthin, which has short latency of action, prompt onset of peak action and rapid dissipation, can be used intravenously in very small incremental doses which may expose unsuspected digitalis toxicity by producing arrhythmias. This test is not without hazard, needs very careful supervision and has not yet been fully assessed. 'Digitoximetry' is another experimental approach yet to be assessed clinically. In this method an electrical stimulus is delivered to the heart in diastole and in the digitalised animal will result not in a single propagated response but in a repetitive ventricular response.

'LOADING' DOSES VERSUS 'MAINTENANCE' DOSES IN 'DIGITALISATION'

The question is frequently raised as to whether digitalisation with loading doses of digoxin is really necessary. This depends upon how quickly a therapeutic response is desired. Marcus et al (1966) using tritiated digoxin have shown quite clearly that, with loading doses, full therapeutic levels of 1.2 - 1.4 ng/ml were achieved in 24 hours whereas without loading doses and using 0.5 mg digoxin daily orally, it took 6 days to reach the same level. However, from the experimental work which has been done (see Mason et al, 1969) one would expect that even small doses of digoxin, producing low levels of plasma digoxin, very probably produce appreciable inotropic effect, though this effect will usually increase if the plasma level rises to sub-toxic levels. Thus in critical clinical situations fraught with hazard from potential digitalis toxicity very small doses of digoxin would nevertheless be expected to produce a beneficial inotropic and therapeutic action.

REFERENCES

Beller, G. A., Smith, I. W., Abelmann, W. H., Haber, H., Grahame-Smith, D. G. and Wood, W. B. (1971) New England Journal of Medicine, **284**, 989

Binnion, P. F., Morgan, L. M., Stevenson, H. M. and Fletcher, E. (1969) British Heart Journal, **31**, 636

Bertler, A. and Refors, A. (1970) Clinical Pharmacology and Therapeutics, **11**, 665

Braunwald, E., Bloodwell, R. D., Goldberg, L. I. and Morrow, A. G. (1961) Journal of Clinical Investigation, **40**, 52

Brooker, G. and Appelman, M. M. (1968) Biochemistry, **7**, 4182

Burnett, G. H. and Conklin, R. L. (1968) Journal of Laboratory and Clinical Medicine, **71**, 1040

Butler, V. P. Jr. and Chen, J. P. (1967) Proceedings of the National Academy of Sciences of the USA, **57**, 71

Chung, E. K. (1969) Digitalis Intoxication. Excerpta Medica Foundation, Amsterdam

Doherty, J. E. (1968) American Journal of the Medical Sciences, **255**, 382

Doherty, J. E. (1972) In 'Basic and Clinical Pharmacology of Digitalis', (Ed.) B. H. Marks and A. M. Weissler, page 230. Charles C. Thomas, Springfield, Illinois, USA

Doherty, J. E. and Perkins, W. H. (1966) Annals of Internal Medicine, **64**, 489

Doherty, J. E., Perkins, W. H. and Flanigan, W. J. (1967) Annals of Internal Medicine, **66**, 116

Fisch, G. and Knoebel, S. B. (1970) Progress in Cardiovascular Disease, **12**, 383

Grahame-Smith, D. G. and Everest, M. S. (1969) British Medical Journal, **1**, 286

Greenberger, N. J. and Caldwell, J. H. (1972) In 'Basic and Clinical Pharmacology of Digitalis'. (Ed.) B. H. Marks and A. M. Weissler. Charles C. Thomas, Springfield, Illinois, USA. page 15

Heizer, W. D., Smith, T. W. and Goldfinger, S. E. (1971) New England Journal of Medicine, **285**, 257

Hurwitz, N. and Wade, O. L. (1969) British Medical Journal, **1**, 531

Jelliffe, R. W. (1968) Annals of Internal Medicine, **69**, 703

Kahler, R. L., Thompson, R. H., Buskirk, E. R., Frye, R. L. and Braunwald, E. (1962) Circulation, **27**, 397

Lancet (1972) Editorial **ii**, 311

Lee, K. S. and Klaus, W. (1971) Pharmacological Review, **23**, 193

Lindenbaum, J., Mellow, M. H., Blackstone, M. O., Butler, V. P. (1971) New England Journal of Medicine, **285**, 1344

Lowenstein, J. M. and Corrill, E. M. (1966) Journal of Laboratory and
Clinical Medicine, **67**, 1048
Lown, B., Hagemeijer, F., Barr, I. and Klein, M. (1972) In 'Basic and
Clinical Pharmacology of Digitalis'. (Ed.) B. H. Marks and A. M.
Weissler. Charles C. Thomas, Springfield, Illinois, USA. page 299
Marcus, F. I. (1972) In 'Basic and Clinical Pharmacology of Digitalis'.
(Ed.) B. H. Marks and A. M. Weissler. Charles C. Thomas, Springfield,
Illinois, USA. page 243
Marcus, F. I., Burkhalter, L., Cuccia, C., Pavlovich, J. and Kapadia, G.
G. (1966) Circulation, **34**, 865
Mason, D. T., Spann, J. F. and Zelis, R. (1969) Progress in Cardiovascula
Disease, **11**, 443
Mason, D. T. and Braunwald, E. J. (1963) Journal of Clinical Investigation,
42, 1105
Okita, G. T. (1972) In 'Basic and Clinical Pharmacology of Digitalis'. (Ed.)
B. H. Marks and A. M. Weissler. Charles C. Thomas, Springfield,
Illinois, USA. page 181
Shaw, T. R. D., Howard, M. R. and Hamer, J. (1972) Lancet **ii**, 303
Smith, T. W., Butler, V. P. Jr. and Haber, E. (1969) New England Journal
of Medicine, **281**, 1212
Sonnenblick, E. H., Williams, J. F., Glick, G., Mason, D. T. and
Braunwald, E. (1966) Circulation, **34**, 532
Williams, J. F. Jr. and Braunwald, E. (1965) American Journal of Cardiolog
16, 534
Wotman, S., Bigger, J. T. Jr., Mandel, I. D. and Barthestone, H. J.
(1971) New England Journal of Medicine, **285**, 871

The Treatment of Mild Hypertension
GEOFFREY ROSE

WHY CONTROVERSIAL?

There are reasons both good and bad why the treatment of mild hypertension should be a matter of controversy. It is clearly wise to be most cautious about advocating a life-time of drugs for symptomless persons, especially where they form a sizeable proportion of the population. The idea is inherently repugnant. In addition, no one can say, in the absence of controlled trials extending over many years, what may be the long-term hazards of hypotensive drugs: for every one of these drugs has, besides its hypotensive effect, other influences on basic metabolic or neurological functions. The possibility cannot be refuted now — and maybe not for many years, if ever — that there are subtle ill-effects of chronic hypokalaemia, or of persistent β-sympathetic blockade, or from the changes in carbohydrate and uric acid metabolism which result from thiazide diuretics. Taking known risks in medicine is painful enough: naturally we resist even more the taking of unknown risks. (It should, however, be recognised that in therapeutics this situation is actually the rule rather than the exception.)

There is also a less worthy reason for the controversy: the evidence that the condition needs to be treated at all is epidemiological and not clinical. We are used to treating patients who come with symptoms and seek our help; but mild hypertension is symptomless. In the natural course of events the subject is unaware of its presence, and gets no warning of impending cerebrovascular accident or myocardial infarction. Yet these risks are substantially increased by increments of blood pressure far short of those which would earn a clinical diagnosis of hypertension (Dawber & Kannel, 1961). Thus, for example, for middle-aged men with a diastolic pressure of 95mm the standardised mortality ratio (all causes) is doubled. These hazards of symptomless hypertension would not easily be suspected from hospital experience, and ignorance of them seems to be common.

EVIDENCE ON THE VALUE OF TREATMENT

When a sick patient seeks our help, we feel a strong pressure on us to attempt some form of alleviation: for one thing, the risks in acute illness tend to be high, and we feel correspondingly justified in taking some risks with an uncertain treatment. The situation is different when it is the doctor who takes the initiative, advising emotional and physical interference in the life of an uncomplaining individual. Here it is not sufficient merely to have evidence that the condition if untreated is dangerous: one must have some positive evidence that 'treatment' is better than 'no treatment'.

In the case of malignant hypertension there was no need for controlled trials to demonstrate that the prognosis was improved by hypotensive drugs (Rosenheim, 1954). The demonstration of benefit, however, becomes increasingly difficult as one descends the scale of pressure. Over many years the cumulative risk from even mild hypertension becomes large: among 100 untreated men aged 30 years whose diastolic pressure is 100mm, 30-40 more deaths can be expected to occur by the age of 60 than among 100 men with a diastolic pressure of 75mm. But this corresponds to an average mortality excess of only c.1% per year, and alleviation of this risk, although very desirable, could only be demonstrated by large controlled therapeutic trials.

The US Veterans Administration group reported very striking evidence of therapeutic benefit in their controlled trial in more severe hypertension (Veterans Administration Co-operative Study Group on Anti-hypertensive Agents, 1967), paralleling the results of a previous trial in this country

Table I. Results of the Veterans Administration controlled trial of treatment of hypertension (diastolic pressure 90-114mm)

Complication	Control (N=194)	Treated (N=186)
DEATHS		
Stroke	7	1
Coronary heart disease	11	6
Other	3	3
Total	21	10
NON-FATAL		
Stroke	13	4
Coronary heart disease	2	5
Cardiac failure	11	0
Estimated 5 year incidence of all complications	55%	18%

(Hamilton et al, 1964). They proceeded with a further randomised controlled trial conducted among 380 men, of average age 51.3 years, whose diastolic pressures at entry showed sustained elevation to 90-114mm. A randomly selected half of the patients were treated with hydrochlorothiazide, reserpine (0.2mg daily) and hydralazine (75mg daily); the remainder received indistinguishable placebo tablets. Follow-up continued for from 1 to $5\frac{1}{2}$ years, until the termination of the trial (Veterans Administration Co-operative Study Group, 1970).

Table I summarises the main findings. The trial was stopped when it appeared that the total mortality among the treated patients had been halved. At this point the reduction in cerebrovascular accidents (the commonest major complication in this trial) was both large and significant, but there was no statistically significant reduction in myocardial infarction. This finding has been widely misunderstood, many people who should know better saying that this trial has demonstrated that the treatment of hypertension does not reduce the incidence of myocardial infarction. The fact is that, at the time when the trial had to be stopped, the number of cases of coronary heart disease was still too small to permit proper assessment. For fatal coronary events nevertheless the difference, such as it was, favoured the treated group (6 deaths, as compared with 11 among the controls). One would much liked it to be possible to continue the trial for a longer period, but this was precluded by the high incidence of strokes in the control group.

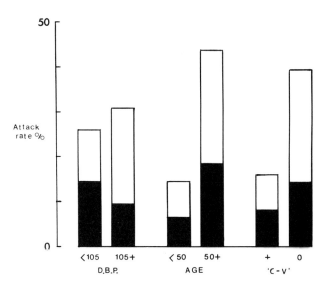

Figure 1. Attack rates of hypertensive complications among control (clear area) and treated (solid area) patients according to the presence or absence of certain initial risk characteristics: diastolic blood pressure (DBP), age, and initial cardiovascular complications (C-V). (Veterans Administration Trial, 1972)

Further analysis of the results from this trial (Veterans Administration Co-operative Study Group, 1972) has shown that treatment benefit was not the same in all sub-groups (Figure 1). The proportionate reduction in the incidence of complications did not differ very greatly, and hence the absolute reduction in risk — which is what matters most — was greatest in the high-risk sub-groups, ie those with pre-existing cardiovascular complications, the older subjects, and those with higher levels of pressure.

The Veterans Administration trial seems to provide irrefutable evidence that, among the patients they studied, the balance of benefit lay strongly with treatment. The uncertainty lies in identifying a corresponding group of our own patients: the incidence of complications in the trial was higher than we might normally have expected among patients with diastolic pressures of 90 to 115mm: it was clearly not dealing with a category which we could really describe as 'mild hypertension'. The frequency and nature of the complications correspond more to those of a pressure range perhaps about 10mm higher, as measured casually under the ordinary conditions of outpatients clinics.

The situation with regard to evidence on the benefits of treating mild hypertension might then be summarised like this:

1. At the upper end of this pressure range we have strong evidence of major benefit among middle-aged men, and some less strong evidence (Hamilton et al, 1964) for women.

2. At the lower end of the 'mild hypertension' range, and among old people, we have evidence of tne dangers of the untreated condition, but little evidence one way or the other on how treatment affects prognosis.

A PRACTICAL POLICY

Further and much larger controlled trials are now being mounted in this country and in the United States, based on cases of mild hypertension detected by some form of population screening; but it will be five years or more before their findings are available to us, so that in the meantime we have to try to work out a reasonable provisional policy. What follows is simply one man's opinion on a complex and uncertain situation.

Identifying the Cases

It is now agreed that the more severe grades of symptomless hypertension should be treated, but that there are large numbers of undetected cases (not to mention the large numbers of known cases that are nevertheless untreated or inadequately treated). This establishes the case for screening: all young and middle-aged adults (say, under the age of 65) should have their blood pressures checked every few years. In the course of looking for these more severe cases, we shall inevitably identify the much larger numbers of milder hypertensives.

Blood pressure is a labile characteristic. Even under standardised conditions of measurement the within-subject standard deviation of diastolic pressure averages 8mm, and sometimes it can be as much as 20mm. This means that a single reading is a very poor guide: it can easily be 15mm above or below the individual's mean level for those particular circumstances, and hence multiple readings are obligatory before treatment can be started. Unfortunately we know next to nothing of the periodicity of blood pressure fluctuations, and so it is anybody's guess as to whether readings to characterise an individual should be separated by days or weeks. My own practice in screening — and it is admittedly arbitrary — is to record two pairs of duplicate readings on separate days; if the mean of all four values exceeds the treatment level, the subject is recalled after an interval of a week or more, treatment being started if the cut-off level is still exceeded.

And what is this cut-off point? That is a thoroughly nasty question. On the one hand some kind of general guideline is necessary, and for me that figure is at present a mean diastolic pressure (based on muffling — phase 4 — as the end-point) of 100mm: in other words, the evidence suggests to me that the balance of benefits lies with treatment in most such cases. But on the other hand, such a rule-of-thumb approach should not be applied rigidly, for two different kinds of reason.

(1) Your reading of 100mm may not mean the same as my reading of 100mm. The use of disappearance of sounds rather than muffling as the diastolic end-point can account for an average systematic difference of about 4mm, which corresponds to an approximately two-fold difference in the prevalence of 'mild hypertension'. The conditions, both emotional and physical, in which pressure is measured can account for an additional 10-15mm difference. This seems the most likely reason why the control group in the Veterans Administration trial experienced a much higher complication rate than we would have expected from patients with such levels of pressure. We have a long way to go in calibrating our standards of blood pressure measurement. At the present we are blandly tolerating a state of uncertainty over the quality of basic clinical measurement which would cause an outcry if it occurred in a chemical pathology laboratory.

(2) A given level of blood pressure does not constitute the same risk for everyone. It is more hazardous for men than women, and very much more hazardous for smokers and for others with additional coronary risk factors (eg hypercholesterolaemia, diabetes). In the short term it is much more hazardous for older people, and for those with any existing atherosclerotic or hypertensive complications.

(3) Conversely, for some patients intervention is unusually hazardous.

223

Mental breakdown, overt or covert, may follow the news that 'your blood pressure is high'. Adherence to treatment varies, and erratic or erroneous consumption of tablets may well be worse than no treatment at all.

Putting these various thoughts together, I suggest that between the ages of 40 and 65 a sustained diastolic pressure of 100mm or more should generally be taken as indicating treatment, but that this general guide should be modified in individual cases. It will need to be raised or lowered according to the local circumstances and standards of measurement. It can be lowered a little in those with associated coronary risk factors or evidence of established cardiovascular disease; and it can be raised somewhat in women, the young, those with evidence of mental instability and those judged less likely to adhere to treatment. On the whole one treats a certain level of risk rather than a certain level of pressure. Over the age of 65 it is uncertain whether symptomless hypertension should be treated except in those who have had a stroke: controlled trials are much needed.

Investigation Before Treatment?

In mild hypertension the yield of correctable underlying causes is extremely low (Gifford, 1969), except perhaps in young persons or those with a history suggesting renal disease or phaeochromocytoma. In general, therefore, there is no call for investigation other than urine testing, unless the individual case arouses suspicions.

Hypotensive Drugs

The policy advocated here would imply a large increase in the number of patients receiving hypotensive treatment. This is a strong argument for preferring drugs which can be given in something approaching a fixed dosage, with relatively long intervals between visits. One is committing patients to potentially a lifetime of treatment with drugs whose long-term effects are unknown; to keep the uncertainties as small as possible, one should avoid drugs which have not already been widely used for several years.

From the patient's point of view the all-important need is to avoid side-effects. It is easier than one might suppose to induce a symptomless person to take tablets, provided that they do not upset him, but few will exchange fitness for symptoms. Less important, but still desirable, is that treatment should if possible need to be taken only once or at most twice a day, and that there should be only one kind of tablet.

These various arguments point strongly at present towards a thiazide diuretic as the basis of treatment. This is not to say that the possibility has been excluded that their metabolic effects might actually aggravate atherosclerosis; but there is no direct evidence that this is so, and on all other counts the thiazides score strongly. They should be avoided in those with pre-existing diabetes or hyperuricaemia, but Kohner et al (1971) could find no evidence in non-diabetic patients of an effect on glucose tolerance. The question of potassium supplementation has been much debated, but one can say that clinically apparent hypokalaemia is extremely rare in these cases, and that anyway the potassium dosage commonly in use does little to correct the deficit (Down et al, 1972). On the other hand, the effects of chronic hypokalaemia are unknown.

The full hypotensive effect of thiazides may take some weeks to develop, so that a decision to add a stronger drug should not be hurried. The choice of a second-line drug is controversial, but lies chiefly between a small dose of reserpine (up to 0.25mg daily) or α-methyldopa. The latter has the disadvantages of multiple daily doses and a higher incidence of symptomatic side effects (Gibb et al, 1970). Reserpine got a bad name in this country because of its ability to induce suicidal depression, but this danger is extremely remote if patients with any depressive tendency are excluded, if the dose is small, and if patients are warned to report at once if they experience depression.

The Heart Disease Prevention Project is a controlled trial of the prevention of coronary heart disease in collaboration with medical departments in British industry (Rose, 1970), and one of the preventive measures used is the detection and treatment of hypertension. The trial continues, but in the preliminary stages 200 men were classed as eligible for treatment of their mild hypertension (systolic pressure 160-199mm, based on a mean of four screening readings). When re-examined by the occupational physician, 60% of these cases were now found to be below the treatment level. In the remainder bendrofluazide 10mg daily was prescribed. In all but 3% of the men the subsequent systolic pressures were maintained below 160mm, and even in these it was sufficient to add a small dose of reserpine. One concludes that there need be little difficulty in getting symptomless individuals to take hypotensive treatment, and that simple drugs in fixed doses are generally sufficient.

Duration of Treatment

Must treatment, once started, be continued for life? This is a question which no one can answer. At present we must assume that the answer is generally 'yes', but a controlled trial in Japan (Chiba et al, 1965) found that a hypotensive effect of thiazides could still be detected nine months after stopping a three months course of treatment. Miall and Lovell (1967) have suggested that there may be a 'vicious circle' feedback, whereby hypertension tends progressively to aggravate itself: possibly a period of hypotensive treatment might interrupt the feedback, having the set point for blood pressure at a lower level. This is a very important question, but still largely hypothetical.

Other Treatment

If this account has given the impression that drug therapy is the most important feature in managing mild hypertension, then that would have been a serious error. It may be our chief means of preventing stroke, but it is not our best hope of preventing coronary heart disease, and it is this which is the chief danger confronting the patient with mild hypertension. The finding of symptomless hypertension identifies a person with a much increased coronary risk, and the best hope of improving prognosis is likely to be by energetic attention to a cholesterol-lowering diet, abandonment of cigarettes, regular physical exercise and the control of obesity. Control of the blood pressure is only one part of the management of the patient with hypertension.

REFERENCES

Chiba, Y., Fukuda, Y., Kondo, K., Sokuma, K., Morioko, M., Jitsukama, H. and Imai, T. (1965) Japanese Circulation Journal, **29**, 719

Dawber, T. R. and Kannel, W. B. (1961) Modern Concepts of Cardiovascular Disease, **30**, 671

Down, P. J., Polak, A., Rao, R. and Mead, J. A. (1972) Lancet, **ii**, 721

Gibb, W. E., Malpas, J. S., Turner, P. and White, R. J. (1970) Lancet, **ii**, 275

Gifford, R. W. (1969) Millbank Memorial Fund Quarterly, **47**, 170

Hamilton, M., Thompson, E. N. and Wiesniewski, T. K. M. (1964) Lancet, **i**, 235

Kohner, E. M., Dollery, C. T., Lowy, C. and Schumer, B. (1971) Lancet, **1**, 986

Miall, W. E. and Lovell, H. G. (1967) British Medical Journal, **2**, 660

Rosenheim, M. L. (1954) British Medical Journal, 2, 1181

Rose, G. (1970) Transactions of the Society of Occupational Medicine, 20, 109

Veterans Administration Co-operative Study Group on Anti-hypertensive Agents (1967) Journal of the American Medical Association, 202, 1028

Veterans Administration Co-operative Study Group on Anti-hypertensive Agents (1970) Journal of the American Medical Association, 213, 1143

Veterans Administration Co-operative Study Group on Anti-hypertensive Agents (1972) Circulation, **45**, 991

Prevention and Treatment of Urinary Tract Infection in Women

A W ASSCHER

Antibacterial agents effective in the treatment of urinary tract infection have been available for more than 35 years. Although the morbidity associated with urinary tract infections has been much reduced, it still continues to be a major problem. Logan and Cushion (1958) noted that 11 per 1,000 consultations in general practice are on account of symptoms which suggest urinary tract infection. The formation of lay organisations which seek a better deal for women plagued by recurrent cystitis further illustrates our therapeutic limitations. The mortality associated with infections of the urinary tract appears to have been even less influenced by the introduction of antibacterial agents than the morbidity. Kessner and Florey (1967) did not observe any decline in deaths attributable to infections of the kidney over the period 1950 to 1964 and Parsons et al (1972) found that chronic pyelonephritis was the cause of kidney failure in 21.2% of patients accepted for treatment by European dialysis and transplant centres.

In this paper, the two major problems in the management of women with urinary tract infection will be examined, namely how to minimize morbidity and how to avoid mortality.

REDUCTION OF MORBIDITY FROM URINARY TRACT INFECTION

Most women with urinary tract infection present with frequent painful micturition. In about half of them, a positive urine culture is obtained (Mond et al, 1965). Since the usual source of these urinary pathogens is the normal bowel flora (Grüneberg et al, 1968), primary prevention of recurrent attacks of bacterial cystitis is unlikely to be successful because it would necessitate bowel sterilization. Secondary prevention must, therefore, be relied upon. Stamey et al (1971) showed that the onset of bacterial cystitis is preceded by colonisation of the perineal floor with the same strain of Escherichia coli which is later recovered from the urine. This would suggest that recurrent bouts of bacterial cystitis are associated with a breakdown of the defensive mechanisms of the perineal floor. These observations have prompted the use of antiseptic applications to the perineal floor in order to reduce the morbidity resulting from recurrent bouts of cystitis. In the hands of some investigators (Landes et al, 1970) such measures have proved successful.

The ascent of micro-organisms to the bladder is thought to be facilitated by the shortness of the female urethra, the existence of a retrograde flow of urine in the female urethra, the fact that infection may be present in the female analogue of the prostate gland (peri-urethral glands) and the possibility that the organisms may enter the bladder during bathing, or perhaps most important of all, as a result of sexual intercourse.

An opportunity recently arose to obtain pre- and post-sexual intercourse mid-stream urine specimens from a medical practitioner who had for some years suffered from recurrent attacks of frequency and dysuria following sexual intercourse. This patient had been most carefully instructed in urine collection technique and on many occasions had been shown to have a negative urine culture. We were able to show by the dip-slide technique that a 6-hour post-intercourse specimen contained a pure growth of 10^3 E. coli per ml, whereas the pre-intercourse specimen had shown no growth. Clearly observations of this kind must be extended, but the difficulties are obvious. The role of sexual intercourse in the pathogenesis of the frequency and dysuria syndrome is well known to clinicians as implied in the term 'honeymoon cystitis'. The frequency and dysuria syndrome is more commonly precipitated by sexual intercourse in the younger than in the older woman. This may be on account of their greater sexual activity but poor sexual technique may also be a contributing factor. Asscher (1973) showed that 83% of a group of 36 women in whom the symptoms of cystitis were precipitated by sexual intercourse were relieved of their symptoms by emptying the bladder after intercourse and taking a single dose of an antibacterial agent at this time.

In patients in whom such a relationship does not exist, other precipitating factors may be discovered and attended to. The onset of symptoms may be related to the menstrual periods, childbirth, previous gynaecological operations or instrumentation of the urinary tract or the use of an intra-uterine contraceptive devise or diaphragm. In some 50% of the patients, however, no precipitating factor was obvious. In these patients, provided urine culture is positive, the approach to treatment should depend on whether or not one is dealing with a relapse of infection, ie a recurrence of infection due to the same organism which was isolated before treatment, or a reinfection, ie a recurrence due to a different micro-organism from that originally isolated. Relapses which account for about 15% of all recurrences, signify ineffective treatment, whereas reinfections indicate failure of the host defensive mechanisms. If facilities for serotyping urinary pathogens are not available, the simplest method of telling whether one is dealing with a relapse or reinfection is to study the timing of the recurrence. Relapses usually occur within six weeks of stopping treatment whereas reinfection occurs later. The approach to treatment of these two types of recurrence should be different. Thus, with relapsing infection, an attempt should be made to eradicate infection once and for all by high dosage treatment using bactericidal agents. Should this fail, long-term suppressive therapy with urinary antiseptics or low doses of antibacterial agents may prove successful in ridding the patient of recurrent symptoms. Reinfections may be dealt with as they arise and the patient should be given an antibacterial agent to take home with instructions to take a one week course of the drug at the first sign of symptomatic reinfection. At the same time she should send an inoculated dip-slide to the laboratory so that in case of failure to respond to treatment a further course of treatment may be prescribed on the basis of the sensitivity of the infecting micro-organism to antimicrobial agents.

The value of screening for and treating asymptomatic infections in reducing morbidity must also be considered. The outcome of these asymptomatic infections in pregnancy has been extensively studied. Some 20% of women who enter pregnancy with asymptomatic infection later develop symptomatic infection either during pregnancy or the puerperium. This risk is largely avoided if the asymptomatic bacteriuria (a.s.b.) is eradicated (Kass, 1960). This relationship of a.s.b. in early pregnancy to the emergence of symptomatic infection at a later stage of pregnancy has received widespread confirmation (Whalley, 1967) and forms the basis for advocating bacteriuria screening in antenatal clinics. It would clearly be an advantage if treatment of a.s.b. in pregnancy could be confined to the 20% of pregnant bacteriuric women who go on to develop symptomatic infection. As yet there is no reliable means of doing this. The value of screening non-pregnant women for a.s.b. in the prevention of morbidity is much less clear since the natural history of a.s.b. in the non-pregnant woman differs from that in the pregnant woman in two important aspects (Asscher et al, 1969). Firstly, bacteriuria in non-pregnant women shows a high spontaneous cure rate and secondly, although bacteriuria in the non-pregnant woman predisposes to urinary symptoms these are milder than in the pregnant woman and are usually confined to the lower urinary tract. Asscher et al (1969) showed that in the non-pregnant woman with a.s.b. a short course of treatment did not lead to a lasting cure and that the reinfections which followed 'successful' treatment were more commonly associated with a bout of symptoms than the persistent infections in untreated bacteriuric subjects. It seems, therefore, that the bacteria in the urinary tract of asymptomatic adult bacteriuric women are living in a kind of peaceful symbiosis with their host and are better left undisturbed.

PREVENTION OF MORTALITY FROM URINARY TRACT INFECTION

To achieve a reduction in the mortality from chronic pyelonephritis requires a thorough understanding of the pathogenesis of the condition. In this discussion the term chronic pyelonephritis will be used to refer to kidneys which bear localised scars, each of which overlies a dilated calyx. This juxtaposition of dilated calyx and scar enables recognition of the disease by means of excretion urography. Our studies of the pathogenesis and prevention of chronic pyelonephritis started with the assumption that bacterial infection of the urinary tract is at the root of the problem. The introduction of quantitative urine culture by Kass (1956) was a great step forward. It enabled population screening for urinary tract infection because the distinction between bacterial contamination and infection of the urine could be made without the need for catheterisation or suprapubic bladder aspiration. Contaminants which are added to the urine during or after voiding are present in small numbers providing the urine is cultured immediately or cooled to $4^{o}C$ to prevent multiplication of organisms in the urine after it is voided. In contrast, when infection exists, organisms are present in large numbers because of rapid bacterial multiplication in the bladder urine. High numbers of bacteria (usually more than 10^{5} organisms per ml of urine) therefore indicate the presence of bacteria above the internal urethral orifice and this state is referred to as 'significant' bacteriuria. It is possible to detect significant bacteriuria by various means, both bacteriological and chemical (for review see Asscher, 1970). The dip-slides introduced by Guttman and Naylor (1967) provide the most convenient and reliable method available at present.

In 1965 a long term study of the natural history of women with significant bacteriuria was started (Sussman et al, 1969). The objectives were to determine with what frequency significant bacteriuria leads to kidney damage, rise of blood pressure and impairment of kidney function and to establish whether treatment suitable for use on a large scale would affect the natural history. At the Royal Infirmary in Cardiff, 3,587 female visitors, aged 21-65, were screened for significant bacteriuria. In 3% the presence of bacteriuria was established, and each of the bacteriuric women was matched with a control of identical age, parity and civil state. Comparison of the bacteriuric and control women revealed that the bacteriurics gave a past history of symptomatic infection more frequently than the controls. Also the blood pressure and serum urea of the bacteriuric subjects were significantly raised. It was shown that 12 of the 93 bacteriuric women in whom excretion urograms were performed had pyelonephritic scars, whereas only 1 of the 50 controls showed such a scar. Pyelonephritic scars and bacteriuria are, therefore, correlated but to establish a causal relationship it is necessary to show the formation of new scars on long-term follow-up and to establish that eradication of the bacteriuria prevents renal scarring. The effect of treatment is

RESPONSE TO TREATMENT

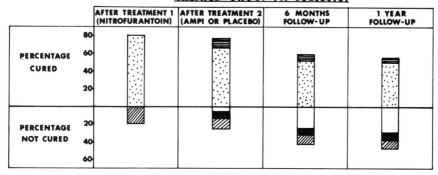

Figure 1. Effect of treatment on asymptomatic significant bacteriuria
(By kind permission of the Editor of the British Medical Journal)

shown in Figure 1. After a one week course of treatment with Nitrofurantoin 50mg four times daily followed by a further week of Ampicillin 500mg four times daily given to the non-responders, 80% of the subjects were cured. Unfortunately, recurrences proved to be common and after one year had elapsed only half of the subjects initially cured were still cured. It will be noted from Figure 1 that many of the untreated bacteriuric women developed a spontaneous cure, so much so that by the end of the first year of the follow-up, the difference between the cure rate in the treated and untreated groups was no longer significant. It follows that a short course of treatment, such as that which might be used on a national scale, does not alter the natural history of significant bacteriuria.

Recently a five year follow-up of our bacteriuric and control populations was completed (Asscher et al, 1973). Neither blood pressure nor serum urea showed changes greater than those which could be attributed to ageing and not a single instance of new pyelonephritic scar formation was encountered. Progressive kidney damage was noted in three of the bacteriuric women, all of whom had had persistent bacteriuria and obstructive uropathy throughout the follow-up period. The conclusion drawn from these observations was that bacteriuria in the adult woman is a benign condition provided it is not associated with obstructive uropathy. Although this conclusion receives support from the observations of Freedman (1972) it cannot be more than tentative because our follow-up is short and the population may not have been of sufficient size and in any case it is never possible to prove the absence of a phenomenon.

In recent years (Waters et al, 1970) we also carried out a retrospective study of the natural history of urinary tract infection. This study was based on the fact established by Mond et al (1965) that some 50% of women who present to their general practitioners with symptoms of urinary tract infection are found to have significant bacteriuria. We decided, therefore, to compare kidney function in women with a past history suggesting 'cystitis', with that of women who had had no such symptoms. The particular test of renal function we selected was urinary concentrating power, since defect of concentrating power is a sensitive indicator of renal involvement in urinary tract infection (Winberg, 1958). In a defined population of 2,933 women, aged 21-65, we found that concentrating power declined with age and that the rate of decline was similar in women with and without a past history of 'cystitis'. This finding supports the view that the long term natural history of significant bacteriuria is benign. One valuable clue emerged from this study, namely, that the urinary concentrating power in women who dated the onset of urinary symptoms to their childhood, was significantly impaired. This would suggest that urinary tract infection in childhood may have more serious consequences than in the adult. A second type of retrospective study (Asscher et al, 1971) supported this concept. It was shown that women with scarred kidneys and bacteriuria dated the onset of urinary symptoms more frequently to the childhood period than bacteriuric subjects in whom the excretion urogram had shown no abnormalities.

In an experimental model (Asscher & Chick, 1972) it was shown that kidneys which grow rapidly as a result of compensatory hypertrophy following unilateral nephrectomy, are more susceptible to the effects of ascending infection than fully hypertrophied kidneys. Thus both clinical and experimental observations lead to the conclusion that the scarred pyelonephritic kidney arises in childhood — a conclusion which is in keeping with the findings of Smellie and Normand (1968).

It seems, therefore, that if a young girl with kidney scars reaches womanhood she is unlikely to develop further kidney damage, provided her blood pressure remains normal and there is no obstructive uropathy. The likely explanation for the association between pyelonephritic scarring and bacteriuria which is noted in the adult (see above), is that most women probably acquire bacteriuria at some stage in their lives, usually the condition is transient, but if abnormalities of the urinary tract exist the bacteriuria may persist, possibly because of impairment of urinary drainage. Thus screening for bacteriuria will identify subjects with urinary tract abnormalities even though in the adult these abnormalities are neither aggravated nor produced by bacteriuria. This is an important concept since it enables us to reassure women with bacteriuria that they are unlikely to develop progressive kidney damage and even less likely to require dialysis and/or kidney transplantation. It also follows that asymptomatic episodes of infection in the absence of obstructive uropathy will not require treatment. The clinical management of urinary tract infection in the adult woman should, therefore, consist of exclusion of obstructive uropathy, treatment of symptomatic episodes and regular measurement of blood pressure, since rise of blood pressure is more likely to produce kidney damage than recurrent bacteriuria.

To return to the pathogenesis and prevention of chronic pyelonephritis. If we are to be successful in prevention it seems likely that we must turn to the young. Kunin et al (1960) showed that in 1.2% of 5-year old schoolgirls significant bacteriuria was found and that even at this age pyelonephritic scars were a common finding. It may be that screening for urinary tract infection amongst 5-year olds is already too late to prevent scars. Perhaps we should aim to screen nursery school populations. The problem here is that the younger the child the more difficult it is to obtain a 'clean' urine specimen, since we cannot resort to suprapubic aspiration for epidemiological studies. Another problem in screening schoolgirls for bacteriuria is that each year 0.32% of the population acquires bacteriuria (Kunin, 1968). If treatment of bacteriuria is, therefore, shown to be of preventive value, the whole of our schoolgirl population would have to be screened at regular intervals to detect new cases as they arise. This would be a massive undertaking unless a simple, reliable and economic technique for screening could be established. This technique would have to be acceptable to schoolgirls, parents, school health authorities and bacteriologists alike. In October, 1971, we set out to tackle the problem. Two surveys were started in Oxford and Cardiff, and the details of these will appear shortly (Asscher et al, in preparation). Briefly, in Cardiff, screening is carried out in an 'optimal' fashion with the use of a mobile laboratory. The laboratory is staffed by two nurses, it visits each of the schools in the city in turn and all schoolgirls aged 5-11 have clean catch urine specimens collected under strict supervision of the nurses. Dip-slides are inoculated and incubated on the spot. Girls showing a positive result are asked to provide a second specimen and if this is positive, general practitioners and parents are informed and the child and her parents are invited to attend the hospital clinic for full investigation including excretion urography and a micturating cystogram. Thereafter, the children are allotted to treatment or non-treatment groups. The effect of treatment will be judged by comparing the incidence of scarring and the extent of kidney growth over a four year period in the treated and untreated groups.   The hospital procedure in Oxford is identical with that in Cardiff, but the screening procedure in Oxford is a more practical one and could readily be applied on a national scale. In Oxford, the girls are given dip-slides to take home, together with an explanatory letter addressed to their parents. They are also given a container with boric acid preservative. The dip-slides and urine specimens are then collected from the school the following day. The results of our first year's experience indicate that there is little difference between the optimal and expensive method used in Cardiff and the method adopted in Oxford. Another encouraging feature of the Oxford/Cardiff study is that the older girls have a higher prevalence of pyelonephritis scars than the younger ones.   These findings raise our hopes that treatment of asymptomatic infections in schoolgirls will reduce the incidence of chronic pyelonephritis, raised blood pressure and impairment of kidney function in later life.

REFERENCES

Asscher, A. W. (1970) Early diagnosis paper No. 8.   Office of Health
    Economics, London
Asscher, A. W. (1973) in 'Planned Antibiotic Therapy'.   (Ed) A. M. Geddes
    and J. D. Williams.   Churchill Livingstone, London & Edinburgh. Page 93
Asscher, A. W. and Chick, S . (1972) British Journal of Urology, **44**, 202
Asscher, A. W., Chick, S., Radford, N., Waters, W. E., Sussman, M.,
    Evans, J. A. S., Campbell, H., Evans, K. T. and Williams, J. E. (1973)
    in 'New Developments in Urinary Tract Infection'.   (Ed) W. Brumfitt and
    A. W. Asscher.   Oxford University Press, London (in press)
Asscher, A. W., Chick, S. and Waters, W. E. (1971) Postgraduate Medical
    Journal. September Supplement, **47**, 28
Asscher, A. W., Sussman, M., Waters, W. E., Evans, J. A. S.,
    Campbell, H., Evans, K. T. and Williams, J. E. (1969) British Medical
    Journal, **1**, 804
Freedman, L. R. (1972) in 'Abstracts of plenary sessions and symposia'.
    Vth International Congress of Nephrology, Mexico City, **1**, 25
Grüneberg, R. N., Leigh, D. A. and Brumfitt, W. (1968) in 'Urinary Tract
    Infection'.   (Ed) F. O'Grady and W. Brumfitt.   Oxford University Press,
    London.   Page 68
Guttmann, D. E. and Naylor, G. R. E . (1967) British Medical Journal, 3, 343

Kass, E. H. (1956) Transactions of the Association of American Physicians, **69**, 56

Kass, E. H. (1960) in 'Biology of Pyelonephritis'. (Ed) E. L. Quinn and E. H. Kass. Little Brown and Co., Boston. Page 399

Kessner, D. M. and Florey, C. V. (1967) Lancet, ii, 979

Kunin, C. M. (1968) Pediatrics, **41**, 968

Kunin, C. M., Southall, I. and Paquin, A. J. (1960) New England Journal of Medicine, **263**, 817

Landes, R. R., Melnick, I., and Hoffman, A. A. (1970) Journal of Urology, **104**, 749

Logan, W. P. D. and Cushion, A. A. (1958) 'Morbidity Statistics from General Practice'. Volume I. General. Studies on medical and population subjects, No.14. HMSO, London

Mond, N. C., Percival, A., Williams, J. D. and Brumfitt, W. (1965) Lancet, **1**, 514

Parsons, F. M., Brunner, F. P., Gurland, H. J. and Harlen, H. (1972) in 'Proceedings of the European Dialysis and Transplant Association' Volume IX. (Ed) J. S. Cameron, C. S. Ogg and D Fries. Pitman Medical, London. Page 3

Smellie, J. M. and Normand, I. C. S. (1968) in 'Urinary Tract Infection'. (Ed) F .O'Grady and W. Brumfitt. Oxford University Press, London. Page 123

Stamey, T. A., Timothy, M., Millar, M. and Mihara, G. (1971) California Medicine, **115**, 1

Sussman, M., Asscher, A. W., Waters, W. E., Evans, J. A. S., Campbell, H., Evans, K. T. and Williams, J. E. (1969) British Medical Journal, **1**, 799

Waters, W. E., Elwood, P. C., Asscher, A. W. and Abernethy, M. (1970) British Medical Journal, **2**, 754

Whalley, P. J. (1967) American Journal of Obstetrics and Gynecology, **97**, 723

Winberg, J. (1958) Acta paediatrica, **47**, 635

The Treatment of Mild, Late Onset Diabetes Mellitus

R J JARRETT

I shall begin this discussion by considering the semantics of its title. Accepting the ambiguity of 'late onset', what is meant by 'mild' and by 'diabetes mellitus'? This concern with semantics is not mere pedantry, but, as I shall attempt to demonstrate, is not only pertinent but essential to any rational discussion of therapy.

Firstly, what is diabetes? We have national, European and international organisations devoted to its study, so it presumably exists. However, none of these bodies can provide a precise, dictionary definition. Any definition must at present be in terms of blood glucose levels, which leads us into the question of the relationship between hyperglycaemia and the clinical syndrome of diabetes. Apart from the relatively few conditions known to cause diabetes by direct insult to the pancreatic beta cells, we do not know whether diabetes is a single condition with a number of contributing causes or a syndrome, expressed as hyperglycaemia, with multiple aetiology and, possibly, diverse biochemical, clinical and pathological accompaniments. This uncertainty is exemplified by the wealth of adjectives (Tables Ia and Ib) which are used to define diabetes. Even this long list is not complete. Is the natural history of all these types the same, or even similar?

Table Ia. Terminology of diabetes

| Preclinical | Intermediate | Overt | | |
		Aetiological	Temporal	Biochemical
'Constituted as'	Chemical	Idiopathic	Juvenile onset	Ketoacidosis-prone
Potential	Borderline	Primary	Growth onset	Ketoacidosis-resistant
Latent	GTT	Secondary	Maturity onset	
Prediabetic	Premellitic		Adult onset	
Presymptomatic	Survey		Gestational	

Table Ib. Terminology of Diabetes – Clinical

Symptomatic	Labile	Lipoatrophic
Asymptomatic	Brittle	Lipoplethoric
Insulin sensitive	Stable	J-type
Insulin resistant	Severe	
Insulin dependent	Mild	
Non-insulin dependent	Florid	

Classical diabetes mellitus, that is the dramatic, wasting disease described by classical authors, is not considered mild and is not usually of late onset. The term mild properly refers to the degree of hyperglycaemia and the related symptomatology, but is a misnomer as I shall later show, in relation to the long term complications. This kind of diabetic may present because of symptoms, such as thirst, polyuria, weight loss and genital pruritus, but is nowadays more likely to be discovered because of routine screening of urine and, more recently, of blood. A not inconsiderable number are discovered because of diabetic complications - often via the ophthalmologist, who sees diabetic retinopathy in a patient presenting with deterioration of vision. In the Birmingham clinic (Soler et al, 1969), 7.5% of newly diagnosed diabetics already had some diabetic retinopathy, the relative frequency increasing with age. Although screening of the urine of patients presenting to hospital or general practice and even screening for glycosuria in people having routine medical examinations does not lead, so far as one knows, to many diagnostic problems, the screening of blood glucose on an epidemiological scale has given results which have undermined the conventional concept of diabetes.

In 1962, the combined Department of Medicine at Guy's Hospital and the Medical Officer of Health and staff of Bedford carried out a Diabetes Survey within the Borough (Sharp et al, 1964). The first part of the Survey consisted of testing for glycosuria in urine specimens passed about an hour after a carbohydrate-rich Sunday breakfast. Those positive – about 4% of the total – were recalled for a modified glucose tolerance test. From the co-operating population, including the glycosurics, a stratified random sample was selected for full, two-hour oral glucose tolerance tests. The results for the women – those for the men were very similar – are shown in Figure 1. Two main points emerge from these histograms. Firstly, in no age group is it possible to discern levels of blood glucose which discriminate between normals and diabetics. Secondly, if one should apply diagnostic levels without distinction of age, then the prevalence of diabetes would increase, with age, to a maximum in the seventh decade, though the peak age of **incidence** of diabetes is nearer 50 years. These findings concur with other studies both in this country and elsewhere (College of General Practitioners, 1963; Gordon, 1964).

237

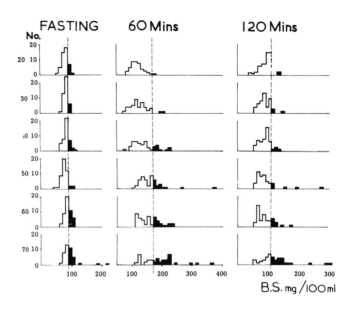

Figure 1. Blood sugar levels during a 50 g oral glucose tolerance test (zero, 60 and 120 minutes only) in the women of the Bedford random population sample. The upper row represents the age group 20-29 years and succeeding rows the decades up to and including 70-79 years. Vertical, interrupted lines indicate arbitrary upper limits of normality - 90, 180 and 120 mg/100 ml respectively

There is thus a practical problem in identifying diabetes; also, having made a diagnosis, in deciding which particular therapy to employ. In the asymptomatic, survey diabetic is there any justification in imposing treatment anyway? At Bedford, a pragmatic definition of diabetes was employed using the blood glucose level two hours after the 50 g oral glucose load. If 200 mg/100 ml or above, the individual was referred for treatment. If between 120 and 199 mg/100 ml the label 'borderline diabetes' was applied and the individual, after due explanation of what was involved, enrolled in a follow-up study, including a therapeutic trial, which is still continuing. Some justification for this division has emerged subsequently. Thus, approx mately 7% of the new diabetics, so-defined, had some degree of diabetic retinopathy at diagnosis. Five years later, the frequency had increased to 24% and amongst those were patients with florid retinopathy, some with actual visual impairment (Keen & Jarrett, 1971). The borderline diabetics, on the other hand, initially had a prevalence of retinopathy of 1%, rising to 3% five years later. In no case was this more than a few micro-aneurysms visible with the ophthalmoscope and all were near the upper cut-off level of blood sugar or were quite severely hypertensive. After ten years of follow-up we have yet to see convincing clinical retinopathy in someone initially a borderline diabetic, even though an appreciable number have crossed the arbitrary divide into the category of diabetes.

Even for the survey diabetic, then, there is an appreciable risk of retinopathy and visual impairment, which, one might hope, therapy might prevent or delay. In the clinical diabetic, admitting the distinction is not absolute, called mild on the basis of the degree of hyperglycaemia or symptomatology, retinopathy is a major risk. Sorsby (1966) found that diabetic retinopathy accounted for about 7% of all new blind registrations (Table II) and that, in middle aged people, it was second only to myopic chorio-retinal atrophy in frequency. More recently, the Committee on Blindness of the British Diabetic Association (1967-9) found that increased registrations for diabetic retinopathy had led to its becoming the single most common cause of blindness in the middle aged. The same committee also found considerable under-registration, particularly in the elderly. Even so, Sorsby's data (Table III) showed that almost half of the registrations for diabetic retinopathy were in people over the age of seventy. The so-called mild diabetic of late onset has something like a ten-fold excess risk of becoming blind from diabetic retinopathy compared with the risk of non-diabetics becoming blind from all causes (Caird et al, 1969). Further, the progression to blindness in the older diabetic is about twice as fast as in the juvenile onset type.

Table II. Causes of blindness in England and Wales (after Sorsby 1966). (same cause in both eyes; 1955-1962)

	Average number per year	Percentage of total
Senile macular lesions	2,615	27
Senile cataract	2,195	22
Glaucoma	1,225	13
Myopic chorioretinal atrophy	814	8
Diabetic retinopathy	671	7
All other causes	2,254	25

Table III. Average number of new blind registrations attributed to diabetic retinopathy (after Sorsby, 1966)

Age	15-29	30-49	50-59	60-69	70+	Total
Males	3	28	26	48	48	153
Females	2	18	60	188	250	518

The other excess risk run by the late onset diabetic is from the morbidity and mortality associated with atherosclerosis. This has been demonstrated in several investigations (see Jarrett, 1971), amongst which the Framingham study is notable. In this prospective study, in which both diabetics and non-diabetics were derived from the same population, there was an excess mortality amongst the diabetics from 'sudden death', cardiac infarction and cerebral vascular disease (Garcia et al, 1973). There was also an increased incidence of non-fatal events affecting coronary, cerebral and peripheral arteries. There is evidence from three epidemiological studies — Framingham (Gordon & Kannel, 1972) and Tecumseh (Epstein, 1967 in the USA and from Bedford (Jarrett, 1971) in this country that the lesser degrees of glucose intolerance — borderline or chemical diabetes — also are associated with an enhanced risk of episodes of arterial disease. It may be, though evidence is scarce on this point, that there is some dissociation of risk between the lesser and greater glucose intolerance — borderline diabetes and diabetes, respectively — the latter incurring the risk of microvascular disease as well as atherosclerosis, the former, at least in the short term, incurring the atherosclerosis risk only. If this dissociation is confirmed then it has important implications with regard to both aetiology and therapy. Whereas hyperglycaemia may be the prime aetiological agent in retinopathy, it is clearly one among many risk factors, and may not be an independent one, associated with atherosclerosis.

TREATMENT OF LATE ONSET DIABETES

In the symptomatic patient, the justification for treatment is obvious. In the asymptomatic subject, particularly when his degree of glucose intolerance/ hyperglycaemia is not very great, the justification rests largely upon the risks of arterial disease discussed above and the possibility of prevention, although blindness is a risk in the more hyperglycaemic among them. It is here that we enter upon difficult and disputed territory.

The first problem is that of remission of diabetes. The return to normal of glucose tolerance after weight loss in the obese is a familiar phenomenon. However, spontaneous remission also occurs. O'Sullivan and Hurwitz (1966) studied 83 women found to have glucose tolerance tests diagnostic of diabetes by the fairly stringent criteria of the US Public Health Service. These patients were followed for several years without specific treatment, although they were 'advised of the benefits of normal weight'. Spontaneous remissions to normal glucose tolerance were frequent, both in obese and non-obese women. Two-thirds of those with remissions experienced no change in weight, or even gained weight! We have a similar experience at Bedford. Many people have returned to normoglycaemia irrespective — or despite — the treatment they have received. Because of this apparently spontaneous change, any assessment of therapy becomes very difficult and controls are essential.

It seems probable, though again there is little data, that the greater the glucose intolerance, the smaller the possibility of spontaneous remission.

It seems likely that these are the people who are at greater risk both in the short and long term and in whom justification for treatment may also be greater. However, many of these people are asymptomatic. At Bedford, 60% of those with two hour blood sugars exceeding 200 mg/100 ml were without symptoms, even on direct questioning before the blood sugar was known (Keen, 1966). Even amongst those with blood sugar levels exceeding 300 mg/100 ml, 40% had no symptoms. So, despite the relatively gross hyperglycaemia in these individuals, justification for treatment again often rests only upon the risks associated with the hyperglycaemia. It remains possible, of course, that many of these people would have become sympto-matic eventually, but one does not know how many or how long it would have taken.

TREATMENT AVAILABLE

It is conventional to consider the therapy of late onset diabetes under the headings of diet and drugs. It is also conventional teaching in this country that one begins with dietary therapy – either carbohydrate or calorie restric-tion – and only proceeds to drugs if control of symptoms or blood sugar is not achieved with diet alone, although some authorities have advocated the use of biguanides along with diet in the treatment of the more obese. The conventional wisdom is based upon the well established phenomenon of improved glucose tolerance following weight loss in the diabetic. It is buttressed by the evidence that obesity is associated with an enhanced risk of atherosclerosis and a shortened life span.

The use of drugs, such as the sulphonylureas, is justified by their un-doubted efficacy in lowering the blood sugar and in relieving symptoms; also by the belief that by restoring the elevated blood sugar towards normal the likelihood of long term complications will be reduced. There is, in addition, the evidence from animal experiments that sulphonylureas protect against induced diabetes and, in the partially depancreatised animal, promote the regrowth of the islets (Loubatières, 1957).

These comfortable ideas received a rude shock with the publication of the results of the University Group Diabetes Program (UGDP) long term clinical trial, carried out in the USA (UGDP, 1970 a and b). This was a multi-centre trial of diet recommendation plus one of the following – placebo tablet, tolbutamide, fixed dose of insulin, variable dose of insulin – and was intended to observe the natural history of late onset diabetes and the effect of various treatment regimes upon it. The biguanide, phenformin, was entered into the trial at a later date. The data available at present is largely concerned with mortality and this has aroused tremendous controversy in the USA on both medical and medico-political grounds. The latest news from the battle is that a group of physicians is suing the Food and Drug

Table IV. Causes of death in the UGDP study
(UGDP 1970b)

	Placebo	Tolbutamide	Insulin - fixed dose	Insulin - variable do:
At risk	205	204	210	204
Deaths-all causes	21	30	20	18
Deaths-CV causes	10	26	13	12
Myocardial infarction	0	10	3	2
Sudden death	4	4	4	5
Other heart disease	1	5	1	2
Extracardiac vascular disease	5	7	5	3

Administration (FDA) over its intervention. The controversy arises, ultimately, from the relative mortality figures in the different treatment groups
(Table IV). The overall mortality was higher in the group treated with
tolbutamide, though the difference was not statistically significant. However,
when different **causes** of death were assigned, there was now a significant
excess of deaths ascribed to cardiovascular disease in the tolbutamide group.
In a preliminary report on the phenformin trial (Knatterud et al, 1971), the
cardiovascular mortality was again higher in the group treated with the antidiabetic drug. However, because of the trial design, the insulin treated
groups had to be taken into the comparison. The placebo treated group was
common to both parts of the trial. On the basis of these results, the FDA
has approved the following labelling of the package inserts (FDA, 1972) –

'Because of the apparent increased cardiovascular hazard associated
with oral hypoglycaemic agents, they are indicated in adult-onset, non-
ketotic diabetes mellitus only when the condition cannot be adequately controlled by diet and reduction of excess weight alone, and when, in the judge-
ment of the physician, insulin cannot be employed because of patient
unwillingness, poor adherence to injection regimen, physical disabilities
such as poor vision and unsteady hands, insulin allergy, employment requirements, and other similar factors.'

This is, in effect, a recommendation to use the oral agents only under
the most exceptional circumstances.

In this country, the Committee on Safety of Medicines has not yet taken
any definite stand on the issue and the British Diabetic Association has not
thought it necessary to change its traditional advice. The FDA itself seems
to have a somewhat ambivalent attitude, for it is apparently prepared to
support further studies of the long term effects of oral antidiabetic agents in
other countries. Presumably, such trials would be difficult to carry out in
the USA after the FDA's warning.

The UGDP trial has been subjected to more criticism and analysis, from both pro- and anti- positions, than any other clinical trial in their relatively short history. The two chief reasons for this are, I think, that the results were against most clinical expectation and that the intervention of a government agency in patient management occurred **before** the results were generally available to the profession. This led to much ill feeling against the FDA, which extended to the trial itself. As a result, much of the discussion concerning the trial has been intensely partisan in nature.

Usually, when there is controversy about clinical trials, it is possible to compare the results of one with several others. However, ten year therapeutic trials are not common. In our own study at Bedford (Keen & Jarrett, 1970), the duration of observation is the same or longer as that in the UGDP, but we have a different starting population – unselected, except for the level of blood sugar, more homogeneous and treated with a lower dose of tolbutamide – 1 g/day against 1.5 g/day. We find no significant difference in either overall mortality, or mortality ascribed to cardiovascular disease, between groups treated with tolbutamide and those without (Figure 2). Further, the mortality is slightly higher in the placebo treated groups. As there was not a significant excess of deaths from all causes in the tolbutamide treated patients in the UGDP study, I am not sure that the two investigations differ in their results. If one believes that they do, then is any difference due to different populations, to different drug doses or merely to chance?

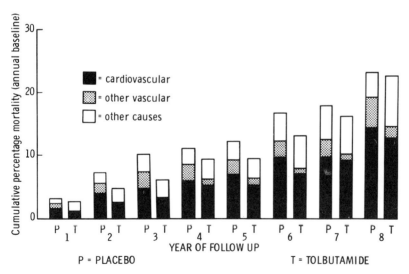

Figure 2. Cumulative percentage mortality amongst the borderline diabetics for the first eight years of the Bedford follow-up. The comparison is of the two groups placebo ± diet against the two groups tolbutamide ± diet

The third prospective, **randomised** trial of tolbutamide is very different in that the population studied was composed of survivors of a first and recent myocardial infarct (Paasikivi, 1970). They were also Swedish! Overt diabetics were excluded; among the remaining patients, intravenous glucose tolerance ranged from the clearly normal to the clearly diabetic. Tolbutamide appeared to protect against fatal and non-fatal infarction over the first eighteen months of follow-up, an advantage which had been largely lost by five years, and which was greatest in those with impaired glucose tolerance. Such is the partisan nature of the tolbutamide controversy that it has been claimed that the greater mortality rate after eighteen months in those treated with tolbutamide, ie. when the tolbutamide group was 'catching up' with the control, is evidence in favour of a malign effect of the drug (Medical Letter, 1970).

What then are we to conclude from the evidence available? Different people have reached and will reach different conclusions. My submission is that any conclusion must be tentative. Taking the three studies together, it seems probably that there is no significant effect of tolbutamide upon overall mortality and I am sceptical of any specific cardiac toxicity. As for cardiovascular morbidity, there is some evidence of a beneficial effect from the British and Swedish studies and possibly in the American one also. However, if one wanted a statistically satisfactory result, one would need much larger numbers of patients to achieve it.

It has been said that the UGDP study disproves the thesis that control of blood sugar is beneficial to the diabetic (Goldner et al, 1971). This notion is derived from the observation that the mortality in the group treated with a variable dose of insulin, with apparently better blood sugar control, did not have better mortality figures than the placebo treated group. However, because of patient selection, the mortality in these groups was better than would be expected from a comparable group of non-diabetics (Cornfield, 1971)! It would have been difficult for insulin, or indeed any other therapy, to improve on this. Similarly, at Bedford, after five years the mortality in the Borderline Diabetics was not significantly higher than in normoglycaemic controls, so a demonstrable beneficial effect of therapy would not be expected. We must wait for the data concerning microvascular disease before we know whether therapy with insulin or antidiabetic drugs did, or did not, have any beneficial effects in the UGDP study. From other studies of diabetic patients there is evidence that diabetic retinopathy is less frequent or less severe in the better controlled (Miki et al, 1969; Kohner et al, 1969), although it has to be admitted that there is little data on adult onset diabetics. While these and similar studies are open to objections or to alternative explanations, it is nevertheless true that there is no study showing that good control **increases** the risk of diabetic retinopathy. The working hypothesis remains a tenable one

With regard to atherosclerotic disease, however, there are other factors to consider. Consider, for instance, the Japanese diabetic. Goto and Fakuhara (1968) reported that in only 6% of a large series of post-mortem examinations of diabetics could death be attributed to coronary heart disease. Comparable figures from Western Europe or the USA would be around 50%. Other diabetic populations have also been shown to have a low prevalence and incidence of coronary artery disease (Shaper et al, 1962; Woolf, 1971; Greenwood & Taylor, 1968). The important point is that these diabetics all come from populations where atherosclerosis is generally uncommon. Thus atherosclerosis need not be an irrevocable accompaniment of diabetes. The corollary is that treatment directed at hyperglycaemia may not be the most effective way of preventing atherosclerosis in the diabetic. An obvious candidate for attention is the level of serum lipids and to talk of diet for diabetics without considering the purpose or the effects of those diets is, to put it mildly unsophisticated. To quote another American group – the Committee on Food and Nutrition of the American Diabetes Association (1971) – 'At the present time, there is not enough evidence to determine to what extent restriction of dietary fat and cholesterol is desirable. However diabetic patients appear to respond to reduction of saturated fat and cholesterol intake with a lowering of circulating cholesterol, as do non-diabetic persons. There is at present no firm evidence that this restriction will retard the development of diabetic complications, particularly atherosclerosis. However, the epidemiologic and experimental evidence relating to atherosclerotic cardiovascular disease also appears to apply to the diabetic patient. Reduction of serum lipids can be accomplished in general by limitation of calories, saturated fat, and cholesterol intake. Specifically, since most diabetics are obese, hypertriglyceridaemia when present responds to calorie restriction, as in non-diabetic patients. Diabetic patients who already have hyperlipidaemia may be more prone to develop atherosclerosis and therefore deserve particular attention to dietary management. '

Small groups of adult diabetics have been successfully maintained on low cholesterol, low fat diets for varying periods of time and with significant lowering of serum cholesterol levels (Van Eck, 1959; Stone & Connor, 1963). Van Eck also reported the clearing of retinal exudates, a phenomenon noted by others during therapy with clofibrate, which lowers serum lipid levels (Duncan et al, 1968; Harrold et al, 1969). However, even if such therapies prove to be beneficial in the long term, I do not need to remind you of the problems in inducing patients to adhere to even the relatively simple, carbohydrate restricted diet.

I began by questioning my title. I hope I have convinced you that it is wrong to refer to any kind of diabetes mellitus as mild, without acknowledging

the special connotation. My second thesis was that diabetes is not a precise
entity and may contain under the umbrella of hyperglycaemia a number of
conditions with different natural histories. Where symptoms are absent,
the case for treatment rests upon the prevention or amelioration of the two
varieties of arterial disease. An iconoclast might say, with some justification, that at present we can do neither of these things. I submit that there is
some evidence that we can do both and that there are rational therapies,
which must be tested, which may well prove to be more effective than the
traditional ones. What is certain is that mild, late onset diabetes is a subject requiring a great deal more research.

ACKNOWLEDGEMENTS

The Bedford Study is supported by a grant from the Department of Health
and Social Security. It also depends on the hard work and good will of many
people in Bedford and at Guy's Hospital. The opinions above are my own,
but I am grateful to my colleague Professor Harry Keen for the continuing
discussion which helps to clarify them.

REFERENCES

Caird, F. I., Pirie, A. and Ramsell, T. G. (1969) Diabetes and the Eye.
  Blackwell Scientific Publications, Oxford
College of General Practitioners, (1963) British Medical Journal, 2, 655
Committee on Blindness, British Diabetic Association 1967-1969, published
  by the British Diabetic Association
Committee on Food and Nutrition of the American Diabetes Association
  (1971) Diabetes, 20, 633
Cornfield, J. (1971) Journal of the American Medical Association, 217, 1676
Duncan, L. J. P., Cullen, J. F., Nolan, J., Ireland, J. T., Clarke, B. F.
  and Oliver, M. F. (1968) Diabetes, 17, 458
Epstein, F. H. (1967) Circulation, 36, 609
FDA Drug Bulletin, May 1972
Garcia, M. J., McNamara, P., Gordon, T. and Kennel, W. B. (1973) New
  England Journal of Medicine. In press
Goldner, M. G., Knatterud, G. L. and Prout, T. E. (1971) Journal of the
  American Medical Association, 218, 1400
Gordon, T. (1964) Vital and Health Statistics, Series 11, No 2
Gordon, T. and Kannel, W. B. (1972) Journal of the American Medical
  Association, 221, 661
Goto, Y. and Fukuhara, N. (1968) Diabetes (Japan) 11, 197
Greenwood, B. M. and Taylor, J. R. (1968) Tropical and Geographical
  Medicine, 20, 1
Harrold, B. P., Marmion, V. J. and Gough, K. R. (1969) Diabetes, 18,
  285
Jarrett, R. J. (1971) Acta Diabetologica Latina 8, Supplement 1, 7
Keen, H. (1966) Proceedings of the Royal Society of Medicine, 59, 1169
Keen, H. and Jarrett, R. J. (1970) In 'Atherosclerosis: Proceedings of the
  Second Symposium', (Ed) R. H. Jones, Springer-Verlag, New York,
  page 435
Keen, H. and Jarrett, R. J. (1971) Lancet, ii, 379
Knatterud, G. L., Meinert, C. L., Klimt, C. R., Osborne, R. K. and
  Martin, D. B. (1971) Journal of the American Medical Association,
  217, 777

Kohner, E. M., Dollery, C. T. and Bulpitt, C. J. (1969) Diabetes, **18**, 691
Loubatieres, A. (1957) Annals of the New York Academy of Sciences, **71**, 4
Medical Letter on Drugs and Therapeutics (1970) **12**, 97
Miki, E., Fukuda, M., Kuzuya, T., Kosaka, K. and Nakao, K. (1969) Diabetes, **18**, 773
O'Sullivan, J. B. and Hurwitz, D. (1966) Archives of Internal Medicine, **117**, 769
Paasikivi, J. (1970) Acta Medica Scandinavica, Supplement **507**, 1
Shaper, A. G., Lee, K. T., Scott, R. F., Goodale, F. and Thomas, W. A. (1962) American Journal of Cardiology, **10**, 390
Sharp, C. L., Butterfield, W. J. H. and Keen, H. (1964) Proceedings of the Royal Society of Medicine, **57**, 193
Soler, N. G., Fitzgerald, M. G., Malins, J. M. and Summers, R. O. C. (1969) British Medical Journal, **3**, 567
Sorsby, A. (1966) Reports on Public Health and Medical Subjects, No **114**, HMSO, London
Stone, W. B. and Connor, W. E. (1963) Diabetes, **12**, 127
University Group Diabetes Program (1970a) Diabetes 19, Supplement **2**, 747
University Group Diabetes Program (1970b) Diabetes 19, Supplement **2**, 789
Van Eck, W. F. (1959) American Journal of Medicine, **27**, 196
Woolf, N. (1971) In 'Blood Vessel Disease in Diabetes Mellitus' (Ed) K. Lundbaek and H. Keen. Il Ponte, Milan, page 14

PART IV

HAEMATOLOGY
Chairman: Dr C A CLARKE

The Role of the Red Cell in Oxygen Transport

A J BELLINGHAM

INTRODUCTION

It is now over seventy years since the oxygen dissociation curve of blood was first described. During this period it has fascinated investigators in many disciplines but only in recent years has this primary function of the red cell; oxygen transport, become so well understood. The molecular biologists have unravelled the anatomy of the haemoglobin molecule and demonstrated its molecular physiology. Meanwhile biochemists and physiologists have demonstrated the interplay between haemoglobin function and the 'milieu interieur' of the red cell which is essential for the red cell's adaptive role in oxygen transport.

HAEMOGLOBIN

The haemoglobin molecule is a tetramer consisting of four polypeptide chains, two α containing 141 amino acids and two β containing 146 amino acids. Attached to each chain is a haem group which is capable of reversibly binding with oxygen. Hence each molecule of haemoglobin can bind four molecules of oxygen. Due to this tetrameric structure, haemoglobin has the ability to increase its oxygen affinity as it takes up oxygen giving rise to the sigmoid oxygen dissociation curve, so important for its physiological function. In contrast the monomeric molecule myoglobin has a hyperbolic oxygen dissociation curve. This increase in oxygen affinity as haemoglobin binds oxygen is the result of reorientation of the chains within the tetramer. In the deoxy or low affinity conformation, the β-chains are approximately 7 angstrom further apart than in the oxy or high affinity conformation (Perutz, 1970). Any factor which tends to stabilize the deoxy conformation lowers the oxygen affinity and conversely stabilizing of the oxy-conformation increases the oxygen affinity. Although many factors alter the oxygen affinity (Figure 1), pH, temperature and pCO_2 are of particular physiological importance. The increase in P50 (see Fig. 1) accompanying a decrease in pH (Bohr Effect) and increase in temperature are well known and standard factors are in use for these effects (Severinghaus,

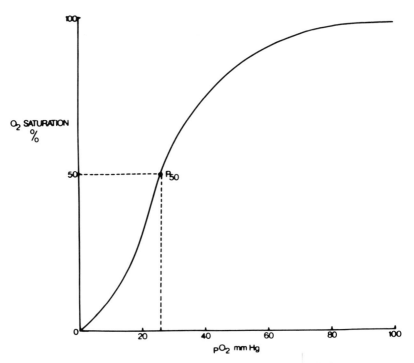

Figure 1. The normal oxygen dissociation curve of whole blood at pH 7.4, temperature 37°C. The position of the curve is characterised by the partial pressure of oxygen at 50% saturation (P50) which is normally 27 mm Hg. Therefore an increase in P50 is a decrease in oxygen affinity

1966). The effect of pCO_2 on P50 was originally thought to be due to its effect on pH but it is now clear that it produces an independent decrease in oxygen affinity due to carbamate formation (Roughton, 1970). The effect of pCO_2 is, by contrast, small relative to that of pH and temperature. However, it was the discovery of the action of phosphate esters on haemoglobin function, particularly 2,3-diphosphoglycerate, in 1967 by Chanutin and Curnish, and Benesch and Benesch, which has led to our current better understanding of red cell physiology.

2,3-DIPHOSPHOGLYCERATE

2,3-diphosphoglycerate (DPG) is a metabolic intermediate of the main glycolytic (Embden-Meyerhof) pathway of the red cell and is normally present in a high concentration (5 mM) peculiar to the red cell. Although discovered in 1925 when its high concentration was noted, the function of DPG within the red cell remained subject to much speculation until 1967.

DPG binds in equi-molar proportions with deoxy haemoglobin stabilizing this conformation and hence reducing the oxygen affinity. Studies using modified and abnormal haemoglobins and more recently X-ray diffraction have shown that DPG binds specifically between the two β-chains in the deoxy conformation to the residues: histidines β^{143} and β^{2}, lysine β^{82} and the amino terminal valine (Bunn & Briehl, 1970; Arnone, 1972). The gap between the β-chains in the oxy conformation is smaller not leaving room for the DPG molecule and hence binding does not occur. Oxygen and DPG may therefore be considered as competitive binders for haemoglobin, the binding of oxygen to haemoglobin releases DPG and conversely the binding of DPG releases oxygen. As might be expected the effect of DPG on haemoglobin is modified by various factors. Increasing pH, temperature and pCO_2 all reduce the DPG effect on oxygen affinity. However, within the ranges usually encountered these changes of DPG effect are relatively small and probably have only minor physiological significance.

The maintenance and the detailed mechanism involved in alterations of the concentration of DPG in the red cell are still not completely resolved.

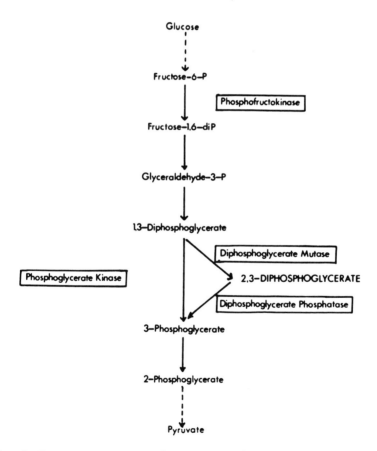

Figure 2. The main glycolytic pathway (Embden-Meyerhof) of the red cell. The enzymes in boxes are those mainly responsible for controlling the DPG concentration in the red cell

253

Physiologically the red cell concentration of DPG is modified predominantly by pH and hypoxia although changes in plasma phosphate may also have an effect. Increasing pH increases DPG concentration by raising glycolytic rate mainly by its effect on the activity of phosphofructokinase (PFK) (Rose & Warms, 1966). The final controlling factor of DPG concentration is the balance of activities between the three enzymes involved in the Rapoport Luebering bypass, ie phosphoglycerate kinase (PGK), diphosphoglycerate mutase (DPGM) and diphosphoglycerate phosphatase (DPGP) (Figure 2). Normally only 20% of the 1,3-diphosphoglycerate is metabolised through 2,3-diphosphoglycerate. Increasing pH both increases the activity of the DPGM and reduces the activity of DPGP so predisposing to an increase in DPG. However, the pH dependence of PGK has not been fully defined and the importance of altered activity of PGK in determining DPG level is unknown. Therefore, pH dependent changes in DPG are largely due to the effect of glycolysis at the PFK step and secondly to alteration of the balance of the activities of the enzymes in the Rapoport Luebering shunt.

The mechanism by which hypoxia causes an increase in DPG is even more uncertain. The increase in deoxy haemoglobin causes a rise in intracellular pH and hence will act through the steps outlined above. The increase in the deoxy haemoglobin in the red cell will also result in an increased binding of DPG and remove product inhibition on DPGM leading to further synthesis of DPG. Rapoport et al (1972) in a recent review suggest that the first mechanism is likely to be the predominant one. The effect of inorganic phosphate in increasing DPG is probably due to its release of inhibition by ATP on the PFK reaction (Rapoport et al, 1972).

OXYGEN TRANSPORT BY BLOOD

The red cell is but one link in a chain that transports oxygen from the atmosphere to the tissues. The transport by blood is dependent on both the quantity of haemoglobin present and the characteristics of the haemoglobin's reaction with oxygen. This physiological role of blood can therefore best be shown graphically by using oxygen content as the ordinate rather than percentage saturation when depicting the oxygen dissociation curve (Figure 3). Owing to the sigmoid shape of the curve, the normal arterial oxygen tension (90-100 mm Hg) is on the flat upper part and arterial oxygen content is minimally altered by shifts in the curve. By contrast, venous oxygen tensions are on the steep part and venous oxygen content is very dependent on oxygen affinity. Hence the adaptive role of blood in oxygen transport is by modulating tissue oxygen delivery.

Alterations in oxygen affinity may occur independently or alongside the other adaptive mechanism of blood, namely increase in haemoglobin concentration. This latter mechanism is well known but represents a slower form

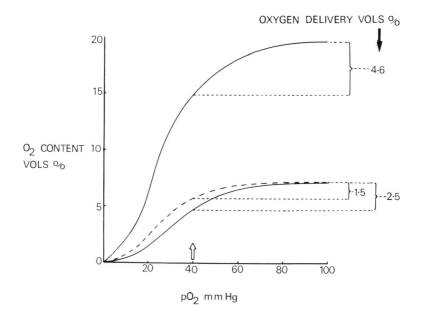

OXYGEN DELIVERY VOLS %

O₂ CONTENT VOLS %

pO₂ mm Hg

Figure 3. The oxygen dissociation curves of a normal subject (P50 = 27 mm Hg, Hb 13.4 G/100ml) and a patient with pernicious anaemia (P50 = 33.8 mm Hg, Hb 5.7 G/100 ml, and DPG 8.8 mM). Both are shown as solid lines. The interrupted line is the dissociation curve at the same oxygen capacity as the patient but without an increase in P50. The shift of dissociation curve has increased oxygen delivery at normal mixed venous oxygen tensions, as shown by the arrow, by approximately 65%

of adaptation, being dependent on an increased production of red cells. The DPG mediated changes in oxygen affinity are faster, having a half time of 10-12 hours. The pH and temperature dependent changes in oxygen affinity are of course immediate. However, it must be remembered that some factors, notably pH, have not only this direct effect on oxygen affinity but also an indirect effect due to their ability to modify DPG concentration. Hence, the resulting in vivo oxygen affinity in any adaptive process is frequently the result of the interaction of several factors.

PHYSIOLOGICAL ADAPTATIONS OF OXYGEN AFFINITY

Foetal Blood

Perhaps one of the severest adaptations that occurs is during birth when the foetus moves rapidly from a low environmental pO₂ (approximately 25 mm Hg) at the placental bed to atmospheric oxygen tensions in the lungs. In order to secure an adequate oxygen uptake at these low oxygen tensions, foetal blood has a high oxygen affinity with a P50 of 20-22 mm Hg. However, Allen et al (1953) showed that while there were differences between foetal and adult blood, purified Hb-F and Hb-A had similar oxygen affinities and they suggested that the difference in whole blood was due to the environment of the haemoglobin within the red cells. This difference could not be ascribed directly to DPG, however, as the concentration of DPG in both cord and adult blood is similar (Hjelm, 1969). Tyuma and Shimizu then showed in 1969 that the increase in P50 of Hb-F by DPG is less than the increase in P50 of Hb-A by the same amount of DPG. Furthermore, with the elucidation of the binding site of DPG to haemoglobin, such a reduced DPG effect would be expected as the γ-chains present in Hb-F lack the β^{143} histidine residue involved in the binding of Hb-A to DPG. Hence by switching from Hb-F to Hb-A the oxygen affinity is reduced whilst maintaining a similar DPG concentration. This adaptive process in the human contrasts with that in birds which on hatching raise the level of inositol pentaphosphate (the organic phosphate in chick red cells with a function similar to DPG) whilst keeping the haemoglobin type constant.

Hypoxia

The increase in P50 with anaemia was described as long ago as 1930. The increase in DPG which brings about this decreased oxygen affinity was demonstrated in 1970 by Torrance et al who showed that the severity of anaemia was proportional to the increase in both DPG and P50. This shift of the curve clearly makes a significant contribution to maintaining tissue oxygenation (Figure 3). Indeed, even within the normal population, the haemoglobin concentration is inversely related to the DPG (Hjelm, 1969). Cardiac disease, both congenital cyanotic (Oski et al, 1970) and ischaemic (Woodson et al, 1970), is associated with an increase in DPG and P50 which is proportional to the severity of the condition. A raised DPG is also found in thyrotoxicosis where, although an adaptive mechanism in increasing oxygen availability, it is probably not mediated in the same way as other hypoxic conditions since in vitro studies have shown that thyroxine directly stimulates red cell glycolysis, increasing DPG (Snyder & Reddy, 1970).

pH Disturbance

Guest and Rapoport (1939) first showed that acidosis is accompanied by a low DPG. With the discovery of the action of DPG on oxygen affinity it became clear that acidosis had two conflicting actions. Firstly by the Bohr effect it decreases oxygen affinity while secondly by its effect on red cell metabolism and hence reducing DPG it increases oxygen affinity. Similar but opposite arguments can be made for alkalosis. In studies on subjects with induced acidosis and alkalosis and in patients with diabetic ketoacidosis the alteration in DPG is such that the two actions on the oxygen affinity counteract one another and the in vivo P50 remains within the normal range (Bellingham et al, 1971). Owing to the difference in time for a DPG and pH effect on oxygen affinity (see above) this compensatory mechanism has important implications in the management of severe acidosis. If the acidosis is corrected rapidly there will be an immediate decrease of the in vivo P50 so impairing oxygen delivery until the DPG concentration readjusts to the new pH (Bellingham et al, 1970).

Rapid changes in pH, however, can have an advantageous role. In acute exercise the acidosis and rise in body temperature both occur too rapidly for a change in DPG to occur. Hence there is a pH and temperature mediated decrease of in vivo oxygen affinity facilitating oxygen delivery. At maximum oxygen consumption these changes reduce the required increase in blood flow by about 10% (Shappell et al, 1971). However, whether other adaptive changes occur in more prolonged exercise, eg as in marathon runners, is yet to be reported.

Hypoxia with pH Disturbance

In adapting to disturbances of oxygen transport the alterations to DPG often represent a response to more than one factor. Perhaps one of the best studied changes in oxygen affinity is that during adaptation to altitude. Although the increase in P50 with increasing altitude was well known, Lenfant et al (1968) showed that this rise in P50 corresponded with the increase in DPG. The same workers went on to show that the DPG response is due in part to the respiratory alkalosis and in part to the hypoxia. By inducing an acidosis with acetazolamide during ascent they found a reduced DPG response (Lenfant et al, 1971). However, when allowance is made for the plasma pH the in vivo oxygen affinity is still decreased. Unlike anaemia the advantage of the reduced oxygen affinity is not so clear cut. On exposure to altitude the arterial oxygen tension falls and approaches the steep part of the dissociation curve where any reduction of oxygen affinity reduces the arterial as well as the venous oxygen content, hence the increase in arterial-venous oxygen difference that usually occurs with a reduction in oxygen affinity is reduced. The decrease in oxygen affinity is therefore only a minor adaptive process at altitude (Lenfant et al, 1971).

In chronic respiratory disease hypoxia is commonly associated with an acidosis due to CO_2 retention. The acidosis and hypoxia both act to alter DPG in opposite ways. The resulting DPG concentration is therefore dependent on the severity of both the hypoxia and the acidosis, thus explaining the variable values reported. Similar to the situation at altitude, however, it seems that the in vivo oxygen affinity is reduced to a degree dependent on the severity of the hypoxia (Edwards, 1971). Again, these patients have a lowered arterial oxygen tension, hence the decreased oxygen affinity has a small adaptive role to play, particularly when compared to the advantage gained from the secondary polycythaemia.

In renal failure three factors affect the DPG concentration: hypoxia of anaemia, acidosis and increase in plasma inorganic phosphate. Inorganic phosphate is known to stimulate glycolysis and hence raise the DPG in vitro. The DPG level has been reported to be affected by the inorganic phosphate concentration in uraemic patients but it is difficult in these studies to be sure that the alteration in DPG is solely due to phosphate. In uraemia it is probable that inorganic phosphate mediated changes in DPG are minor compared to those due to pH and anaemia.

Stored Blood

Several workers have shown that storage of blood in acid citrate dextrose (ACD) causes a rapid fall in DPG and P50. By the end of the first week of storage DPG falls some 60-70% and hence the oxygen delivery capacity of the blood is severely reduced. Various methods have been investigated in an attempt to either maintain DPG levels for a longer period or regenerate DPG by incubating with additives prior to transfusion. The storage of blood in citrate phosphate dextrose (CPD) results in improved maintenance of DPG and P50 (Dawson et al, 1971), particularly for the first week of storage, and yet maintains the other functions of stored blood satisfactorily. The use of various additives such inosine, phosphate and pyruvate result in regeneration of DPG but have the attendant risk of introducing infection and in the case of inosine an element of toxicity. As DPG is regenerated after transfusion in about 24 hours this loss of oxygen transport function is temporary and only becomes clinically significant when large volumes of blood (in excess of 6 units) are used in, for instance, major accidents, heart surgery and exchange transfusions. It would seem at present logical to switch to CPD as a storage medium which is well tried and free of the risks of additives.

CONCLUSIONS

The discovery of the action of DPG on haemoglobin function, coupled with our better understanding of the molecular mechanisms involved, have opened a new era of red cell physiology. One of the most exciting prospects is the possible therapeutic control of DPG and P50 in such conditions as ischaemic heart disease and with improved knowledge of red cell metabolism this may not be too far in the future.

REFERENCES

Allen, D. W., Wyman, J. and Smith, C. A. (1953) Journal of Biological
  Chemistry, **203**, 81
Arnone, A. (1972) Nature, **237**, 146
Bellingham, A. J., Detter, J. C. and Lenfant, C. (1970) Transactions of
  the Association of the American Society of Physicians, **83**, 113
Bellingham, A. J., Detter, J. C. and Lenfant, C. (1971) Journal of Clinical
  Investigation, **50**, 700

Benesch, R. and Benesch, R. E. (1967) Biochemical Biophysics Research
Communications, **26**, 162
Bunn, H. F. and Briehl, R. W. (1970) Journal of Clinical Investigation,
49, 1088
Chanutin, A. and Curnish, R. R. (1967) Archives of Biochemistry and
Biophysics, **121**, 96
Dawson, R. B., Kocholaty, W. F. and Gray, J. L. (1971) Transfusion,
10, 299
Edwards, M. J. (1971) Abstract: Aspen Conference
Guest, G. M. and Rapoport, S. (1939) American Journal of Diseases of
Children, **58**, 1072
Hjelm, M. (1969) Försvarsmedicin, **5**, 195
Lenfant, C., Torrance, J. D., English, E., Finch, C. A., Reynafarje, C.,
Ramos, J. and Faura, J. (1968) Journal of Clinical Investigation,
47, 2652
Lenfant, C., Torrance, J. D. and Reynafarje, C. (1971) Journal of Applied
Physiology, **30**, 625
Oski, F. A., Gottlieb, A. J., Miller, W. W. and Delivoria-Papadopoulos, M.
(1970) Journal of Clinical Investigation, **49**, 400
Perutz, M. F. (1970) Nature, **228**, 726
Rapoport, S., Maretzki, D., Schewe, Ch. and Jacobasch, G. (1972) Alfred
Benzon Symposium IV, Munksgaard, 527
Rose, I. A. and Warms, J. V. B. (1966) Journal of Biological Chemistry,
241, 4848
Roughton, F. J. W. (1970) Biochemistry, **117**, 801
Severinghaus, J. W. (1966) Journal of Applied Physiology, **21**, 1108
Shappell, S. D., Murray, J. A., Bellingham, A. J., Woodson, R. D. and
Lenfant, C. (1971) Journal of Applied Physiology, **30**, 287
Snyder, L. M. and Reddy, W. J. (1970) Science, **169**, 879
Torrance, J., Jacobs, P., Restrepo, A., Esback, J., Lenfant, C. and
Finch, C.A. (1970) New England Journal of Medicine, **283**, 165
Tyuma, E. and Shimizu, K. (1969) Archives of Biochemistry and Biophysics,
129, 404
Woodson, R. D., Torrance, J. D., Shappell, S. D. and Lenfant, C. (1970)
Journal of Clinical Investigation, **49**, 1349

Disorders of Haemoglobin Synthesis

D J WEATHERALL

The object of this review is to classify broadly the genetic and acquired
disorders of haemoglobin synthesis. In order to fully appreciate their
pathophysiology it is necessary to describe briefly the structure and synthesis of normal human haemoglobin. It is beyond the scope of this article to
deal with this subject in detail and the reader is referred to several recent
reviews for more extensive coverage (Weatherall & Clegg, 1969; 1972).

THE STRUCTURE AND SYNTHESIS OF HUMAN HAEMOGLOBIN

Structure

Human haemoglobin (Hb) shows heterogeneity at all stages of development.
In foetal life the main component is Hb F and after birth this is replaced,
almost completely, by the adult haemoglobins, Hb A and Hb A_2. In normal
adults Hb A makes up the major part of the haemoglobin complement and
Hb A_2 comprises about 2.5% of the total.

All the human haemoglobins have a similar structure. They are globular
proteins which consist of 4 globin chains, each associated with one haem
molecule. All the human haemoglobins share one pair of globin chains, the
α-chains; in Hb F these are paired with γ-chains ($\alpha_2 \gamma_2$), in Hb A with β-
chains ($\alpha_2 \beta_2$), and in Hb A_2 with δ-chains ($\alpha_2 \delta_2$) (Figure 1). The four
chains fit together in a complex three dimensional structure with the haem
groups lying in deep pockets in the surface of the molecule. The way in
which this structure is related to the function of haemoglobin as an oxygen
carrier has been reviewed recently (Perutz et al, 1968; Perutz, 1970).

Haem is a tetrapyrrole which consists of an iron atom coordinated to
four pyrrole rings through their respective nitrogen atoms. The β positions
of the pyrrole rings are joined to each other through methane bridges and
these, together with the pyrrole rings, form an extended conjugated ring structure. The iron atom is bound in coordination with each of the pyrrole rings
leaving two other ligand-binding sites. One of these is bound to a histidine
residue of the globin chain while the other is the binding site for oxygen in
the oxyhaemoglobin form.

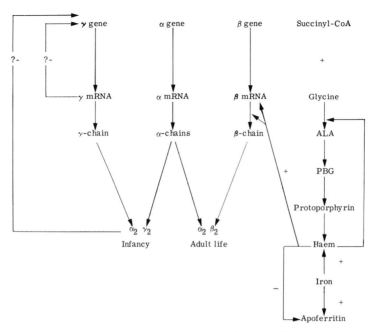

Figure 1. A schematic representation of the control of haemoglobin synthesis; + indicates stimulation, - indicates inhibition. ALA (δ-aminolaevulinic acid), PBG (porphobilinogen) and protoporphyrin are the main intermediates in the haem pathway

Synthesis

The synthesis of haemoglobin is achieved by the synchronous production of the haem and globin components through distinct metabolic pathways. The rate of globin and haem production is so regulated that there is no excess of either component during erythroid maturation.

The structure of the constituent globin chains of haemoglobin is directed by separate pairs of genes as shown in Figure 1. The genetic information which determines the order of amino acids in these chains is stored in their respective genes in the sequence of nucleotide bases which constitute their DNA. The genetic code consists of a series of triplets of bases which direct the insertion of a particular amino acid. This information has to be fed into the cytoplasm of the cell and this is achieved by the production of a form of RNA called messenger RNA (mRNA) which, because of the rules of base pairing, has a base composition exactly complementary to that of the DNA strand from which it is copied. Protein synthesis is achieved by the transfer of amino acids to the messenger template on small transfer RNA (tRNA) molecules which have three bases, the anticodon, which fit into the appropriate bases in the messenger RNA. A specific codeword is required for initiation of globin chain synthesis and the appropriate transfer RNA, together with the ribosomes which hold the growing chain in place, and various protein initiation factors, together form an initiation complex (Crystal et al, 1972). The chains are synthesised as the ribosomes move along the messenger and each amino acid is put into its correct place and joins the end of the growing chain until a codeword is reached which reads 'end chain', whereupon the completed chain drops off the messenger and the ribosomes return to the cellular pool for further protein synthesis. The production of α and β-chains is almost synchronous.

Haem is synthesised in a completely separate pathway; starting with glycine and activated succinate from the Krebs cycle the first important intermediate in the pathway, delta aminolaevulinic acid (ALA), is produced. There follows a series of condensations with the production of ring structures and various porphyrin intermediates before the production of protoporphyrin is completed (Figure 1). Iron is incorporated into the protoporphyrin ring and the resulting haem molecule rapidly combines with a single globin chain. The globin chains then come together to produce the completed haemoglobin molecule.

Some of these interactions are shown in Figure 1. Haem appears to be the central controlling molecule in this system since it can control its own rate of production by feedback inhibition of ALA synthetase, the rate-limiting enzyme in the haem pathway. It is also involved in determining the rate of globin chain synthesis, probably by limiting the rate at which new chains are initiated. Thus the molecule is synthesised through different pathways which are beautifully synchronised to produce a final product and no excess of intermediates en route.

DISORDERS OF HAEMOGLOBIN SYNTHESIS

Disorders of haemoglobin synthesis fall into two main groups (Table I). First there are the genetically determined abnormalities of globin or haem production which cause a variety of anaemias or other clinical syndromes due to abnormal haemoglobin function. The second group are the acquired conditions which interfere with haemoglobin synthesis. These result from either a deficiency of one of the substances required for normal haemoglobin production or from an acquired inability of the red cell precursor to synthesise haem or globin in the presence of adequate amounts of precursor substances.

GENETIC DISORDERS OF HAEMOGLOBIN SYNTHESIS

Globin

There are two main groups of genetic disorders of globin synthesis. First there are conditions which result from a genetically determined alteration in the structure of the haemoglobin molecule. These usually follow a single

262

Table I. Disorders of haemoglobin synthesis

Genetic disorders of haemoglobin synthesis

(1) GLOBIN
     The thalassaemia syndromes
(2) HAEM
     X-linked sideroblastic anaemia
     Autosomal sideroblastic anaemia
(3) IRON TRANSPORT
     Atransferrinaemia

Acquired disorders of haemoglobin synthesis

(1) DEFICIENCY STATES
     Iron
     Pyridoxine
(2) ANAEMIA OF CHRONIC DISORDERS
(3) SIDEROBLASTIC ANAEMIA
(4) LEUKAEMIA, MYELOPROLIFERATIVE and
     RELATED DISORDERS

amino acid substitution in one of the globin chains which results in either instability of the molecule or in its disordered function (Perutz & Lehmann, 1968). Occasionally such structural haemoglobin variants result from a deletion of one or more amino acids due to unequal genetic crossing over during meiosis. The second group of disorders of globin synthesis, the thalassaemias, result from a reduced rate of production of one or more of the globin chains (Weatherall & Clegg, 1972). This causes imbalanced chain production, a hypochromic anaemia and ineffective erythropoiesis with a shortened red cell survival due to precipitation of the globin chain which is produced in excess.

Structural haemoglobin variants The structural haemoglobin variants are summarised in Table II. The commonest clinical disorder which results from a single amino acid substitution is a haemolytic anaemia; this may occur in several ways. First the amino acid substitution may so alter the properties of the haemoglobin molecule that it causes distortion of the red cell with a shortened cell survival. Thus the mutation in sickle-cell anaemia results in a change in the molecular configuration during deoxygenation such that long stacks of molecules are formed and this process leads to the sickling deformity of the red cell. In the haemoglobin C disorders the substitution alters the solubility of haemoglobin so that the red cell becomes more rigid and hence is subject to destruction during its passage through the reticulo-endothelial system. There are also a variety of haemoglobin variants due to

263

Table II. Diseases due to structural haemoglobin variants

CHRONIC HAEMOLYTIC ANAEMIA

        Altered molecular configuration :- Hb S

        Altered solubility :- Hb C

        Altered molecular stability :- Hb Köln etc

DRUG INDUCED HAEMOLYTIC ANAEMIA

        Increased susceptibility to oxidation :- Hb Zürich

HEREDITARY CYANOSIS

        Permanent methaemoglobinaemia :- Hbs M

        Reduced oxygen affinity :- Hb Kansas

HEREDITARY POLYCYTHAEMIA

        High oxygen affinity :- Hb Chesapeake etc

HYPOCHROMIC ANAEMIA

        Low rate of synthesis :- Hb Lepore

                             Hb Constant Spring

substitutions at critical areas inside the molecule or in the haem pocket, all of which result in molecular instability (White & Dacie, 1971). In these conditions the unstable haemoglobin precipitates in the cell producing a red cell inclusion or Heinz body. If the precipitation is rapid these bodies may be formed in the bone marrow and cause intramedullary destruction with ineffective erythropoiesis, whereas if the cells pass into the peripheral blood the rigid Heinz bodies are removed in the spleen or reticuloendothelial system with subsequent damage to the red cell membrane. Affected patients have chronic haemolytic anaemia with jaundice and the passage of dark urine due to the breakdown of haem products from the precipitated haemoglobin material.

Another important group of haemoglobin variants are those which result in abnormal oxygen transport. The haemoglobin Ms are a group of structural variants in which a mutation near the haem-attachment results in the formation of a permanent bond with the iron of the haem molecule in the oxidised (Fe^{+++}) state. This causes permanant methaemoglobinaemia and congenital cyanosis. There is another group of haemoglobin variants in which the amino acid substitution causes diminished haem-haem interaction with the production of a high oxygen affinity haemoglobin molecule (Weatherall, 1969). In this case each unit of blood gives up less oxygen to the tissues; this causes an increased production of erythropoietin and a mild polycythaemia. Such patients present with congenital polycythaemia.

Finally there are a group of structural haemoglobin variants which cause clinical disorders because they are synthesised slowly and therefore cause chain imbalance similar to that seen in thalassaemia (vide infra).

The Thalassaemias

These are by far the commonest genetic disorders of haemoglobin production and cause a massive public health problem in the Mediterranean region and South-east Asia. There are two main groups of thalassaemias, the α and β-thalassaemias, depending on whether the synthesis of α - or β-chains is reduced (Table III).

Table III. Thalassaemia

β-THALASSAEMIA

A heterogenous group of disorders of β- or δ- and β-chain production.

Common in Mediterranean, Middle East, India and Far East.

Severe anaemia with high level of HbF in homozygotes.

Mild anaemia with raised HbA_2 or HbF in heterozygotes.

α-THALASSAEMIA

A heterogenous group of disorders of α-chain production.

Common in S E Asia, Middle East and parts of Mediterranean.

In severest form causes picture of hydrops foetalis.

Milder form (due to interacting 2 genes) occurs in adults as HbH disease.

Carrier states not recognisable in adult life.

There are several forms of β-thalassaemia. In some cases there is a diminished production of β-chains while in others there is a total absence of β-chain synthesis. There is a further subclass in which δ-chain synthesis is also abnormal, called the $\delta\beta$-thalassaemias. In homozygous state for these conditions there is severe anaemia from about the third month of life requiring repeated blood transfusion, and death occurs commonly in early life from anaemia or infection. If these children survive the first few years they usually die in the second decade from the results of iron overload due to repeated blood transfusion. In the heterozygous states there is a mild anaemia which becomes worse during periods of stress such as pregnancy. Although these diseases are found most commonly in Mediterranean and Oriental races they occur in every population. In a recent review of 85 British β-thalassaemia heterozygotes a history of repeated anaemia of pregnancy was common and many of the patients had been investigated and treated for refractory anaemia for many years because the diagnosis was not suspected. This resulted in much anxiety and there was evidence of iron overload in patients who had long-term iron therapy (Knox-Macaulay et al, 1973). The clinical picture together with the findings of a hypochromic blood film and large amounts of foetal haemoglobin makes the diagnosis of the homozygous state relatively easy. In the heterozygotes there is mild anaemia with hypochromic red cells and a normal serum iron level. In β-thalassaemia the haemoglobin A_2 levels is elevated while in δ β-thalassaemia there is a high level of haemoglobin F with normal levels of haemoglobin A_2.

There are several types of α-thalassaemia gene. Most of the α-thalassaemia disorders result from the interaction of three distinct genes; α-thalassaemia 1, α-thalassaemia 2 and the gene for haemoglobin Constant Spring (Hb CS), an α-chain haemoglobin variant which occurs commonly in South East Asia and causes a reduced rate of α-chain production (Weatherall & Clegg, 1972). The homozygous state for the α-thalassaemia 1 gene produced a total absence of α-chain synthesis and death in utero with a clinical picture of hydrops feotalis. The heterozygous state for the α-thalassaemia 1 and 2 genes, or for α-thalassaemia 1 and HbCS genes, is compatible with survival into adult life. Affected patients have a hypochromic anaemia and because of the deficiency of α-chains produce excess β-chains which form β_4 molecules or Hb H. This haemoglobin is unstable and precipitates, causing intracellular inclusion bodies and a shortened red cell survival. These varieties of haemoglobin H disease are extremely common in South East Asia and some Mediterranean races and have been seen in people of every background including several British families.

Current evidence suggests that many of the thalassaemia syndromes result from a reduced rate of mRNA production for the affected chain; the reason for this abnormality is unknown.

Haem

Genetic abnormalities of haem production are uncommon. It is possible, although far from certain, that the X-linked hypochromic anaemias associated with ring sideroblasts in the bone marrow (vide infra) result from genetic abnormalities of haem synthesis (Mollin & Hoffbrand, 1968). However, it appears that this disorder is not always X-linked and there may be congenital sideroblastic anaemias with an autosomal mode of inheritance (Weatherall et al, 1970). These conditions are easily diagnosed by the finding of an iron-refractory hypochromic anaemia with ring sideroblasts in the bone marrow in a young child. There are no associated abnormalities of the haemoglobin pattern. Some of these patients make an incomplete response to pyridoxine therapy. They develop a considerable degree of iron overload as they get older (vide infra).

Iron Transport

Congenital iron deficiency due to absence of transferrin is a very rare condition and there has been only one reported family (Heilmeyer et al, 1961).

ACQUIRED DISORDERS OF HAEMOGLOBIN SYNTHESIS

Deficiency States

By far the commonest acquired disorder of haemoglobin synthesis is simple iron deficiency anaemia. In addition there appears to be a form of sidero-blastic anaemia (vide infra) which is due to an acquired pyridoxine deficiency usually associated with either malabsorption or excessive utilisation due to haemolysis (Mollin & Hoffbrand, 1968). In addition there may be a group of young adults who develop a sideroblastic anaemia which is responsive to pyridoxine but in several cases the clinical response has only been transient suggesting that there is another underlying metabolic deficiency.

The anaemia of chronic disorders

This type of anaemia is found commonly in clinical practice in association with infection, malignant disease, rheumatoid arthritis, renal disease and other chronic disorders (Cartwright, 1966). It is extremely important to recognise the various components of this syndrome as the finding of this type of blood picture nearly always points to the presence of an underlying disease. The pathophysiology of this anaemia is not yet fully understood but it seems to result from the interaction of several factors including a reduced rate of cellular proliferation due to inefficient erythropoietin production, a defect in haemoglobin synthesis with the production of slightly hypochromic red cells, a slightly shortened red cell survival and a failure of transport of iron from the reticuloendoethelial system into the developing red cell precursor (Cartwright & Lee, 1971). The clinical features are summarised in Table IV. These include a mild hypochromic anaemia, a low serum iron level with a low total iron binding capacity, increased iron stores in the storage elements of the marrow but a reduction of iron-containing red cell precursors (sideroblasts) and a raised red cell protoporphyrin level. When this picture is encountered the patient should be fully investigated for one of the disorders mentioned above.

Table IV. The anaemia of chronic disorders

(1) Moderate reduction in haemoglobin and PCV.
(2) Normochromic or slightly hypochromic red cells.
(3) Low serum iron. Low iron binding capacity.
(4) Reduced sideroblasts; increased storage iron.
(5) Increased erythrocyte protoporphyrin.

The acquired sideroblastic anaemias

A clinical classification of these important disorders is shown in Table V.

Normal red cell precursors have iron granules scattered throughout their cytoplasm and are called sideroblasts. In the various refractory anaemias such as thalassaemia there may be increased amounts of iron in these cells but this is distributed normally in the cytoplasm. However, there are a group of anaemias in which there is a large amount of iron

267

Table V. Sideroblastic anaemia

CONGENITAL
X-linked
Non X-linked
ACQUIRED
Primary
Secondary
Specific Mitochondrial Toxins
Lead
Alcohol
Chloramphenicol
Pyridoxine Deficiency
Non-Specific
Malignancy
Collagen Disease
Pre-Leukaemia
Myeloproliferative Disease

distributed abnormally in a ring round the nucleus; such precursors are known as abnormal ring sideroblasts. The sideroblastic anaemias are defined therefore as a group of refractory hypochromic anaemias in which there is an abnormally large proportion of ring sideroblasts in the bone marrow (Mollin & Hoffbrand, 1968). They occur either as an idiopathic group with an onset in late life or secondary to specific or nonspecific toxins. The genetic sideroblastic anaemias were considered in an earlier section.

Idiopathic acquired sideroblastic anaemias (Table VI)

These disorders present as refractory anaemias in the older age groups (MacGibbon & Mollin, 1965). The peripheral blood film tends to be dimorphic with normochromic and hypochromic populations but the overall picture is not very hypochromic and usually there are normal or just subnormal MCHC values. The white cell count and platelet count may be slightly reduced. There are no abnormal physical signs; the spleen is not enlarged usually. The bone marrow shows erythroid hyperplasia with large numbers of ring sideroblasts. Although there have been reports of response to various haematinics, including large doses of pyridoxine, in the author's experience these anaemias are refractory to all treatment and patients are best maintained with blood transfusion, if the anaemia is symptomatic. Occasionally secondary folic acid deficiency occurs and a trial of folate therapy is worthwhile in all cases.

Table VI. The clinical characteristics of congenital and acquired sideroblastic anaemia

Acquired sideroblastic anaemia	
Age	40 years +
Splenomegaly	Unusual
Sex	Equal
Blood film	Dimorphic. Mild Hypochromia
MCHC	30-34%
MCV	100-120 fl
Serum Fe	Normal or high
TIBC	Normal or low
WCC + Platelets	May be reduced
Marrow	Ring Sideroblasts ++

Congenital sideroblastic anaemia	
Age	Childhood
Sex	Usually male
Splenomegaly	Usual
Blood	Dimorphic. Hypochromia ++
MCHC	24-28%
Serum Fe	Normal or high
TIBC	Normal
WCC + Platelets	Normal
Marrow	Ring Sideroblasts ++

Secondary acquired sideroblastic anaemias (Table VI)

A variety of mitochondrial toxins will produce a secondary acquired sideroblastic reaction. These include alcohol, lead, chloramphenicol and the antituberculous drugs. The finding of a sideroblastic anaemia should always provoke an intensive search for the exposure to any of these toxins. The sideroblastic reaction is usually reversible if the toxin is removed although patients who have been treated with chloramphenicol may go on to develop hypoplastic or aplastic anaemia. A sideroblastic reaction may also be the first indication of an underlying myeloproliferative disorder such as leukaemia or myelosclerosis and a proportion of patients who present apparently with an idiopathic acquired sideroblastic anaemia go on to develop one of these disorders.

Although the findings outlined above suggest that this type of anaemia results from the production of a cell line in which there is defective synthesis of haem, no definite abnormality in the haem synthetic pathway has been demonstrated.

Other acquired disorders of haemoglobin synthesis

A variety of ill-understood changes in haemoglobin pattern occur in such conditions as aplastic anaemia, the myeloproliferative disorders and the leukaemias. These include the reactivation of Hb F production, changes in the level of Hb A_2 and, in erythroleukaemia, the production of Hb H. These conditions have been discussed in detail by Weatherall and Clegg (1972).

Diagnosis of iron-refractory hypochromic anaemia (Table VII)

The first step in this common clinical problem is to make sure that there is genuine failure of response to iron. This can usually be achieved by simple clinical and haematological studies but if there is any doubt the marrow iron stores should be assessed by a bone marrow aspiration suitably stained for iron. If the anaemia is hypochromic and free iron is present in the marrow then one is dealing with one of the conditions outlined in this review. Using bone marrow preparations stained adequately for iron it is possible to categorise these conditions into the anaemias of chronic disorders or the sideroblastic anaemias. Once having established either of these groups the next step is to find the underlying cause, if possible. If the anaemia falls into neither of these categories then full studies for the haemoglobinopathies should be undertaken.

Table VII. Diagnosis of iron-refractory hypochromic anaemia

---

(1) Is it really iron deficiency? Serum Fe. Marrow Fe.

(2) If not:-

    (a) Is it anaemia of chronic disorders? Serum Fe. TIBC

                                            Marrow Fe.

                  If so, why?

    (b) Is it sideroblastic? Serum Fe. Marrow Fe.

        If so, primary (genetic or acquired) or secondary?

    (c) Is it a haemoglobinopathy? Serum Fe. Marrow Fe.

                                Hb analysis

REFERENCES

Cartwright, G. E. (1966) British Journal of Haematology, **21**, 147

Cartwright, G. E. and Lee, G. R. (1971) California Medicine, **102**, 222

Crystal, R. G., Nienhuis, A. W., Elson, N. A. and Anderson, W. F. (1972) Journal of Biological Chemistry, **247**, 5357

Heilmeyer, L., Keller, W., Vivell, O., Keiderling, W., Betke, K., Wohler, F. and Schultze, H. E. (1961) Deutsche medizinische Wochenschrift, **86**, 1745

Knox-Macaulay, H. H. M., Weatherall, D. J., Clegg, J. B. and Pembrey, M. E. (1973) In preparation

MacGibbon, B. H. and Mollin, D. L. (1965) British Journal of Haematology, **11**, 59

Mollin, D. L. and Hoffbrand, A. V. (1968) Recent Advances in Clinical Pathology series **5**, 273

Perutz, M. F. (1970) Nature, **228**, 726 and 734
Perutz, M. F. and Lehmann, H. (1968) Nature, **219**, 902
Perutz, M. F., Muirhead, H., Cox, J. M., Goaman, L. C. G., Matthews,
F. S., McGandy, E. L. and Webb, L. E. (1968) Nature, **219**, 29
Weatherall, D. J. (1969) New England Journal of Medicine, **280**, 604
Weatherall, D. J. and Clegg, J. B. (1969) Progress in Hematology, **6**, 261
Weatherall, D. J. and Clegg, J. B. (1972) The Thalassaemia Syndromes,
Blackwell Scientific Publications Ltd., Oxford
Weatherall, D. J., Pembrey, M. E., Hall, E. G., Sanger, R., Tippett, P.
and Gavin, J. (1970) Lancet **ii**, 744
White, J. M. and Dacie, J. V. (1971) Progress in Hematology, **7**, 69

Recent Advances in Megaloblastic Anaemia

I CHANARIN

PHYSIOLOGY AND PATHOLOGY OF FOLATE ABSORPTION

Folic acid is a relatively complex molecule comprising a double-ringed structure, the pteridine ring, para-aminobenzoic acid and glutamic acid (Figure 1).

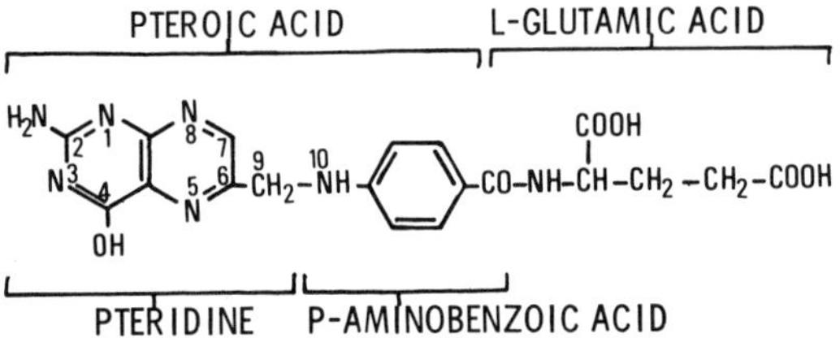

Figure 1. Pteroylglutamic acid

Cellular folate is more complex (Figure 2) insofar as:

i)   The pteridine ring is normally reduced by the addition of hydrogens to give tetrahydro- (but occasionally dihydro-) pteroylglutamic acid. This renders the compound very susceptible to oxidative cleavage, particularly when combined with heat as in cooking food.

ii) Cellular folate has not one, but a chain of glutamic acid residues. Thus, rat liver folate has 5 glutamic acids, ie it is a pentaglutamate. A normal mixed diet has 75-90% of polyglutamate forms of folate.

iii) Folate functions in the transport of single carbon units in purine and pyrimidine synthesis. Most folates thus have an additional carbon unit either as a -CHO (formyl) or -CH$_3$ (methyl) group.

By contrast with cellular folate which is a reduced polyglutamate, folate in body fluids, plasma and CSF, is a monoglutamate — invariably 5, methyltetrahydrofolate. Transport of folate, for example, from food to portal blood

272

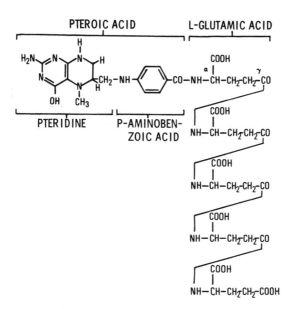

Figure 2. Methyltetrahydropteroyl-pentaglutamate

therefore involves removal of the glutamic acid chain so that a monoglutamate appears in the plasma and entry into the cell is followed by reconstitution of the glutamic acid chain.

Food folate is a mixture of **monoglutamates** in various states of reduction, that is, dihydro- and tetrahydro- forms with formyl or methyl substituents, and **polyglutamates** of various chain lengths also with formyl or methyl substituents.

Intestinal absorption of dietary folate involves conversion of the various folate analogues into 5, methyltetrahydropteroylglutamic acid. The steps are:

1) Removal of the glutamic acid chain. The lysosomal enzyme, folate conjugase, which removes the glutamic acid residues, has a pH optimum of 4.5 and is not active above pH 5.5. Thus, it is inactive at the normal pH found in the small intestinal lumen and removal of peptide chain presumably occurs in the intestinal cell.

2) Dihydrofolate is further reduced to tetrahydrofolate since if dihydrofolate is given orally only tetrahydro- forms appear in blood.

3) A single carbon unit is added as formate and this is, in turn, reduced to the methyl form. Finally, 5, methyltetrahydropteroyl-glutamic acid is transferred to portal blood.

Pteroylglutamic acid, the pharmacological form of folate is not a normal substrate for the enzyme, dihydrofolate reductase, and when pteroylglutamic acid is given orally it passes into the portal blood largely unchanged. Reduction and methylation of some of this compound occurs in the tissues, but the bulk is normally excreted into the urine either unchanged or after cleavage of the molecule.

MALABSORPTION OF FOLATE

This may occur in: Coeliac disease (commonly)
Tropical sprue (commonly)
Dermatitis herpetiformis (commonly)
Crohn's disease (if extensive)
Partial gastrectomy (rarely)

Transient impairment of absorption may occur after excessive alcohol intake. There are claims that folate malabsorption may occur in women taking the contraceptive pill and patients on anticonvulsant drugs. Two patients have been recorded where there was a specific failure to absorb folate in the absence of other evidence of intestinal malabsorption (Luhby et al, 1961; Lanzkowsky et al, 1969).

FOLATE AND ORAL CONTRACEPTIVES

Shojania et al (1968,1969) reported that women taking oral contraceptives had reduced serum and red cell folate levels. There soon followed a number of case reports of women with megaloblastic anaemia due to folate deficiency where the cause was alleged to be the oral contraceptive (Paton,1969; Streiff, 1969,1970; Necheles & Snyder,1970; Toghill & Smith,1971; Ryser et al,1971 Wood et al,1972). Finally, the mechanism whereby the oral contraceptives produced folate deficiency was postulated as an interference with the enzyme, folate conjugase, which split the glutamic acid chain from folate polyglutamate and hence induced malabsorption of folate (Streiff,1969,1970; Necheles & Snyder,1970; Streiff & Greene,1970). These claims were based on in vivo absorption tests with folate polyglutamate in women on oral contraceptives.

Now to consider each of these factors in turn.

Shojania et al (1969) found that women taking oral contraceptives for more than one year had a mean serum folate of 3.9ng/ml as compared to 5.8 in controls. Those on the pill had a mean red cell folate of 107ng/ml as compared to 186 in controls and a urinary formimino-glutamic acid excretion of 8.6 μmole/hour as compared to 4.3 in controls. Attempts to confirm these observations by Spray (1968), Maniego-Bautista and Bazzano (1969), McLean et al (1969), Castrén and Rossi (1970), Kahn et al (1970), Pritchard et al (1971) and Stephens et al (1972) all failed.

In the clinical case reports of megaloblastic anaemia attributed to oral contraceptives, some of the patients had poor dietary histories, while others had abnormal jejunal biopsies suggesting intestinal malabsorption (Toghill &

274

Smith, 1971). Many cases, however, were not fully investigated and in these coeliac disease remains a possibility. This has emerged as the diagnosis in a significant number of women initially thought to have megaloblastic anaemia due to oral contraceptives (Shojania et al, 1969).

The results of in vitro tests to demonstrate that 'the pill' acts as an inhibitor of the enzyme, folate conjugase, are difficult to interpret.   No satisfactory substrate is available.   The usual substrate is a crude concentrate prepared from yeast.   The source of the enzyme has been an extract of a jejunal biopsy specimen, but animal extracts have been used.   Nor does assay of folic acid released by microbiological assay represent a sensitive method of reading the result.

In vivo tests have usually been carried out after inadequate preparation of the patient.   In particular, other than in the study by Stephens et al (1972), patients have not been saturated with folic acid before the test and this has led to misleading results (Streiff, 1969, 1970; Necheles & Snyder, 1970). When

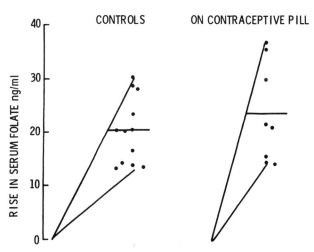

Figure 3. Peak folate blood level after an oral dose of 20μg folate polyglutamate (from yeast) per kg in women on the contraceptive pill and in controls (Stephens et al, 1972)

absorption tests were carried out after proper precautions there was no difference in the manner in which women taking or not taking oral contraceptives absorbed folate polyglutamate (Figure 3).

Finally, we have measured the red cell mean corpuscular volume (MCV) in women on 'the pill' and in controls and obtained essentially identical results in both groups.

In conclusion, it remains unproven whether oral contraceptives have any effect on folate metabolism and if they do, whether such an effect is manifest only on the basis of underlying nutritional deficiency or a malabsorption state.

FOLATE AND ANTICONVULSANT DRUGS

The mechanism whereby anticonvulsant drugs such as diphenylhydantoin interfere with folate metabolism and give rise to a megaloblastic anaemia remains unknown. A number of reports indicate that anticonvulsants interfere with the absorption of pteroylglutamic acid and hence exert their effect by preventing absorption of dietary folate-monoglutamates (Meynell, 1966; Dahlke & Mertens-Roesler, 1967; Hepner et al, 1970; Benn et al, 1971). Others have reported that malabsorption is restricted to polyglutamate forms of folate (Streiff & Rosenberg, 1967; Hoffbrand & Necheles, 1968; Rosenberg et al, 1968). The mechanism suggested was that drugs used as anticonvulsants interfered with the action of folate conjugase in splitting folate polyglutamate. However, careful studies by Baugh and Krumdieck (1969) using synthetic folate polyglutamate as substrate failed to show that phenytoin had any effect in preventing human intestinal, liver or brain conjugase in splitting polyglutamate.

Another mechanism suggested by Benn et al (1971) was that phenytoin interfered with folate absorption by producing an alkaline intestinal pH. Direct measurement of intra-luminal pH, however, failed to show that phenytoin had any effect (Doe et al, 1971) and, in fact, alkalis such as bicarbonate enhance folate absorption (Perry & Chanarin, 1972).

Observations on man have failed to confirm that phenytoin has any effect on intestinal folate absorption (Perry & Chanarin, 1972). It is thus unlikely that the effect of phenytoin is produced at the level of the small gut. Other suggestions are that it induces hepatic enzyme activity and hence enhances catabolism of folic acid (Maxwell et al, 1972), that it functions as an antagonist in a manner similar to methotrexate (Girdwood & Lenman, 1956) and that it may hinder folate transport by interfering with protein binding (Klipstein, 1964) or by other means (Woodbury & Kemp, 1971).

TROPICAL SPRUE

In this disorder there are reports that folate polyglutamate is malabsorbed and that the absorption of monoglutamate is not affected to the same extent. Thus, Hoffbrand et al (1969) found that after 200µg oral folic acid there was a mean rise in serum folate of 11.8ng in controls and 9.4ng in untreated sprue. With oral yeast polyglutamates there was a rise of 12.7ng in controls and only 2.4ng in sprue. Higher serum folate levels were obtained after oral polyglutamate in patients with treated tropical sprue (9.5ng/ml).

Jeejeebhoy et al (1968) reported similar results using larger doses of

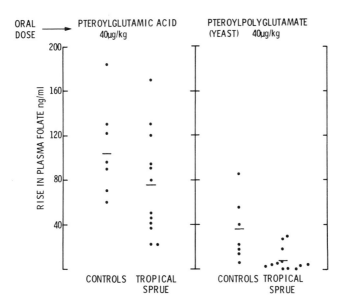

Figure 4. The absorption of pteroylglutamic acid and folate polyglutamate (equivalent to 40μg/kg) in controls and patients with tropical sprue (Jeejeebhoy et al, 1968)

folate (40μg/kg). Pteroylglutamic acid was absorbed in a relatively normal manner, but yeast polyglutamate was absorbed poorly by patients with tropical sprue (Figure 4). Both these studies were carried out after adequate saturation of the patients with folate and suggest that the cause of folate deficiency in tropical sprue is, indeed, failure to utilise folate from the polyglutamate component of the diet. If correct, it emphasises that the polyglutamate component is an important part of dietary folate and that the view put forward recently that only the monoglutamates in a diet are available for absorption is incorrect.

The mechanism whereby folate polyglutamate is malabsorbed in sprue is obscure because folate conjugase activity in jejunal biopsy specimens from patients with sprue is generally normal.

Finally, since, unlike coeliac disease, the ileum is affected with equal severity in tropical sprue, it raises the possibility as to whether polyglutamate is not absorbed at a more distal area of the small gut than monoglutamates.

CO-TRIMOXAZOLE AND MEGALOBLASTIC ANAEMIA

Generally, the combination of trimethoprim with sulphamethoxazole is an extremely safe and effective drug combination.

There are, however, occasional reports of adverse effects on the blood associated with Septrin or Bactrim medication. These range from neutropenias and thrombocytopenias to more severe pancytopenias.

Figure 5 shows the changes in the blood of a young Indian girl who had a severe megaloblastic anaemia due to nutritional vitamin B12 deficiency. She was treated with oral vitamin B12. Urine examination confirmed a urinary tract infection and trimethoprim-sulphamethoxazole was added. The reticulocytes started to rise following the start of oral vitamin B12, reached 10%, and then to our surprise not only did they decline but neutrophil and platelet levels fell rapidly. Initially there appeared to be no obvious reason for failure

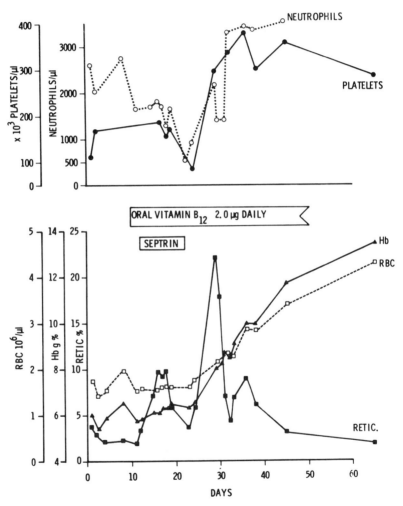

Figure 5. The effect of septrin on the haematological response of a patient with nutritional vitamin B12 deficiency to oral vitamin B12. Note the reversal of the response associated with septrin and recovery following septrin withdrawal

278

of haemopoiesis. There was a second rise in reticulocytes, this time exceeding 20% and recovery of platelets and white cells. The second reticulocyte peak was reached exactly five days after the end of the septrin course and it was evident that septrin was responsible for these changes.

Subsequently we have treated three other patients with megaloblastic anaemia with the appropriate haematinic substance and in each case septrin interfered to a greater or lesser extent with the normal haematological response.

Minor megaloblastic changes due to folate deficiency and sometimes to vitamin B12 deficiency are relatively common. Such patients are unusually susceptible to the toxic effects of trimethoprim sulphamethoxazole medication. It seems likely that the adverse reactions recorded in relation to this drug have arisen on such a basis. Infection, particularly urinary tract infection, is a common accompaniment of megaloblastic anaemia. It is clear that neither Septrin nor Bactrim should be used in such patients.

ALCOHOL AND MEGALOBLASTIC ANAEMIA

Alcohol in adequate amounts acts as a marrow toxin. The commonest manifestation, as seen by the haematologist, is macrocytosis measured on the Coulter counter, usually in the presence of a normal haemoglobin concentration.

The changes in the blood were demonstrated in the experimental study carried out by Eichner and Hillman (1971). There is depression of all marrow elements with a fall in red cells, white cells, platelets and reticulocytes. There is also a fall in the serum folate concentration and a rise in the serum iron level. All these changes recover with alcohol withdrawal.

The marrow in about 60% of patients shows megaloblastic changes, pathological sideroblasts and vacuolation of cells. These changes are also reversed by alcohol withdrawal unless severe folate deficiency has supervened.

Other changes, equally transient, are malabsorption of vitamin B12 (Lindenbaum et al, 1970) and folic acid (Halsted et al, 1967) as well as fat and xylose (Roggin et al, 1969).

REFERENCES

Baugh, C. M. and Krumdieck, C. L. (1969) Lancet, ii, 519
Benn, A., Swan, C. H. J., Cooke, W. T., Blair, J. A., Matty, A. J. and Smith, M. E. (1971) British Medical Journal, 1, 148
Castrén, O. M. and Rossi, R. R. (1970) Journal of Obstetrics and Gynaecology of the British Commonwealth, 77, 548
Dahlke, M. B. and Mertens-Roesler, E. (1967) Blood, 30, 341
Doe, W. F., Hoffbrand, A. V., Reed, P. I. and Scott, I. M. (1971) British Medical Journal, 2, 669
Eichner, E. R. and Hillman, R. S. (1971) American Journal of Medicine, 50, 218
Girdwood, R. H. and Lenman, J. A. R. (1956) British Medical Journal, 1, 146

Halsted, C. H., Griggs, R. C. and Harris, J. W. (1967) Journal of Laboratory and Clinical Medicine, **69**, 116

Hepner, G. W., Aledort, L. M., Gerson, C. D., Cohen, N., Herbert, V. and Janowitz, H. D. (1970) Clinical Research, **18**, 382

Hoffbrand, A. V. and Necheles, T. F. (1968) Lancet, **ii**, 528

Hoffbrand, A. V., Necheles, T. F., Maldonado, N., Hortas, E. and Santini, R. (1969) British Medical Journal, **2**, 543

Jeejeebhoy, K. N., Desai, H. G., Borkar, A. V., Deshpande, V. and Pathare, S. M. (1968) American Journal of Clinical Nutrition, 21, 994

Kahn, S. B., Fein, S., Risberg, S. and Brodsky, I. (1970) American Journal of Obstetrics and Gynecology, **108**, 931

Klipstein, F. A. (1964) Blood, **23**, 68

Lanzkowsky, P., Erlandson, M. E. and Bezan, A. I. (1969) Blood, **34**, 452

Lindenbaum, J., Rybak, B., Gerson, C. D., Rubin, E. and Lieber, C. S. (1970) Clinical Research, **18**, 385

Luhby, A. L., Eagle, E. J., Roth, E. and Cooperman, J. M. (1961) American Journal of Diseases of Children, **102**, 482

McLean, F. W., Heine, M. W., Held, B. and Streiff, R. R. (1969) American Journal of Obstetrics and Gynecology, **104**, 745

Maniego-Bautista, L. P. and Bazzano, G. (1969) Journal of Laboratory and Clinical Medicine, **74**, 988

Maxwell, J. D., Hunter, J., Stewart, D. A., Ardeman, S. and Williams, R. (1972) British Medical Journal, **1**, 297

Meynell, M. J. (1966) Lancet, **i**, 487

Necheles, T. F. and Snyder, L. M. (1970) New England Journal of Medicine, **282**, 858

Paton, A. (1969) Lancet, **i**, 418

Perry, J. and Chanarin, I. (1972) Gut, **13**, 544

Pritchard, J. A., Scott, D. E. and Whalley, P. J. (1971) American Journal of Obstetrics and Gynecology, **109**, 341

Roggin, G .M., Iber, F. L., Kater, R. M. H. and Tabon, F. (1969) Johns Hopkins Medical Journal, **125**, 321

Rosenberg, I. H., Godwin, H. A., Streiff, R .R. and Castle, W. B. (1968) Lancet, **ii**, 530

Ryser, J. E., Farquet, J. J. and Petite, J. (1971) Acta Haematologica, **45**, 319

Shojania, A. M., Hornady, G. and Barnes, P. H. (1968) Lancet, **i**, 1376

Shojania, A. M., Hornady, G. and Barnes, P. H. (1969) Lancet, **i**, 886

Spray, G. H. (1968) Lancet, **ii**, 110

Stephens, M. E. M., Craft, I., Peters, T. J. and Hoffbrand, A. V. (1972) Clinical Science, **42**, 405

Streiff, R. R. (1969) Clinical Research, **17**, 345

Streiff, R. R. (1970) Journal of the American Medical Association, **214**, 105

Streiff, R. R. and Greene, B. (1970) Clinical Research, **18**, 418

Streiff, R. R. and Rosenberg, I. H. (1967) Journal of Clinical Investigation, **46**, 1121

Toghill, P. J. and Smith, P. G. (1971) British Medical Journal, **1**, 608

Wood, J. K., Goldstone, A. H. and Allen, N. C. (1972) Scandinavian Journal of Haematology, **9**, 539

Woodbury, D. M. and Kemp, J. W. (1971) Psychiatria Neurologia Neurochirurgia, **74**, 91

Coagulation and Fibrinolysis in Liver Disease

P T FLUTE

Normal haemostasis depends on the concerted interaction and proper functioning of blood vessels, of platelets, and of the enzyme systems of coagulation and fibrinolysis which control the formation and removal of fibrin. In liver disease any one, and usually more than one, of these mechanisms may be disturbed, and bleeding is a frequent and often troublesome complication (Ratnoff, 1963; Walls & Losowsky, 1971).

Abnormalities of blood vessels and platelets, though frequent in liver disease, seem to be of less clinical importance than abnormalities of fibrin formation and removal. An increase in capillary fragility, indicated by a positive tourniquet test, has been observed in many patients with liver disease (Hedenberg & Korsan-Bengtsen, 1962), but does not correlate with the incidence of serious bleeding. Raised pressure in the portal venous system will contribute to bleeding from anatomical lesions of the vessels, oesophageal varices or collaterals in other sites. Thrombocytopenia is common, but seldom severe (Spector & Corn, 1967), counts below $50,000/\mu l$ being unusual. When the spleen is enlarged due to portal hypertension, sequestration and destruction of platelets within it may be the cause of the thrombocytopenia (Penny et al, 1966). Another cause is increased consumption due to intravascular coagulation, and functional abnormalities of the platelets which may be found have been attributed to the presence of fibrinogen/fibrin degradation products (FDP) in the circulation (Thomas et al, 1967). Thrombocytopenia may also be found in the unusual cases of bone marrow aplasia complicating liver disease (Levy et al, 1965).

Since the liver plays the dominant role in the production of plasma-proteins, it is in the regulation of fibrin formation that the most important defects are found. The liver produces the coagulation factors (Olson et al, 1966), and probably synthesises protein inhibitors of both coagulation and fibrinolysis, and plasminogen, the important precursor of the fibrinolytic enzyme plasmin. In addition, the liver is the site for clearance from the circulation of the active enzymes of both coagulation and fibrinolysis and their products (Spaet et al,1961; Deykin,1966; Wessler et al,1967). Defects of synthesis may be complicated by intravascular coagulation with accelerated consumption of platelets and coagulation factors, and by accelerated fibrinolysis, usually secondary to intravascular coagulation but perhaps sometimes primary. Circulating anticoagulants have also been described and it is possible that in liver disease abnormal fibrinogens may be synthesised to further complicate the coagulation anomalies.

DEFECTIVE SYNTHESIS OF COAGULATION FACTORS

Few patients with significant liver disease will fail to show evidence of decreased synthesis of coagulation factors. Prolongation of the one-stage prothrombin time in liver disease was first described by Quick et al (1935). Many subsequent studies have linked hepatic resection (Almersjö et al,1967), interruption of the arterial supply to the liver (Almersjö et al,1968), and hepato-cellular disease to reduced production of coagulation factors. Although the prothrombin time is insensitive to reductions in prothrombin itself and may therefore fail to reveal the early mild defects (Mindrum & Glueck,1959), it remains the single most important coagulation test in judging the prognosis in patients with hepato-cellular disease (Cook & Sherlock,1965).

A clear distinction must be drawn between defective synthesis of the vitamin K-dependent clotting factors and those which do not require this vitamin. Obstructive jaundice, with lack of bile salts in the intestine, gives defective absorption of the fat-soluble vitamin K and reduced synthesis of Factors VII, IX, X and prothrombin (II), and thus parallels the defect found with other causes of vitamin K deficiency — steatorrhoea, high intestinal fistulae, and haemorrhagic disease of the newborn. A similar type of defect is produced by the oral anticoagulants of the dicoumarol group. In obstructive jaundice the concentration of the other coagulation factors is normal, except that the plasma fibrinogen concentration is often increased. In hepato-cellular disease including cirrhosis and acute hepatic necrosis there is, in contrast, a much broader spectrum of coagulation factor deficiencies (Rapaport et al,1960; Donaldson et al,1969). Low levels of Factor V are found (Ratnoff,1963), in addition to a fall in plasma concentration of the vitamin K-dependent factors. Rapidly falling levels of Factor V and a value less than 50% of normal indicate a particularly poor prognosis in hepatitis (Owren, 1949; Anderson,1967). Decreased levels of Factor XI have been reported in patients with advanced cirrhosis (Rapaport,1961), as have subnormal levels of Factor XII (Jurgens,1962). Although there is no direct evidence that Factor XIII is synthesised by the liver its plasma concentration is often low in chronic hepato-cellular disease and the change is directly proportional to changes in the concentration of serum albumin, often taken as an index of liver protein synthesis (Walls & Losowsky,1969).

In some patients with hepatitis, or with hepatic tumour, Factor V may actually be increased, as may Factor VIII (Zetterqvist & von Francken, 1963; Deutsch, 1965). Factor VIII undergoes marked changes in activity in both physiological and pathological states of 'stress'. There is a rapid rise of Factor VIII activity following exercise or the administration of adrenaline (Prentice et al, 1972), and in states of chronic intravascular coagulation (Penick et al, 1966), although low levels of Factor VIII activity are characteristic of the severe acute forms (Merskey et al, 1967). Traces of thrombin may be responsible for activation of both Factor V and Factor VIII during intravascular coagulation (Rapaport et al, 1963); although other explanations must be considered, this may be the cause of the elevated levels in liver disease.

FIBRINOGEN METABOLISM IN LIVER DISEASE

The plasma concentration of fibrinogen depends on the balance between synthesis and catabolism of the protein, taking into account shifts between the intra-vascular and extra-vascular compartments and primary changes in plasma water. There is very good evidence that the liver is the normal site of fibrinogen synthesis and that it can easily account for the total body content of fibrinogen (Olson et al, 1963; Straub, 1963; Peppers et al, 1964). However, many authors are agreed that an actual fall in the plasma concentration of fibrinogen is found only in the most severe examples of hepato-cellular disease (Ratnoff, 1963; Walls & Losowsky, 1971; Flute, 1971). It appears that the production of fibrinogen can be increased considerably to maintain the plasma concentration even at a time when there is defective synthesis of many other coagulation factors, and despite the evidence that the catabolism of fibrinogen is often increased in liver disease.

The normal catabolism of fibrinogen appears to follow a first-order reaction; destruction occurs randomly at a relatively constant rate without regard to the age of the individual molecule. Alone among the plasma proteins so far investigated, the mass of fibrinogen catabolised each day appears to be a constant fraction of the total amount in the circulation (McFarlane et al, 1964). Any increase in this fractional catabolic rate suggests an unusual method of breakdown, for example intravascular coagulation of fibrinolysis (Regoeczi, 1971). Such increased catabolism of fibrinogen has been demonstrated in cirrhosis of the liver (Tytgat et al, 1971), in acute hepatic necrosis (Rake et al, 1970a), and after transplantation of the liver (Flute et al, 1969). In many of these patients the rate of loss of fibrinogen can be reduced by heparin, which supports the suggestion that the loss is mainly due to intra-vascular coagulation, for which there is a great deal of contributory evidence to be discussed in the next section. In others, particularly patients with cirrhosis, the rate of loss of fibrinogen is sometimes reduced by inhibitors

283

of fibrinolysis (Tytgat et al, 1971).

An increased synthesis of fibrinogen appears to be a characteristic of many types of disease associated with inflammation, infection, or neoplasm (Regoeczi, 1971). This may account for the increased plasma fibrinogen found in obstructive jaundice, with primary or secondary tumours of the liver, or with infections of the biliary tract. Operations on the liver, as with other surgical procedures, also cause a rise in plasma fibrinogen, but this is quantitatively reduced after hepatic resection or de-arterialisation (Almersjö et al, 1968), or after liver transplantation (Flute et al, 1969). Direct measurement shows the increased synthesis after transplantation (Rake et al, 1970b) and in acute hepatic failure (Clark et al, 1973) to match the increased catabolism, unless the hepatic damage is massive.

INTRAVASCULAR COAGULATION

In addition to the increased fibrinogen turnover there is good supporting evidence for intravascular coagulation in acute hepatitis (Rake et al, 1970a; Gallus et al, 1972; Clark et al, 1973). Otherwise unexplained thrombocytopenia and the frequent failure of blood or plasma transfusion to correct the coagulation defects at the expected rate are both best explained by an increased consumption. There are also signs of a secondary increase of fibrinolysis, low plasminogen and raised FDP, similar to those found in other states of intravascular coagulation, and soluble fibrin monomer complexes can often be demonstrated in the plasma by precipitation with protamine (Gurewich & Hutchinson, 1971; Clark et al, 1973). Further supporting evidence of similar changes comes from studies of eleven patients with hepatitis due to Amanita phalloides poisoning (Ménaché et al, 1968), hepatic necrosis induced in Rhesus monkeys by inoculation with yellow-fever virus (Dennis et al, 1969), and in rabbits by galactosamine (Müller-Berghaus & Reuter, 1972).

Intravascular coagulation may also complicate hepatic cirrhosis. Bergstrom et al (1960) observed that the rate of disappearance from the circulation of fibrinogen given parenterally to a patient with hypofibrinogenaemia and cirrhosis was too rapid to be accounted for by haemorrhage or fibrinolysis, and intravascular coagulation was considered the probable explanation. Administration of heparin has been reported to increase the plasma fibrinogen concentration in other patients with cirrhosis, even those with repeated episodes of gastrointestinal bleeding (Zetterqvist & von Francken, 1963; Johansson, 1964; Verstraete et al, 1965). This would be expected if the low fibrinogen in these patients had been due to intravascular coagulation. As already described, these observations were recently fully documented with fibrinogen turnover studies by Tytgat et al (1971). FDP, convincing evidence of increased fibrinolysis secondary to intravascular coagulation, have been a frequent finding in cirrhosis (Das & Cash, 1969; Thomas et al, 1970).

The stimulus to intravascular coagulation could arise from necrotic cells, a constant feature of acute hepatitis and very liable to occur in the centre of regeneration nodules in cirrhosis. It is also possible that infection in the biliary tract, or endotoxins entering from the gut and by-passing the hepatic filter, could act as potent stimuli to intravascular coagulation (Gans et al, 1972). Tissue thromboplastin from necrotic tumour is a further potential stimulus. In addition, the restriction of portal blood flow in cirrhotics (Shaldon et al, 1961) would tend to reduce the reticulo-endothelial cell clearance of activated products of coagulation from the circulation.

The clinical importance of the intravascular coagulation may be two-fold. First, the increased peripheral consumption of platelets and coagulation factors may accentuate any defect in their production, reduce their blood level still further, and thus increase the risk of bleeding. Second, if the mechanisms for the removal of fibrin are inadequate then thrombotic occulsion of the microcirculation may damage many organs. Disseminated intravascular coagulation has been called an intermediary mechanism of disease (McKay, 1965). In acute liver disease, such microthrombosis might be expected to occur within the liver in relation to necrotic cells. The presence of fibrin thrombi within hepatic sinusoids in toxic hepatic necrosis has been well documented by Popper and Franklin (1948). Conceivably, in severe states, thrombosis of the microcirculation of the kidney could contribute to some cases of renal failure. Thrombi in the small vessels of the gastrointestinal tract could result in ischaemic necrosis of the mucosa, and initiate gastrointestinal haemorrhage. However, it must be stressed that these remain hypothetical dangers. It seems that in most cases of cirrhosis, and in many cases of acute hepatic necrosis, compensating mechanisms combine to prevent damage due to actual thrombosis. These protecting mechanisms include the continuing flow of blood, the normal plasma inhibitors of the active enzymes, reticulo-endothelial cell clearance of these enzymes, and accelerated fibrinolysis.

Recently attempts have been made to show the actual sites of fibrin deposition in rats with hepatic necrosis produced experimentally by the administration of carbon tetrachloride (Rake et al, 1973). For this, differential radioactive labelling was used, each rat being injected with ^{131}I-labelled albumin and ^{125}I-labelled fibrinogen; the radioactivity of each organ was analysed at autopsy, using the albumin as a marker for the amount of radioactivity due to blood within the organ and calculating the excess ^{125}I activity not due to blood. Although excess radioactivity, when found, might have been attached to unmodified fibrinogen, to fibrin, or to FDP, these possibilities could not be distinguished. In rats with hepatic necrosis the major accumulation of radioactivity was limited to the liver and spleen, and may have been due to labelled FDP which had been cleared from the general circulation into

the reticulo-endothelial cells of these organs. The other organs were free
from excess radioactivity, and therefore free from significant fibrin deposits,
unless the animal had been pre-treated with tranexamic acid, an inhibitor of
fibrinolysis, in addition to carbon tetrachloride. In these animals, in which
a normal compensating mechanism had been removed, there was excess radioactivity in the kidney and lung in addition to the liver and spleen, and the
animals died before the experiments were complete.

INTRAVASCULAR FIBRINOLYSIS

There is often evidence for an increase in fibrinolysis in liver disease.   It
may, or may not, contribute to the rapid removal of coagulation factors, but
its frequent association with intravascular coagulation should emphasise its
compensatory role and, therefore, the dangers of using fibrinolytic inhibitors
in liver disease.

Decreased lysis time of blood clots has often been reported in liver disease and was first described by Goodpasture (1914). Ratnoff (1949) extended
the early observations to show that rapid plasma clot lysis was often found in
cirrhosis but not in acute hepatitis or obstructive jaundice. Fletcher et al
(1964) suggested that the increased fibrinolytic activity was related to impaired
clearance of plasminogen activator when blood is diverted from the clearing
activity of reticulo-endothelial cells in the liver, and this was confirmed by
Tytgat et al (1968). In other patients circulating plasminogen activator may
be normal, or more commonly reduced, at a time when there is other evidence of local fibrinolysis: an increase in FDP and a decrease in the plasma
concentration of plasminogen. The latter is likely to be due to increased
consumption of this plasmin precursor, but decreased liver synthesis may
contribute to the fall. Astrup et al (1960) found cirrhotic liver to contain an
excess of tissue plasminogen activator.

INHIBITORS OF COAGULATION AND FIBRINOLYSIS

The plasma concentrations of the normal inhibitors of coagulation and also
of fibrinolysis are often reduced in cirrhosis and in hepatitis, though normal
in obstructive jaundice. These reductions could be due to reduced synthesis
by the liver or to excessive consumption by the acceleration of coagulation
and lysis. Thus, reduced levels of anti-thrombin III (Hallen & Nilsson, 1964;
Deutsch, 1965; Von Kaulla & Von Kaulla, 1967) and anti-plasmins (Tytgat et
al, 1968) could perhaps contribute to the increase in coagulation and lysis, or
merely represent one of their effects if the fall is due to increased consumption.

Unusual inhibitors of coagulation may be found in the circulation.   A
frequent finding is a prolonged thrombin clotting time before there is any
reduction of plasma fibrinogen. This could represent the anti-thrombin

effect of elevated FDP concentrations, other unusual inhibitors as yet unidentified, or perhaps synthesis of an abnormal fibrinogen molecule. This has
been suggested by Ratnoff (1954) and demonstrated in hepatic tumour (von
Fetten et al,1969). Very rarely, particularly in association with liver damage due to disseminated lupus erythematosus, specific immunoglobulin
inhibitors to Factor VIII may be found.

THE PRACTICAL ASPECTS

When screening patients with liver disease for possible disorders of coagulation, considerable use should be made of the simple one-stage prothrombin
time. This can be frequently repeated and is an excellent guide for prognosis.
However, even if the prothrombin time is normal, earlier evidence of hepatic
dysfunction may be obtained by demonstrating a low plasma prothrombin by
specific assay. A low Factor IX may also occur before the prothrombin
time is prolonged; this can be detected by a prolonged partial thromboplastin
time. The thrombotest has also been suggested for this purpose. Suggestive,
though non-specific, evidence of intravascular coagulation comes from the
thrombin time. Therefore, a simple triad of tests is the prothrombin time,
partial thromboplastin time, and thrombin time. If any of these is prolonged
it should be repeated on a mixture of normal and patient's plasma in equal
parts, to show whether the prolongation is due to a deficiency or to an unusual
inhibitor. Occasionally, it will be important to know, by specific assay, if
Factor V is decreased in addition to a fall in the Vitamin K-dependent clotting
factors. As with almost every other acquired coagulation disorder liver disease affects multiple coagulation factors, unlike most inherited disorders
which are limited to a single coagulation factor. It should be emphasised
that the degree of coagulation defect bears no direct relationship to the onset
of bleeding. Some patients with severe deficiencies show none of the bleeding
which can be so troublesome in others in whom the defect is far less severe.

The management of the patient depends on the correct identification of
the major mechanisms involved and frequent repetition of the simple screening tests, or even more complicated assays, to monitor the effects of therapy.
Liver biopsy is contra-indicated if the one-stage prothrombin time is abnormal or if there is a severe defect of prothrombin. If the patient is bleeding
or the prothrombin time is prolonged, 10mg of Vitamin K should be given
parenterally daily. Natural K_1 is more effective than the synthetic, water
soluble, derivatives. A better response is to be expected in obstructive
jaundice than with the more extensive coagulation factor deficiencies of
hepato-cellular disease, but Vitamin K should be given even if they are expected since it may achieve partial correction. In hepato-cellular disease
the transfusion of coagulation factors is necessary if the patient is bleeding
or if the prothrombin time is prolonged and the patient is at special risk of

287

bleeding, for example if surgery is contemplated. Fresh-frozen plasma is to be preferred to dried plasma, since it is likely to have a full complement of coagulation factors. In hepatic coma even the transfusion of two litres of fresh-frozen plasma daily, with all the attendant risks of overloading the circulation, usually fails to achieve complete correction of all the abnormalities. For this reason, in specialised units where continuous monitoring is possible, heparin has been combined with transfusion in an attempt to reduce the consumption of coagulation factors. It appears to have improved the ability of the transfusion to return the concentration of coagulation factors towards normal. Measurement of the heparin in the circulation is necessary at least every six hours, since the response is very variable and over-dosage, even for a short period, hazardous. Coagulation factor concentrates are not yet readily available, but their use is being explored. Some of the antifibrinolytic agents, EACA, tranexamic acid, or Trasylol, have been reported to reduce bleeding, but until the significance of possible thrombotic occlusion of the microcirculation has been investigated further they are best avoided altogether in acute liver disease.

ACKNOWLEDGMENT

I wish to acknowledge my debt to Dr Roger Williams, Director of the Liver Unit, King's College Hospital, London, for his assistance and stimulus in many discussions and projects.

REFERENCES

Almersjö, O., Bergmark, S., Engevik, L., Korsan-Bengtsen, K. and Ygge, J. (1967) Scandinavian Journal of Gastroenterology, 2, 204

Almersjö, O., Bengmark, S., Hafström, L. O., Korsan-Bengtsen, K. and Ygge, J. (1968) American Journal of Surgery, 116, 414

Anderson, M. (1967) New Zealand Journal of Medical Laboratory Technology, 21, 155

Astrup, T., Rasmussen, J. and Amery, A. (1960) Nature (London), 185, 619

Bergstrom, K., Blomback, B. and Kleen, G. (1960) Acta medica Scandinavica, 168, 291

Clark, R., Borirakchanyavat, V., Rake, M. O., Shilkin, K. B., Flute, P. T. and Williams, R. (1973) In preparation

Cook, G. C. and Sherlock, S. (1965) Lancet, i, 175

Das, P. C. and Cash, J. D. (1969) British Journal of Haematology, 17, 431

Dennis, L. H., Heinberg, B. E., Crosbie, J., Crozier, D. and Conrad, M. E. (1969) British Journal of Haematology, 17, 455

Deutsch, E. (1965) 'Progress in Liver Disease' Volume 2. (Ed) H. Popper and F. Schaffner. Grune and Stratton, New York. Page 69

Deykin, D. (1966) Journal of Clinical Investigation, 15, 256

Donaldson, G. W. K., Davies, S. H., Darg, A. and Richmond, J. (1969) Journal of Clinical Pathology, 22, 199

Fletcher, A. P., Biederman, O., Moore, D., Alkjaersig, N. and Sherry, S. (1964) Journal of Clinical Investigation, 43, 681

Flute, P. T. (1971) British Medical Journal, 1, 215

Flute, P. T., Rake, M. O., Williams, R., Seaman, M. J. and Calne, R. Y. (1969) British Medical Journal, 3, 20

Gallus, A. S., Lucas, C. R. and Hirsh, J. (1972) British Journal of Haematology, 22, 761

Gans, H., Matsumoto, K. and Mori, K. (1972) Lancet, i, 1181
Goodpasture, E. W.(1914) Bulletin of the Johns Hopkins Hospital, **25**, 330
Gurewich, V. and Hutchinson, E. (1971) Annals of Internal Medicine, **75**, 895
Hallen, A. and Nilsson, I. M. (1964) Thrombosis et Diathesis
  Haemorrhagica, **11**, 51
Hedenberg, L. and Korsan-Bengtsen, K. (1962) Acta medica Scandinavica,
  172, 229
Johansson, S. A.(1964) Acta medica Scandinavica, **175**, 177
Jurgens, J. (1962) Thrombosis et Diathesis Haemorrhagica, **7**, 48
Levy, R. N., Sawitsky, A., Florman, A. L. and Rubin, E. (1965) New
  England Journal of Medicine, **273**, 1118
McFarlane, A. S., Todd, D. and Cromwell, S. (1964) Clinical Science,
  26, 415
McKay, D. G. (1965) 'Disseminated Intravascular Coagulation: an
  Intermediary Mechanism of Disease'. Hoeber-Harper, New York
Ménaché, D., Guillin, M. C., Rueff, G. B., Bismuth, C., Fréjaville, J.P.,
  Sicot, C. and Benhamou, J. P. (1968) Problemes Réanimation, **5**, 499
Merskey, C., Johnson, A. J., Kleiner, G. J. and Wohl, H. (1967) British
  Journal of Haematology, **13**, 528
Mindrum, G. and Glueck, H. I. (1959) Annals of Internal Medicine, **50**, 1370
Müller-Berghaus, G. and Reuter, C. (1972) Thrombosis Research, **1**, 473
Olson, J. P., Miller, L. L. and Troup, S. B. (1963) Blood, **22**, 828
Olson, J. P., Miller, L. L. and Troup, S. B. (1966) Journal of Clinical
  Investigation, **45**, 690
Owren, P. A. (1949) Scandinavian Journal of Clinical and Laboratory
  Investigation, **1**, 131
Penick, G. D., Dejanov, I. I., Roberts, H. R. and Webster, W. P. (1966)
  Thrombosis et Diathesis Haemorrhagica, Suppl.20, 39
Penny, R., Rozenberg, M. C. and Firkin, B. G. (1966) Blood, 27, 1
Peppers, G. F., Goldsworthy, P. D. and Volviler, W. (1964)
  Gastroenterology, 46, 300
Popper, H. and Franklin, M. (1948) Archives of Pathology, **46**, 338
Prentice, C. R .M., Forbes, C. D. and Smith, S . M. (1972) Thrombosis
  Research, **1**, 493
Quick, A. J., Stanley-Brown, M. and Bancroft, F. W. (1935) American
  Journal of Medical Science, **190**, 501
Rake, M. O., Flute, P. T., Pannell, G., Shilkin, K. B. and Williams, R.
  (1973) in preparation
Rake, M. O., Flute, P. T., Pannell, G. and Williams, R. (1970a) Lancet,
  1, 533
Rake, M. O., Williams, R., Freeman, T. and McFarlane, A. S. (1970b)
  Lancet, **11**, 341
Rapaport, S. I. (1961) Proceedings of the Society for Experimental Biology
  and Medicine, **108**, 115
Rapaport, S. I., Ames, S. B., Mikkelsen, S. and Goodman, J. R. (1960)
  New England Journal of Medicine, **263**, 278
Rapaport, S. I., Schiffman, S., Patch, M. J. and Ames, S. B. (1963)
  Blood, **21**, 221
Ratnoff, O. D. (1949) Bulletin of the Johns Hopkins Hospital, **84**, 29
Ratnoff, O. D. (1954) Journal of Clinical Investigation, **33**, 1175
Ratnoff, O. D. (1963) Medical Clinics of North America, **47**, 721
Regoeczi, E. (1971) British Journal of Haematology, 20, 649
Shaldon, S., Chiandussi, L., Caesar, J. and Sherlock, S. (1961) Journal of
  Clinical Investigation, 40, 1346
Spaet, T. H., Horowitz, H. I., Zucker-Franklin, D., Cintron, J. and
  Biezenski, J. J. (1961) Blood, 17, 196
Spector, I. and Corn, M. (1967) Archives of Internal Medicine (Chicago),
  119, 577
Straub, P. W. (1963) Journal of Clinical Investigation, 42, 130
Thomas, D. P., Niewiarowski, S., Myers, A. R., Bloch, K. J. and
  Colman, R. W. (1970) New England Journal of Medicine, **283**, 663
Thomas, D. P., Ream, V. J. and Stuart, R. K. (1967) New England Journal
  of Medicine, **276**, 1344

Tytgat, G., Collen, D., De Vreker, R. and Verstraete, M. (1968) Acta Haematologica, **40**, 265

Tytgat, G. N., Collen, D. and Verstraete, M. (1971) Journal of Clinical Investigation, **50**, 1690

Verstraete, M., Vermylen, C., Vermylen, J. and Vandenbroucke, J. (1965) American Journal of Medicine, **38**, 899

Von Fetten, A., Straub, P. W. and Frick, P. G. (1969) New England Journal of Medicine, **280**, 405

Von Kaulla, E. and Von Kaulla, K. (1967) American Journal of Clinical Pathology, **44**, 678

Walls, W. D. and Losowsky, M. S. (1969) Thrombosis et Diathesis Haemorrhagica, **21**, 134

Walls, W. D. and Losowsky, M. S. (1971) Gastroenterology, **60**, 108

Wessler, S., Yin, E. T., Gaston, L. W. and Nicol, I. (1967) Thrombosis et Diathesis Haemorrhagica, **18**, 12

Zetterqvist, E. and von Francken, I. (1963) Acta medica Scandinavica, **173**, 753

PART V

RESPIRATORY DISEASE
Chairman: Dr J G Scadding

Exercise Induced Asthma

S GODFREY

It has been known for a very long time that patients with asthma often become more wheezy after exertion (Floyer, 1698). This has come to be called exercise induced asthma, but the name is rather unfortunate in the sense that it has been taken by some to imply a specific disease. It must be emphasised that although airways obstruction following exercise may be a prominent symptom, it is not a disease in its own right and only occurs in patients who have other features of bronchial asthma.

Over the years, exercise induced asthma has evoked increasing interest because of the way in which it can be used to provoke a brief, controlled asthma attack. The typical response of an asthmatic to 6 minutes of running is shown in Figure 1. During the early part of exercise, bronchodilation occurs as shown by an improvement in tests of airways obstruction such as the peak expiratory flow rate (PEFR). Towards the end of exercise, or immediately after stopping, bronchoconstriction occurs and the PEFR falls.

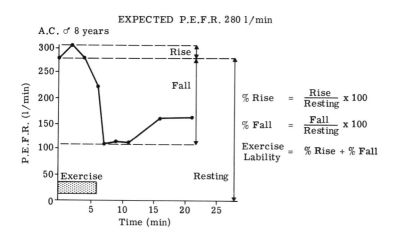

Figure 1. Typical example of exercise induced asthma in children. Peak Expiratory Flow Rate (P.E.F.R.) rises during exercise and falls afterwards. The indices used to calculate the changes are also shown

The severest constriction is reached about 5 to 10 minutes after stopping and then the attack begins to pass off spontaneously. It is convenient to quantitate these phenomena by means of the simple indices also illustrated in Figure 1. It is important to realise that this pattern occurs even if the patient has normal or near normal lung function at the start of the test, and in fact the level of resting lung function has little effect on the percentage fall in PEFR.

The features of exercise induced asthma were described in a series of studies by R S Jones and his colleagues. They found that the pattern was diagnostic of asthma and could be abolished by premedication with isoprenaline (Jones et al, 1962; Jones et al, 1963); they also noted that it persisted into adult life, even though the patient was no longer having clinical attacks (Jones & Jones, 1966). In my own department we have found an abnormal exercise test in 98% of children with clinically diagnosed bronchial asthma, provided that the appropriate type of exercise test is performed, as will be discussed below. The most characteristic feature of the response of the asthmatic is the post-exercise fall in PEFR which occurred in 87% of these children. Total bronchial lability as expressed by the sum of the per cent rise and per cent fall was the only abnormality in a further 11% of children, but it can also be abnormal in children with a past history of infantile wheezy bronchitis (Konig et al, 1972), in the relatives of asthmatic children (Konig & Godfrey, 1973) and in children with cystic fibrosis (Day & Mearns, 1973). For these reasons, studies in asthmatics should concentrate on the post-exercise per cent fall.

Unfortunately, the literature on exercise induced asthma has become confused because different techniques have been used to study the patients. Some investigators have used unquantitated running or stair climbing, others have used progressively increasing bicycle ergometer exercise and yet others have used steady state walking or running on a treadmill (Jones et al, 1962; Davies, 1968; Irnell & Swartling, 1966; Sly et al, 1967; Connolly & Godfrey, 1970). We have carried out a series of investigations in my department into the effects of the type, severity and duration of exercise which have been recently summarised by Anderson et al (1971) and by Silverman and Anderson (1972). We found that for the same severity and duration of exercise, free range running produced more post-exercise constriction than treadmill running, which in turn produced much more than cycling. Swimming and walking hardly produced any effect at all (Figure 2). The severity of post-exercise asthma increased with duration of exercise up to 6 minutes and there was little increase for longer exercise periods; indeed it sometimes decreased after exercise periods of 10 or 12 minutes. The severity also increased with the work done during a 6 minute run up to a level corresponding to about two-thirds of the working capacity of the patient. Above this level the post-exercise fall was not more marked. The results of these

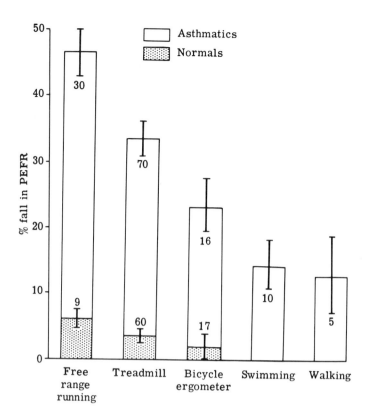

Figure 2. The effects of different types of exercise at similar rates of working on exercise induced asthma. The numbers refer to the number of subjects, and the bars indicate $\pm$ 1 SE

tests have been incorporated in our standard procedure in which the patient is required to run (not walk) on the treadmill for 6 minutes at a heart rate of 170 per minute for children or about 150 per minute for adults.

The effect of different types, duration and severity of exercise described above probably accounts for much of the conflicting literature on this subject, especially since the reproducibility of exercise induced asthma is very poor except for standardised running tests carried out within a week (Silverman & Anderson, 1972). Thus unquantitated stair climbing has been said to produce a diminishing response if repeated throughout the day (McNeill et al, 1966) but we have shown that there is no diminution of effect in carefully controlled tests repeated every 2 hours. Likewise, Katz et al (1971) found exercise induced asthma in only 6 out of 12 asthmatic children studied on a cycle ergometer, and then used the non-constricting asthmatics as their control group.

The effects of different types of exercise have provided a very useful tool for investigating popular theories concerning the patho-physiology of exercise induced asthma. It had often been claimed that exercise induced asthma was due to hyperventilation, low arterial pCO_2 ($PaCO_2$), or lactic acidosis (Herxheimer, 1946; Rebuck & Read, 1968; Seaton et al, 1969). However, it was found that exercise induced asthma was more severe after running compared to cycling, even though the ventilation was higher during cycling, the pCO_2 was lower and the lactate was higher (Silverman et al, 1972). We still have no explanation for the effects of different types of exercise at similar work loads, but the attractive hypothesis that body vibration may be important can no longer be entertained. We studied asthmatic patients during severe whole body vibration and failed to provoke asthma, even though they constricted after running on a treadmill later the same day (Anderson, Godfrey & Andrea, personal observations).

The effect of drugs on exercise induced asthma has proved to be of considerable theoretical and practical value. It has been shown that isoprenaline or other beta adrenergic stimulants block the effect of exercise or reverse the bronchoconstriction if it has already occurred. The theophyllines have a similar effect (Jones et al, 1963). Atropine has a much less predictable response, blocking the asthma in some patients, but not in others (Simonsson et al, 1972) and in fact it is often impossible to distinguish its action from a placebo effect (Silverman, 1972). The two most interesting drugs in relation to exercise induced asthma are disodium cromoglycate and corticosteroids. From the first study by Davies (1968) it has been repeatedly shown that exercise induced asthma provoked by running is prevented by premedication with

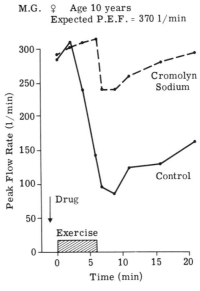

Figure 3. Exercise induced asthma following premedication by a placebo or disodium cromoglycate (cromolyn sodium)

296

cromoglycate in the large majority of asthmatics (Figure 3). My own group has shown that cromoglycate is only effective if given before the exercise and has minimal effect when given after exercise (Silverman & Andrea, 1972). This strongly suggests that it is preventing the release of a chemical transmitter normally liberated by exercise, but that once it is liberated, cromoglycate cannot block its effect. The analogy with antigen provoked asthma is very obvious (Pepys et al, 1968). However, our group has also shown that exercise induced asthma occurs in intrinsic, non-allergic asthmatics and it can also be blocked by cromoglycate in these patients, albeit not quite as well as in extrinsic allergic asthmatics (Silverman & Turner-Warwick, 1972).

In contrast to cromoglycate, corticosteroids and corticotrophin have been shown not to prevent exercise induced asthma (McNeill et al, 1966) and our own studies have confirmed this both for the acute and chronic administration of the drugs (Jaffe, Konig & Godfrey, personal observations). This failure of steroids to block exercise induced asthma has considerable theoretical interest since steroids clearly produce profound clinical benefit in the asthmatic. It is possible that the patients never take enough exercise to provoke severe attacks while on steroids, or else that other factors besides exercise are responsible for the persistence of clinical asthma. In this context it should be noted that steroids do not inhibit immediate (Type I) antigen induced asthma either (Booij-Noord et al, 1972). It is possible that exercise and antigen challenge produce immediate or Type I reactions which are blocked by cromoglycate but not steroids, and these give rise to later Type III reactions

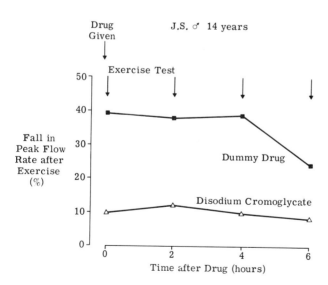

Figure 4. The amount of exercise induced asthma provoked by serial exercise tests following premedication with either a placebo or disodium cromoglycate

in a clinical context, which are blocked by both steroids and cromoglycate. Prevention of the Type I reaction may not be necessary for clinical protection, though we are still evaluating this hypothesis.

Despite the present problem about the clinical significance of exercise induced Type I-like reactions, exercise testing is a very useful method of assessing the duration and extent of protection afforded by drugs like salbutamol or cromoglycate. The exercise test can be repeated every two hours throughout the day without loss of effect and the test drug can be compared with its placebo by giving them as single doses before the first test of each of two days. The immediate protection afforded by the drug and the rate at which this effect diminishes with time can be assessed by following the per cent fall after each test throughout the day (Figure 4). This is a particularly useful method for screening new drugs with bronchodilator, or cromoglycate-like activity.

SUMMARY

Exercise provokes an immediate response in asthmatic subjects resembling Type I asthma. Different types of exercise result in different degrees of constriction, the most potent exercise being running and the least being swimming and walking, even though the work involved is the same. Post-exercise constriction increases with the duration and severity of exercise up to about 6 minutes and two-thirds of the working capacity of the patient. The exercise induced asthma can be blocked by premedication with bronchodilators and cromoglycate but not usually by steroids or atropine. Exercise testing is a very useful method of screening drug action in asthma.

REFERENCES

Anderson, S. D., Connolly, N. and Godfrey, S. (1971) Thorax, 26, 396
Booij-Noord, H., Vries, K. de, Sluiter, H. J. and Orie, N. G. M. (1972)
    Clinical Allergy, 2, 43
Connolly, N. M. and Godfrey, S. (1970) Journal of Asthma Research, 8, 31
Davies, S. E. (1968) British Medical Journal, 3, 593
Day, G. and Mearns, M. B. (1973) Archives of Disease in Childhood
    (in press)
Floyer, Sir J. (1698) 'A Treatise of the Asthma'. R. Wilkins, London
Herxheimer, H. (1946) Lancet, i, 83
Irnell, L. and Swartling, S. (1966) Scandinavian Journal of Respiratory
    Disease, 47, 103
Jones, R. H. T. and Jones, R. S. (1966) British Medical Journal, 2, 976
Jones, R. S., Buston, M. H. and Wharton, M. J. (1962) British Journal of
    Diseases of the Chest, 56, 78
Jones, R. S., Wharton, M. J. and Buston, M. H. (1963) Archives of Disease
    in Childhood, 38, 539
Katz, R. M., Whipp, B. J., Heimlich, E. M. and Wasserman, K. (1971)
    Journal of Allergy, 47, 148
Konig, P. and Godfrey, S. (1973) Archives of Disease in Childhood
    (in press)
Konig, P., Godfrey, S. and Abrahamov, A. (1972) Archives of Disease in
    Childhood, 47, 578

McNeill, R. S., Nairn, J. R., Millar, J. S. and Ingram, C. G. (1966) Quarterly Journal of Medicine, **35**, 55

Pepys, J., Hargreave, F. E., Chan, M. and McCarthy, D. S. (1968) Lancet, **ii**, 429

Rebuck, A. S. and Read, J. (1968) Lancet, **ii**, 429

Seaton, A., Davies, G., Gaziano, D. and Hughes, R. O. (1969) British Medical Journal, **3**, 556

Silverman, M. (1972) MD Thesis, University of Cambridge

Silverman, M., and Anderson, S. D. (1972) Archives of Disease in Childhood, **47**, 882

Silverman, M., Anderson, S. D. and Walker, S. R. (1972) British Medical Journal, **1**, 207

Silverman, M. and Andrea, T. (1972) Archives of Disease in Childhood, **47**, 419

Silverman, M. and Turner-Warwick, M. (1972) Clinical Allergy, **2**, 137

Simonsson, B. G., Skoogh, B. E. and Ekstrom-Jodal, B. (1972) Thorax, **27**, 169

Sly, R. M., Heimlich, E. M., Busser, R. J. and Strick, L. S. (1967) Journal of Allergy, **40**, 93

Extensive Emphysema

PHILIP HUGH-JONES

Emphysema is defined, at least in Britain, in terms of morbid anatomy. The usually accepted definition is one produced at a Ciba Foundation Symposium (1959), namely "a condition of the lung characterized by increase beyond the normal in the size of air spaces distal to the terminal bronchiole, either from dilatation or from destruction of their walls." In the United States the term emphysema is often used in a much wider but less precise sense (Jones et al, 1967) and applied to any patient who complains of chronic breathlessness on exertion — provided he has no specific condition such as tuberculosis, pneumoconiosis, and so on. I shall use it in the strictly morbid anatomical sense, and mainly confine my remarks to **destructive emphysema**, where the walls of the distal air spaces break down, and are not merely dilated.

You will know that pathologists (for example, Leopold & Gough, 1957; Heard, 1959; Reid, 1967) usually classify types of destructive emphysema on the basis of its distribution within the acini of the lung:

1) **Panacinar**, where the air-spaces throughout are enlarged so that all the alveolar structure may disintegrate leaving bullae;

2) **Centri-acinar** (or centrilobular) where the alveoli arising from the respiratory bronchioles in the centre of the lobule are mainly affected, and initially simply dilated;

3) **Peri-acinar** or **paraseptal** with the large air spaces at the edge of the acinus and, where the acinus happens to be against a fibrous interface the bullae are paraseptal;

4) **Irregular** or **scar** type which causes occasional bullae which have no definite distribution within the acinus.

The first two types, peri-acinar and centri-acinar, are the commonest and the most important. It has been suggested that the former is simply an advanced form of the latter (Heard, 1959) but it is now generally accepted that they are two distinct pathological processes; either or both may occur alone or be accompanied by bronchitis.

300

We are now concerned with extensive panacinar emphysema which causes distressing breathlessness on exertion. There is some doubt whether extensive centri-acinar emphysema has nearly as much effect, apart from any bronchitis or bronchiolitis with which it is associated. But the symptom of excessive breathlessness on exertion, which characterises extensive panacinar emphysema, is really just a symptom of **chronic air-flow obstruction** and this symptom also occurs in many cases of chronic bronchitis (with or without any attendant asthma) who do not have significant emphysema at autopsy. Chronic bronchitis, being an inflammation of the airways with increase of their mucus glands and goblet cells (Reid, 1958, 1961) directly causes this air-flow obstruction. Extensive emphysema has no direct effect on the bronchi for it is simply a destruction of the alveoli, but secondarily, as we will discuss, it causes gross functional narrowing of the airways in expiration, and hence the purely expiratory obstruction to air-flow with the resulting symptom of excessive breathlessness on exertion.

It is now well recognised that there is a whole spectrum of chronic non-specific lung disease, manifest with air-flow obstruction and the resultant excessive exertional dyspnoea: on the one hand, pure bronchitis, on the other, pure (or primary) emphysema, but also many cases with chronic bronchitis and different amounts of emphysema (Fletcher et al, 1963). The problem is to assess how much emphysema is present in a given patient. Lung biopsy is impracticable so, because emphysema is defined on the basis of morbid anatomy, we have, in life, to deduce its presence and effects from other diagnostic criteria which we can observe from the living patient.

CLINICAL DIAGNOSIS OF EXTENSIVE EMPHYSEMA

In practice extensive emphysema can be diagnosed with reasonable certainty by a combination of clinical and radiological features, and changes in lung function tests, although all three methods need to be used for success (Simon et al, 1973).

Clinically, there is the non-specific history of progressive exertional dyspnoea. On examination, the chest is held in the inspiratory position and the accessory muscles of breathing are used, mainly to try to further inflate the already inflated chest. There is prolonged expiration — on listening over the larynx with a stethoscope there is the normal inspiration, but a very prolonged time of noisy expiration, often accompanied by lip-pursing. On percussion, the apex beat is difficult to locate and there is diminished superficial cardiac and liver dullness. The heart sounds are very faint (except in the epigastrium) and so are the breath sounds over the lung fields.

Radiologically, (Simon, 1964) there are low flattened diaphragms, a large retrosternal translucent zone seen on the lateral radiograph, and attenuation of the larger intra-pulmonary blood vessels with dilated hilar vessels. Tomography is often a most helpful adjunct in diagnosing the presence of local areas of extensive emphysema. Attenuation of vascular markings needs to be present as well as evidence of overinflation (Simon et al, 1973).

Functionally, in patients with pure (primary) panacinar emphysema and little or no bronchitis, there is a combination of a much reduced forced expired volume ($FEV_{1.0}$) and an FEV_1/FVC often below 45%. The residual volume is increased and so is the total lung capacity, but the former more than the latter because of the very raised resting respiratory level, so that the RV/TLC ratio is raised. There is a reduced transfer of carbon monoxide and a reduced static recoil pressure of the lungs. At rest the arterial oxygen saturation is relatively normal, but the pCO_2 often somewhat reduced (the patients with extensive emphysema and little bronchitis are those often irreverently classified as 'pink puffers' in contrast to the 'blue bloated' patients who have extensive chronic bronchitis, whose resting arterial oxygen saturation is reduced and whose carbon dioxide tension is raised and who, consequently, develop right sided heart failure.

The combination of significant chronic bronchitis with emphysema will naturally modify these function test results.

FUNCTIONAL EFFECTS OF EXTENSIVE EMPHYSEMA

Both ventilation and gas exchange of the lungs are affected. The airways narrow in expiration partly because they are not supported by surrounding intact alveoli, and partly because the reduced static recoil pressure of the lung means that expiratory muscles become active to complete expiration, instead of this phase of breathing being passive from the recoil of the lung stretched during active inspiration, and the transmitted pressure is applied across the walls of the intra-thoracic airways causing their narrowing. Maintenance of the intra-luminal airways pressure, and hence reduction of this narrowing, is one advantage to the patient of lip pursing. Loss of static recoil pressure is the main factor in raising the resting respiratory level of the chest (Comroe et al, 1962).

Although the arterial blood gas tensions are little disturbed at rest (and the patient with severe but pure emphysema is usually symptom free at rest, since his maximum ventilation, although grossly limited, is well above his resting requirements), because of the gross reduction in the effective surface in the lung for gas exchange, the arterial oxygen falls on exercise, in spite of the increased ventilation, and consequently there is severe dyspnoea because of the mechanical limitations for this increased ventilation. This exercise response in extensive pure emphysema contrasts with that of the patient with severe bronchitis and little or no emphysema: he is often desaturated at rest, because of the imbalance between the distribution of gas and blood in the lungs, but actually increases his saturation when his ventilation increases on exercise (Jones, 1966).

AETIOLOGY

Centri-acinar emphysema often occurs in otherwise apparently normal lungs, but it becomes more obvious on histological examination after death if dust pigment is present to outline it (as in the focal emphysema of coal-workers) and may increase with the ball-valve action of bronchiolitis (Leopold & Gough, 1957). Panacinar emphysema is usually confined to the lung apices initially (Ogilvie & Catterall, 1959; Greenberg et al, 1967; Boushy et al, 1968) but it spreads downwards as it progresses. Its distribution may be the key to its pathogenesis from mechanically increased stretch of the lungs at the apices from their suspension within the thorax (West, 1971). But, there was no definite evidence for the aetiology of emphysema until recently, when Eriksson (1964) showed that a particular variety of panacinar emphysema was familial, had a recessive inheritance, was manifest relatively early in life and associated with a dysproteinaemia with a striking deficiency in the amount of $alpha_1$-antitrypsin. Although this deficiency is associated with one particular variety of extensive panacinar emphysema, its occurrence is of such interest that we must consider it in greater detail.

$ALPHA_1$-ANTITRYPSIN DEFICIENCY AND EMPHYSEMA

Since the original paper (Laurell & Eriksson, 1963) clinical, radiographic, and functional studies have confirmed that severe reduction in $alpha_1$-antitrypsin levels, which are manifest in patients homozygous for the gene carrying deficiency, are associated with an onset of breathlessness in the third or fourth decades of life, and extensive emphysema of the lower (Figure 1) rather than the upper parts of the lung (Hutchison et al, 1971; Jones & Thomas, 1971). Since the lower parts of the lungs are normally more perfused with blood than the upper, the suggestion has been made that the factor responsible for the emphysema in $alpha_1$-antitrypsin deficiency is blood borne. Studies with radioactive Xenon-133 in children homozygous for the deficiency, and identified because of their parents having the disease, show that they have diminished blood-flow in the lower parts of their lungs before they develop any symptoms or radiological abnormality (Levine et al, 1970).

How common is $alpha_1$-antitrypsin deficiency as a cause of extensive emphysema, and how severe must the deficiency be to cause the disease? The true frequency of severe deficiency from the homozygous state has not been established in the community but is probably only about 0.06% of the population (Eriksson, 1965) and reports vary depending on the selection of

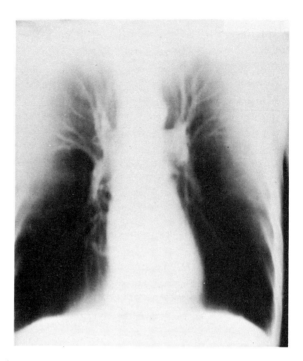

Figure 1. Whole lung tomograph of a patient who is homozygous for α_1-antitrypsin deficiency, showing the bilateral loss of vascular markings at the lung bases accompanied by extensive local emphysema

patients, from between 1% and almost 30% among four different series of patients studied, all of whom had chronic airflow obstruction with severe emphysema (British Medical Journal, 1973). It is probably true that about 15% or 20% of patients with extensive emphysema have it, it can be suspected with confidence in any patient who develops severe breathlessness from the age of 30 or 40 and has extensive emphysema radiologically in the lower parts of the lungs. The heterozygous state, probably about 6-14% of the population (Ostrow & Cherniack, 1972), produces alpha$_1$-antitrypsin levels intermediate between the homozygous deficiency and normal. But various factors, such as infection, alter the antitrypsin levels in the plasma and while the homozygous deficiency state can be identified from the low trypsin inhibitory capacity (TIC) of the blood no precise relationship exists between the TIC levels and the heterozygotes. Moreover, heterozygotes, unlike deficient homozygotes, can increase their TIC levels to normal when stimulated (Kueppers, 1968). Thus identification of heterozygotes is less certain than that of homozygotes and different authors have come to different conclusions about the significance of the partial deficiency of alpha$_1$-antitrypsin, some saying it increases the likelihood of emphysema (Lieberman, 1969; Lieberman et al, 1969; Kueppers et al, 1969; Stevens et al, 1971), others that it does not (Talamo et al, 1968; Welch et al, 1969; Richardson et al, 1969). There now seems little definite evidence that the heterozygous state does predispose to extensive emphysema (Hutchison et al, 1972), there is the possibility that it accelerates the changes in lung elasticity that occur with ageing (Ostrow & Cherniack, 1972), but it may be significant in producing a tendency to chronic bronchitis from other causes, such as cigarette smoking (Falk & Briscoe, 1970; Lieberman, 1972). But the controversy is far from being resolved, and to quote the British Medical Journal (1973) "A solution to this problem may not be found until a sufficient number of obligatory heterozygotes (children of those with unequivocal deficiency) have been studied with a full range of physiological techniques and compared with a group of matched controls."

Another problem is the role of the deficiency in the actual production of emphysema — whether there is a causal relationship or whether it simply acts as a genetic marker. It has been suggested, for example, that a proteolytic enzyme normally inhibited by $alpha_1$-antitrypsin could perfuse the lung in the blood stream, possibly released from disruption of bacteria and leucocytes (Mass et al, 1972). An important practical point is that cigarette smoking seems to hasten the onset of emphysema in patients with the deficiency (Guenter et al, 1968; Hutchison et al, 1971) and some enzyme-deficient non-smokers seem to escape (Guenter et al, 1968; Townley et al, 1970; Jones & Thomas, 1971). If the relationship between the development of extensive emphysema in homozygous $alpha_1$ antitrypsin deficient patients can be established with larger groups of patients (and, incidentally, if the development of chronic bronchitis is related to any partial deficiency) then obviously screening for the deficiency will become of great practical importance. But, much more knowledge is needed before a costly screening procedure could be justified.

TREATMENT OF PATIENTS WITH EXTENSIVE EMPHYSEMA

1. MEDICAL

Because emphysema consists of structural loss of lung substance, there is very little specific medical treatment for the emphysema itself. But, in practice, a great deal can be done for most of the patients who have it by treating what bronchitic or asthmatic element there is and by general measures such as weight reduction and physiotherapy to improve general training and fitness (Figure 2). I would like to stress the need for adequate psychotherapy in managing such patients since stopping cigarette smoking and weight reduction is, in my view, mainly a psychotherapeutic problem, and so is the acceptance of some limitation in exercise capacity.

When all that has been done we are left with a few patients, fortunately

MEDICAL TREATMENT OF PATIENTS WITH CHRONIC AIR-FLOW OBSTRUCTION

1. BRONCHITIC ELEMENT   —   (a) Stop smoking
                              (b) Antibiotics
                              (c) Postural drainage

2. ASTHMATIC ELEMENT   —   Bronchodilator drugs

3. GENERAL MEASURES   —   (a) Weight reduction
                              (b) Breathing and general
                                  exercises
                              (c) Psychotherapy

Figure 2. Medical measures which should be applied to all patients who have extensive emphysema, although they have no bearing on the emphysema itself. Only after general measures, and treatment of any bronchitis or asthma is it reasonable to consider specific treatment of the emphysema itself (see text)

only a few, who remain exceedingly breathless because their disease was either pure extensive emphysema (such as those with $alpha_1$-antitrypsin deficiency) or mostly emphysema. Their help is often exceedingly difficult.

The only other medical measure which can give considerable relief is the use of portable oxygen.

Cotes (1968) working at the MRC Pneumoconiosis Unit has shown that measurement of the resting arterial oxygen tension and its change on exercise is a useful guide to those patients who will benefit from oxygen. And a performance step test is worthwhile, where the subject breathes through a mask without knowing whether he is inhaling normal air or air-enriched with oxygen. Oxygen masks are not easily accepted socially, so that such assessment is important. But, light portable oxygen can be invaluable for some patients and should not be withheld on the argument that it is habit forming!

2. SURGICAL

Only surgery can radically alter the effects of the actual destruction of lung tissue caused by extensive emphysema itself, and there are two possibilities: removal of bullae or lung transplantation.

(1) Removal of bullae

Various surgical procedures have been tried on unfortunate patients who have remained breathless after medical treatment of their extensive emphysema, such as pneumoperitoneum, tracheostomy, etc. But, only the surgical collapse or resection of bullous areas of the lung has stood the test of time and is commonly practised (Knudson & Gaensler, 1965). But, it is not always successful, although we have shown that it can be in carefully selected cases (Hugh-Jones et al, 1966).

It seems, theoretically, that removal of bullae might improve a patient in three ways. Firstly, if healthy lung expands to fill the place left by the bulla, then the elastic recoil pressure of the expanded lung might be greater, there would then be less tendency to expiratory airways collapse and the maximum ventilatory capacity of the lungs might be increased, since greater expiratory gas-flow could be generated (Mead et al, 1967; Pride et al, 1967); secondly, if bullae happen to have significant ventilation (although this is uncommon) they will act as dead-space since blood flow is always sparse in bullous areas; thirdly, if adjacent lung is partly compressed or deflated then it may have a reduced ventilation-perfusion ratio and cause some hypoxia in the arterial blood which would be abolished if this lung were expanded and better ventilated by the removal of adjacent bullous lung. What are the results of such surgery? Firstly, there must be careful selection of patients and operation only recommended to those who are likely to benefit. We believed (Pride et al, 1970) that in general, patients recommended for surgery should be those who (1) after intensive medical treatment are still so breathless that work or everyday activity is irksome or impossible, or (2) in whom consequences of possible pneumothorax would be serious, and (3) when radiology and tests of lung function, including regional tests, show isolated areas of extensive emphysema likely to respond favourably to surgery. We have avoided recommending for operation patients with widespread extensive emphysema without local bullae.

We selected patients with extensive emphysema for surgery who fulfilled these criteria, and of the overall lung function tests paid especial attention to the FEV, the carbon monoxide transfer (Tco), the arterial blood gases at rest and on exercise and the static lung recoil pressure. We find that for regional assessment a combination of lobar sampling at bronchoscopy (Figure 3a & b, measuring lobar tidal volumes and assessing lobar ventilation/blood-flow balance – West, 1960a & b; Hugh-Jones, 1967) combined with radiology (including inspiratory and expiratory films and whole lung tomograms) gives the most useful information about regional function, at present, and that the use of Xenon-133 or other lung scans adds relatively little extra information (Hugh-Jones et al, 1973).

Given such careful selection it is true to say that, in spite of Knudson and Gaensler's (1965) reasonable comment that "it is difficult to believe that a disease characterized by extensive loss of lung parenchyma can be effectively treated by further resection of lung," over two-thirds of patients operated on show definite benefit from removal of bullae, both symptomatically and on function testing, six to nine months after operation and that this improvement is maintained for about three years in most of the patients

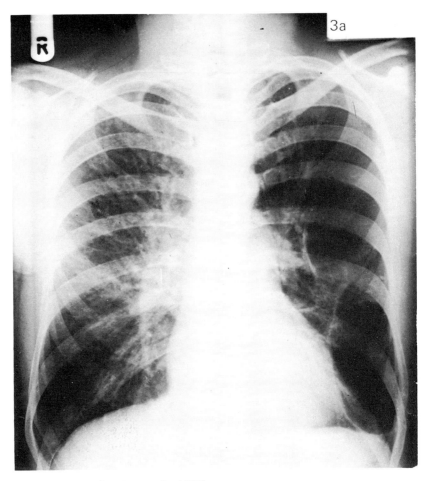

3a

we have studied (Pride et al, 1970).

The most consistent change in function, as the result of surgery, was a rise in resting arterial oxygen saturation of 8 mmHg or more in eight of ten surviving patients out of a consecutive series of eleven studied before and 6-9 months after operation (Figure 4). Three patients showed a rise in FEV_1 of 0.3 litres or more (Figure 5) and there was a fall in arterial CO_2 in five out of seven in whom the pre-operative value was more than 45 mmHg. There were small improvements in ventilation-perfusion balance, but little consistent change in carbon monoxide transfer. Lung elastic recoil pressure at full lung inflation, increased in two patients with the best recoil before operation, but there was no improvement in patients whose elastic recoil pressure was initially low. Nine of the ten patients felt symptomatically

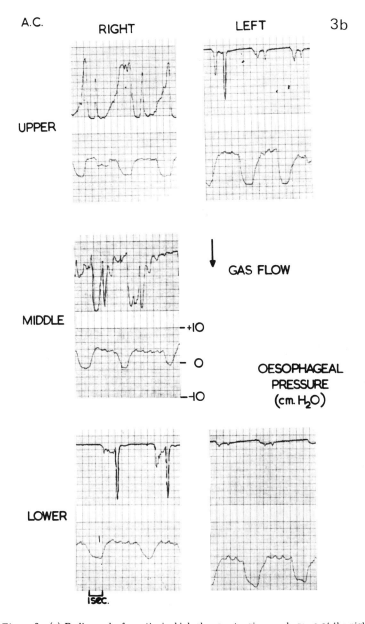

Figure 3. (a) Radiograph of a patient which shows extensive emphysema at the right lower zone, left upper and left lower zones; (b) Bronchoscopic sampling results from this patient, showing mass spectrometer flow tracings with concurrent oesophageal pressure. There is normal gas flow to right upper lobe, some reduction to right middle lobe, very little flow to right lower lobe with trapping in expiration, and negligible gas flow to either lobe of the left lung (for interpretation of such tracings see Hugh-Jones, 1967)

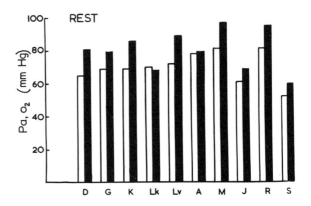

Figure 4. Resting arterial oxygen tensions before (white) and after (black) removal of emphysematous bullae

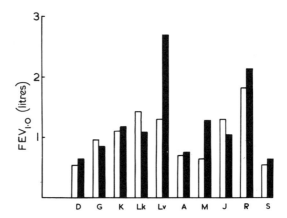

Figure 5. Change in Forced Expired Volume as the result of surgery for emphysema. Before and after, white and black respectively. (**Note**: all patients had had an extensive course of bronchodilator drugs and other medical treatment and their air-flow obstruction was entirely fixed at the time of surgery)

improved and five of them were able to sustain greater exercise loads on a bicycle ergometer. This symptomatic improvement persisted at two to three years after operation in those patients who showed an obvious increase of $FEV_{1.0}$ or resting oxygen tension six months after the operation.

One patient (Lk - Figures 4 & 5) was young and unusual in that regional bronchoscopy showed that he was freely ventilating the bullous areas at his lung apices (Figures 6 & 7). We forecast successful surgery, and indeed he was so pleased with the result of removal of one side (Figure 8) that he came back asking for the other side to be dealt with. But Figure 8 shows development of emphysema at the lung base after removal of the apical bulla

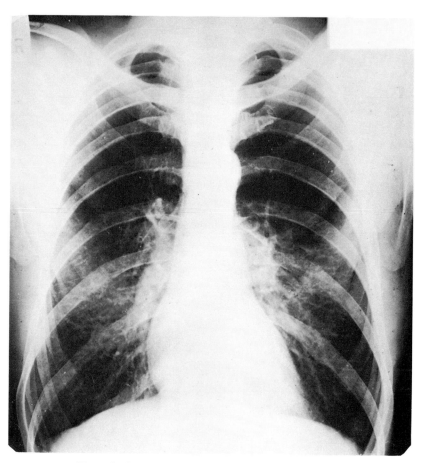

Figure 6. Chest radiograph of patient Lk before operation

LOBAR FUNCTION AT BRONCHOSCOPY
Patient Lk — 28.2.63

		RIGHT	LEFT	
UPPER:	TV(ml)	96	200	
	P max (cmH$_2$O)	7.2	7.0	
	Pattern	B	B	
MIDDLE:	TV(ml)	64		
	P max (cmH$_2$O)	4.5		
	Pattern	Slight B		
LOWER:	TV(ml)	50	80	150
	P max (cmH$_2$O)	7.0	4.0	8.0
	Pattern	-	A + B	

Figure 7. Bronchoscopic sampling results from patient Lk found at the same time
as the radiograph in Figure 6 was taken. It can be seen that a large part of the
tidal volume is going to the right and left upper lobes which are emphysematous.
The 'B' pattern recorded in these lobes, from the mass spectrometer CO_2 and
O_2 tracings shows the lobes to be poorly perfused compared with their ventilation
and hence each is contributory to physiological dead-space

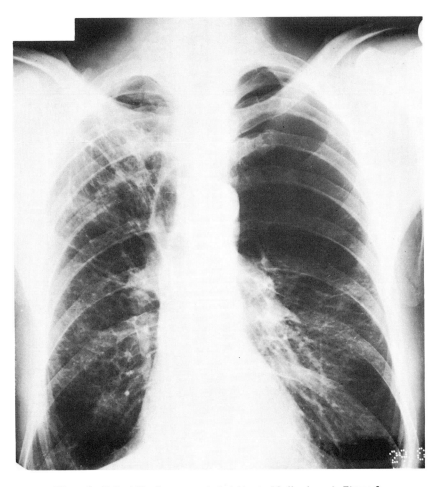

Figure 8. Patient Lk after removal of right apical bulla shown in Figure 6.
Note the apparently satisfactory result on the radiograph except for the
development of emphysema at the right base

and the same sad result happened with the other side so that he became
steadily worse in spite of operation. We view with distrust extensive emphysema with a bilateral upper zone distribution in young men, since in them
the condition seems to spread rapidly down the lungs.

(2) Lung transplantation

Although the longest survival in the world from a clinical lung transplant to
date was about nine months in the patient in Belgium (Derom et al, 1969 &
1971), another transplant for fibrosing alveolitis has been clinically successful, although the patient only survived about two months (Hugh-Jones et al,

1971). It would seem that lung transplantation would be the obvious solution, in the future, for extensive emphysema in young persons such as those with alpha$_1$-antitrypsin deficiency. But it is generally held that if one lung is transplanted in patients with extensive emphysema gross ventilation/perfusion imbalance causes death within days because much of the gas goes to the remaining lung (because of its increased static compliance) while much of the blood flows to the new transplanted lung (because of its lower vascular resistance). Certainly, transplantation of one lung in a young man with extensive emphysema and alpha$_1$-antitrypsin deficiency was fatal (Bates, 1970). However, Professor Veith who has extensive experience in lung transplantation, has recently challenged the accepted view of the cause of blood-gas imbalance after lung transplantation in patients with extensive emphysema, and has maintained that it has often been caused by inadequate immuno-suppression and hence rejection of the transplanted lung, and has possibly demonstrated this view in a recent transplant in a patient with gross chronic air-flow obstruction and extensive emphysema who survived a lung transplant about six weeks (Veith et al, 1972). I, personally, believe from the experience we have had (Hugh-Jones et al, 1971; Cullum et al, 1972) that clinical lung transplantation will succeed and that it can be made to succeed in patients with extensive emphysema. Whether, however, liver transplantation might protect the lungs from damage by reversal of the antitrypsin deficiency, which has been suggested (Sharp, 1971), is an intriguing alternative!

In conclusion, extensive emphysema presents a problem in prevention (possibly by identifying those with genetic abnormalities such as alpha$_1$-antitrypsin deficiency which is the only one known as yet), in assessment (and new techniques with lung scans and flexible bronchoscopes may help enormously), and in medical management and surgical treatment (possibly, in the future, by transplantation).

REFERENCES

Bates, D. V. (1970) New England Journal of Medicine, **282**, 277
Boushy, S. F., Kohen, R., Billig, D. M. and Herman, M. J. (1968) Diseases of the Chest, **54**, 327
British Medical Journal (1973) Leading article, **1**, 1
Ciba Foundation Symposium (1959) Thorax, **14**, 286
Comroe, J. H., Forster, R. E., Dubois, A. B., Briscoe, W. A. and Carlsen, E. (1962) 'The Lung' 2nd Edition. Year Book Medical Publishing Inc., Chicago. Page 165 et seq
Cotes, J. E. (1968) 'Lung Function'. Blackwell, Oxford. Pages 324 & 483
Cullum, P. A., Bewick, M., Shilkin, K., Tee, D. E. H., Ayliffe, P., Hutchison, D. C. S., Laws, J. W., Mason, S. A., Reid, L., Hugh-Jones, P. and Macarthur, A. M. (1972) British Medical Journal, **1**, 71
Derom, F. (1969) Tijdschrift voor Geneeskarde, **25**, 109
Derom, F. (1971) Journal of Thoracic and Cardiovascular Surgery, **61**, 835
Eriksson, S. (1964) Acta medica Scandinavica, **175**, 197
Eriksson, S. (1965) Acta medica Scandinavica, **177**, suppl. 432, 1

Falk, G. A. and Briscoe, W. A. (1970) Annals of Internal Medicine, **72**, 427

Fletcher, C. M., Hugh-Jones, P., McNicol, M. W. and Pride, N. B. (1963) Quarterly Journal of Medicine, **32**, 33

Greenberg, S. D., Boushy, S. F. and Jenkins, D. E. (1967) American Review of Respiratory Diseases, **96**, 918

Guenter, C. A., Welch, M. H., Russell, T. R., Hyde, R. M. and Hammarsten, J. F. (1968) Archives of Internal Medicine, **122**, 254

Heard, B. E. (1959) Thorax, **14**, 58

Hugh-Jones, P., Ritchie, B. C. and Dollery, C. T. (1966) British Medical Journal, **1**, 1133

Hugh-Jones, P. (1967) Bulletin Physio-Path. Respiratoire, **3**, 419

Hugh-Jones, P., Macarthur, A. M., Cullum, P. A., Mason, S. A., Crosbie, W. A., Hutchison, D. C. S., Winterton, M. C., Smith, A. P., Mason, B. and Smith, L. A. (1971) British Medical Journal, **3**, 391

Hugh-Jones, P., Barter, C. E., Laws, J. W. and Crosbie, W. A. (1973) Thorax, **28**, 24

Hutchison, D. C. S., Cook, P. J. L., Barter, C. E., Harris, H. and Hugh-Jones, P. (1971) British Medical Journal, **1**, 689

Hutchison, D. C. S., Barter, C. E., Cook, P. J. L., Laws, J. W., Martelli, N. A. and Hugh-Jones, P. (1972) Quarterly Journal of Medicine, **41**, 301

Jones, M. C. and Thomas, G. O. (1971) Thorax, **26**, 652

Jones, N. L. (1966) Clinical Science, **31**, 39

Jones, N. L., Burrows, B. and Fletcher, C. M. (1967) Thorax, **22**, 327

Knudson, R. J. and Gaensler, E. A. (1965) Annals of Thoracic Surgery, **1**, 332

Kueppers, F. (1968) Humangenetik (Human Genetics), **6**, 207

Kueppers, F., Fallat, R. and Larson, R. K. (1969) Science, **165**, 899

Laurell, C. B. and Eriksson, S. (1963) Scandinavian Journal of Clinical and Laboratory Investigation, **15**, 132

Leopold, J. G. and Gough, J. (1957) Thorax, **12**, 219

Levine, B. W., Talamo, R. G., Shannon, D. C. and Homayoun, K. (1970) Annals of Internal Medicine, **73**, 397

Lieberman, J. (1969) New England Journal of Medicine, **281**, 279

Lieberman, J., Mittman, C. and Schneider, A. S. (1969) Journal of the American Medical Association, **210**, 2055

Lieberman, J. (1972) Chest, **62**, 557

Mass, B., Ikeda, T., Meranze, D. R., Weinbaum, G. and Kimbel, P. (1972) American Review of Respiratory Diseases, **106**, 384

Mead, J., Turner, J. M., Macklem, P. T. and Little, J. B. (1967) Journal of Applied Physiology, **22**, 95

Ogilvie, C. and Catterall, M. (1959) Thorax, **14**, 216

Ostrow, D. N. and Cherniack, R. M. (1972) American Review of Respiratory Diseases, **106**, 377

Pride, N. B., Permutt, S., Riley, R. L. and Bromberger-Barnea, B. (1967) Journal of Applied Physiology, **23**, 646

Pride, N. B., Hugh-Jones, P., O'Brien, E. N. and Smith, L. (1970) Quarterly Journal of Medicine, **39**, 49

Reid, L. (1958) in 'Recent Trends in Chronic Bronchitis'. (Ed) N. C. Oswald. Lloyd-Luke, London

Reid, L. (1961) British Journal of Clinical Practice, **15**, 409

Reid, L. (1967) 'The Pathology of Emphysema'. Lloyd-Luke, London

Richardson, R. H., Guenter, C. A., Welch, M. H., Hyde, R. M. and Hammarsten, J. F. (1969) American Review of Respiratory Diseases, **100**, 619

Sharp, H. L. (1971) Hospital Practice, **6**, 83

Simon, G. (1964) Clinical Radiology, **15**, 293

Simon, G., Pride, N. B., Jones, N. L. and Raimondi, A. C. (1973) Thorax, **28**, 15

Stevens, P. M., Anilica, V. S., Johnson, P. C. and Bell, R. L. (1971) Annals of Internal Medicine, **74**, 672

Talamo, R. C., Allen, J. D., Kahan, M. G. and Austen, K. F. (1968) New England Journal of Medicine, **278**, 345

Townley, R. G. , Ryning, F. , Lynch, H. and Brady, A. F. (1970)
   Journal of the American Medical Association, **214**, 325
Veith, F. J. , Anderson, J. , Koerner, S. K. , Pollara, B. , Attai, L. A. ,
   Steckler, R. , Bardfeld, P. , Nagashima, H. , Boley, S. J. , Siegelman, S. ,
   Bloomberg, A. , Lalezari, P. , Everhard, M. and Gliedman, M. L. (1972)
   Lancet, **i**, 1138
Welch, M. H. , Reinecke, M. F. , Hammarsten, J. F. and Guenter, C. A.
   (1969) Annals of Internal Medicine, **71**, 533
West, J. B. (1960a) Lancet, **ii**, 908
West, J. B. (1960b) Journal of Applied Physiology, **15**, 976
West, J. B. (1971) Lancet, **i**, 839

The Measurement of Closing Volume in Normal Subjects

J M B HUGHES

At some point near the end of a maximal expiration, emptying of the dependent (or lowermost) lung zones ceases while continuing from the upper zones. The lung volume at which this occurs is called the 'closing volume'. It is supposed, though not yet proved, that this change is brought about by closure of some airways. Closing volume (CV) is a relatively easy measurement for investigator and subject. Compared with other tests of uneven pulmonary ventilation it is very sensitive. For example, closing volume changes systematically with age at a greater rate than most other simple respiratory function tests. Because of its sensitivity, the measurement of closing volume may detect respiratory disease in its early, pre-clinical stage. Its simplicity as a test makes it suitable for epidemiological surveys to assess the effects of cigarette smoking or atmospheric pollution on lung function.

THEORY

The rationale behind the measurement of closing volume lies in the non-uniform regional behaviour of lungs which becomes exaggerated at low volumes. Milic-Emili et al (1966), using radioactive gas techniques, showed that up to the first 500ml of gas inspired from the maximum expiratory point (residual volume) in normal subjects seated upright was distributed almost exclusively to the apical regions. Their explanation was that closure of airways at the bottom of the lung had delayed the filling of the lower zones; in terms of overall lung volume they had a higher 'opening volume' than the upper zones. It follows that if a subject starts a vital capacity from maximal expiration with 10 to 300ml of an inert marker gas, there will be a difference in marker gas concentration between apex and base when he reaches full inspiration. Figure 1 shows schematically the concentrations in the upper and lower zones and in the trachea (or mouth) during the subsequent expiration. Provided the two units maintain the same **relative** rates of emptying a uniform concentration in the mixed expired gas will result, but

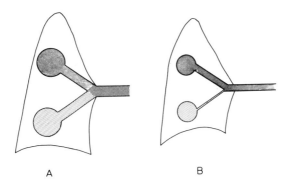

A   B

Figure 1. Schema of marker gas concentrations in upper and lower zones and trachea at
the beginning (A) and end of expiration (B) during the closing volume manoeuvre. Note
that the concentration difference in the common airway changes when emptying of the
lower unit is prevented by closure of its airway (B). (After Mansell et al, 1972)

if the emptying of one ceases (because of closure of its airway, for example)
the concentration in the expirate will abruptly change. Dollfuss et al (1967)
found that not only did the lower lung zones open later than the upper zones
but that they also closed earlier causing a change in expired marker gas
concentration. The marker gas must be introduced at the correct lung volume (residual volume) because it is essential to set up a large concentration
difference between apex and base to obtain a clear signal when their relative
rates of emptying alter.

METHOD

Closing volume can be measured with relatively simple apparatus, as shown
in Figure 2.   During expiration, lung volume is recorded on a spirometer
while an analyser senses the concentration of a marker gas. It is convenient
to plot these signals directly against one another, either on an oscilloscope
or an X-Y plotter.   The subject is instructed to exhale maximally and at
residual volume a bolus of a marker gas is introduced close to the mouth. A
slow inspiration to total lung capacity is made followed by a slow expiration
back to residual volume while lung volume and gas concentration are recorded.
A typical record following a 40ml bolus of argon is shown in Figure 3.   The
first part of the expiration (phase I) contains gas from the anatomic dead
space which is argon-free.   In phase II the remainder of the anatomic dead
space is washed out by alveolar gas, while phases III and IV reflect the
exhalation of alveolar gas only.   Over most of the vital capacity in young
subjects different lung regions maintain approximately the same relative
emptying rates (phase III).   The waves on the trace represent cardiogenic
oscillations — transient variations in lower lobe emptying caused by cardiac

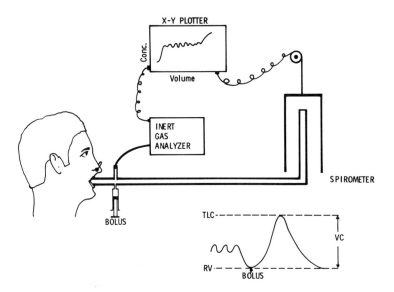

Figure 2. Diagram of apparatus used for measuring closing volume. The subject exhales to residual volume (RV) and pauses while a bolus of a marker gas is given. He inspires his vital capacity (VC) to total lung capacity (TLC) and exhales to RV again while volume and gas concentration are measured

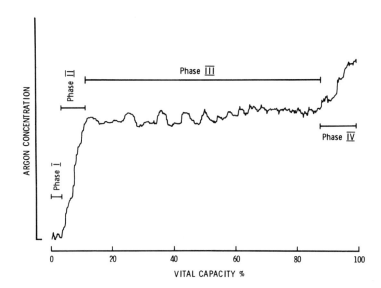

Figure 3. Argon concentration (on an arbitrary scale) plotted against vital capacity per cent in the measurement of Phase IV in a normal man aged 36 years

systole and diastole. Towards the end of expiration, lower zone emptying falls off with a consequent rise in the mixed expired argon concentration at the mouth (phase IV). In phase IV, note that the cardiogenic oscillations have disappeared. Closing volume is the absolute lung volume (often expressed as percent total lung capacity) at which phase IV appears (phase IV volume + residual volume). The volume of phase IV alone is usually measured as a percent of the total capacity; unfortunately 'closing volume' is often used when referring to the volume of phase IV alone.

Many marker gases have been used. Any gas that is safe, poorly soluble in blood, and whose concentration can easily be measured, is suitable. Since expiration is made slowly, the 90% response time of the analyser does not need to be better than 200 m.sec. The original description of phase IV was given by Dollfuss et al (1967) who used 5ml boli of radioactive xenon (about 1 mc activity), and monitored the concentration with a scintillation detector at the mouth. If a mass spectrometer is available a 30-50ml bolus of 100% argon is very suitable (McCarthy et al, 1972). Although the response time of helium analysers is too slow, an ingenious and simple helium detector consisting only of a sensitive pressure transducer was described by Mead and Collier (1959). Greene et al (1972) have shown that it satisfactorily measures phase IV, following the inspiration of 300ml of helium. Phase IV can also be measured with a nitrogen meter following the inspiration of a vital capacity of pure oxygen (Anthonisen et al, 1969/70), although the principle of the method is slightly different. Figure 4 shows diagrammatically the distribution of nitrogen concentration in the lung following the inspiration of a vital capacity of 100% oxygen. Differences in nitrogen concentration at

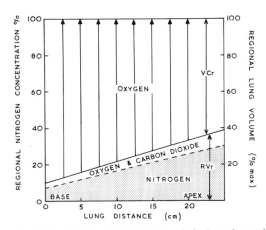

Figure 4. Plot of regional nitrogen concentrations and closing volumes (as per cent regional volume at TLC) against lung distance to illustrate the theory of the single-breath oxygen method for measuring phase IV. Note that there is a four-fold difference of N_2 concentration between apex and base after a maximal inspiration of 100% oxygen

maximal inspiration arise from systematic differences in residual volumes between apex and base (Milic-Emili et al, 1966). The 'bolus method' on the other hand depends on a normal distribution between apex and base of inspiratory 'opening volumes'.

Several comparisons between these methods have been or are being made. As expected, there is good agreement between methods employing the bolus technique — between xenon-133 and helium (Greene et al, 1972) and argon and helium (Freedman & Maberly, 1972). Farebrother et al (1972) and Greene and Travis (1973) have reported that there are differences in normal subjects between closing volume measured with a bolus of argon or helium and a single breath of oxygen. Since the bolus and single breath methods depend on different aspects of lung regional behaviour, these discrepancies are not surprising. Thus it is important that in any survey or study of early disease, normal values for CV should have been obtained by the same technique. For example McCarthy and Craig (1972) recently reported that the CV in normal women (smokers) in Winnipeg was similar to that of normal men (non-smokers) in London. Since the Canadian women were studied with the single breath oxygen test and the men in London with an argon bolus, some of these differences may reflect technique. For the sake of uniformity and to make comparisons between laboratories easier, there is much to be said for using the bolus rather than the single breath oxygen technique. The nitrogen meter can be adapted to measure something closer to a bolus, either by giving 50ml of sulphur hexafluoride (SF6) before the single breath of oxygen (SF6 considerably increases the sensitivity of the meter for nitrogen (Newberg et al, 1972), or by giving 300ml of air before the oxygen (Mansell et al, 1972). A bolus of air should ensure that the nitrogen concentration at the apex is greater than that at the base unless the distribution of residual volumes is extremely abnormal.

In summary, phase IV can be measured with a mass spectrometer (argon), a nitrogen meter, a pressure transducer (helium) or a scintillation detector (radioactive gases). There should be no difficulty in taking the nitrogen meter or pressure transducer on field surveys. A disadvantage of the helium technique is that an assessment of phase III cannot be obtained easily because the changing oxygen and CO_2 concentrations affect the signal. The single-breath oxygen method probably gives different values for phase IV, but these differences will be minimised if a bolus of SF6 or air is given first.

PHASE III

The 'alveolar plateau' as phase III was called will be familiar to all who have used the single-breath oxygen test introduced by Fowler in 1949 to detect uneven ventilation in patients with respiratory symptoms. Fowler recognised phase IV and used it as evidence for the 'first-in last-out' hypothesis of ventilation distribution. In the single-breath test, the slope of phase III, while definitely abnormal in established disease, is often within the normal range in the mild case. The re-emergence of phase IV promises to be of greater value in detecting early disease.

PHASE V

In more elderly subjects a terminal fall in marker gas concentration is often seen (eg Figure 5) giving rise to a fifth phase. Either the mixed expired gas is receiving an additional contribution from the argon-free lower zones (dynamic compression of lower zone airways?) or the most apical part of the lung which empties last has a reduced argon-concentration (inspiration of dead space?). Because phase V disappears when closing volume is measured with a single breath of oxygen (Figure 5) the latter explanation seems more likely. The pattern of inspiration and expiration of the uppermost zones of the lung at low volumes probably changes with age as lung elasticity declines.

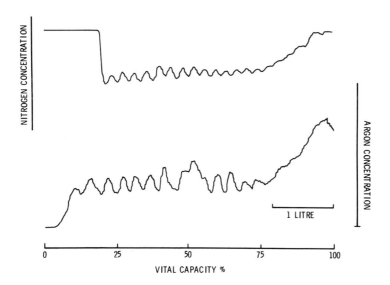

Figure 5. Phase IV measurement in a normal man aged 62 years using argon and (above) a single breath of oxygen. Note the terminal dip (Phase V) in the argon record and the large phase IV compared with the younger subject. The initial portion of the nitrogen record was off-scale

NORMAL VALUES

There are important and systematic changes in closing volume with age. Figure 5 shows a phase IV of 25% VC in a normal man aged 62, compared with 12% in a normal subject aged 36. As a percent of VC phase IV increases from about 8% at age 20 to 20% at age 60. In the erect position the regression line for the increase of phase IV percent VC per year was 0.42 (Leblanc et al, 1970 — xenon-133 marker), 0.36 (McCarthy et al, 1972 — argon) and 0.35 (Collins et al, 1972 — xenon-133). The single breath oxygen method gives a higher regression value of 0.55 (Anthonisen et al, 1969/70). Differences between the seated and the supine posture are small. Bronchodilators have no effect on phase IV (Collins et al, 1972). What are the limits of normality? Leblanc et al (1970) and McCarthy et al (1972) quote 'one standard deviation' of about $\pm 4\%$ of VC at any age for their regression line but Collins et al (1972) believe that this value is an over-optimistic definition of the limits of 'health' and regard $\pm 10\%$ of VC as being more realistic. None of the published reports have studied more than 80 subjects.

REPRODUCIBILITY

In 10 normal subjects, five measurements of phase IV as a volume had a mean coefficient of variation of 11% (Collins et al, 1972). This represents very small variations of phase IV as a percent of VC. There was no significant increase in the variation if measurements were made on two separate days (correlation coefficient 0.88). The measurement of phase IV from the records is liable to observer error. In practice, a straight line of best fit is drawn through phase III and phase IV begins when the expired concentration has left this line 'for good'. Collins et al (1972) found that the correlation coefficient between two observers for phase IV/VC% in 31 subjects was 0.91. Nevertheless in subjects with an abnormal phase III it can be very difficult to distinguish phase IV and there may be differences of over 10% in determination of phase IV/VC% between two observers reading the same record.

EFFECT OF SMOKING

McCarthy et al (1972) found that phase IV/VC% was abnormal in 19 out of 32 smokers who had normal respiratory function tests. When the confidence limits calculated by Collins et al (1972) are applied to their data only 9 out of the 19 are clearly outside the normal range.

EFFECT OF FLOW RATE

Subjects are usually instructed to make a slow initial inspiration from residual volume. Robertson et al (1969) have shown that a rapid inspiration of a bolus of radioactive xenon from residual volume lessens the apex-base concentration differences in normals. In practice the demonstration of phase IV is relatively independent of the inspiratory flow rate provided subjects avoid the fastest flow rates. The effect of flow rate during the expiratory phase is much more important because at high flow rates differences in airways resistance and possibly in pleural pressure distribution change the emptying pattern of the lung. Phase IV increases at high expiratory flow rates and eventually disappears (Jones & Clarke, 1969). Others have found that phase IV is related to the onset of flow limitation (Hyatt & Okeson, 1971) which occurs at higher lung volumes when flow is high. Flow limitation coincides with a sharp rise in transpulmonary pressure which may compress, though not close, lower zone airways and reduce emptying of these regions. Fortunately for those who wish to measure closing volume, phase IV is independent of flow and occurs before the lungs reach flow limitation if expiratory flows are kept at 0.6 litres per second or less (Travis et al, 1972).

RELATION OF CLOSING VOLUME TO RESIDUAL VOLUME

Closing volume defines the lung volume at which the lowermost zones reach their residual volume. In other words CV measures regional residual volume. The RV/TLC ratio increases at a rate of about 0.35% per year (Needham et al, 1954) whereas CV/TLC increases at a rate of 0.54% per year (Leblanc et al, 1970). Thus an index of regional RV (closing volume) appears to be a more sensitive index of the effects of age on the lung than the measurement of overall residual volume. Interestingly the increase of phase IV/VC% per year is the same as the increase of RV/TLC ratio per year. An increase in residual volume is thought to be one of the earliest demonstrable abnormalities of lung function in those who subsequently develop chronic bronchitis with airways obstruction (Bates et al, 1966). If a much simpler measurement such as closing volume was shown to be analogous to residual volume, this would argue strongly for the substitution of CV for residual volume for the detection of pre-clinical disease.

RELATION OF CLOSING VOLUME TO
FUNCTIONAL RESIDUAL CAPACITY (FRC)

From the point of view of gas exchange, this relationship may be very important. If phase IV begins at a volume above the end expiratory level (FRC), the dependent parts of the lung will not be ventilated for part of the breath. Since 'opening volumes' occur at higher lung volumes than closing volumes (Holland et al, 1968) the lowermost parts of the lung may remain closed throughout a tidal breath, opening up only after a deep inspiration. Blood flowing to these regions will not be oxygenated. Leblanc et al (1970) showed that closing volume exceeded FRC at the age of 65 years in the upright position and at age 44 years (because FRC is less) in the supine position. Because FRC varies with posture and CV does not, those with a high closing volume (heavy smokers, for example) may be particularly liable to hypoxaemia while asleep. Several groups have shown that arterial-oxygen tension (PaO_2) falls with increasing age (Mellemgaard, 1966; Sorbini et al, 1968).

The effect of change of posture on PaO_2 is of interest. Normally PaO_2 is greater in the supine than the seated position (Bjurstedt et al, 1962), reflecting a higher cardiac output and better matching of ventilation to perfusion, but in the elderly (Ward et al, 1966) and in young smokers (Streider & Kazemi, 1967) the opposite is the case. These results can be explained by an abnormally high closing volume which exceeds FRC in the supine position. Craig et al (1971) have correlated changes in the alveolar-arterial oxygen-tension difference in different postures with the level of closing volume relative to FRC.

EXPLANATION FOR PHASE IV

The most plausible explanation is that phase IV is associated with closure of airways which starts in the dependent parts of the lung where tissue and airway distending pressures are least (Daly & Bondurant, 1963). Nobody has demonstrated directly airway closure in normal man, but Hughes et al (1970) have observed closure of terminal bronchioles in dog lungs at low volumes. Nunn et al (1965) demonstrated hypoxaemia in man breathing at low lung volumes; lower zone atelectasis occurred when pure oxygen rather than air was breathed. Burger and Macklem's (1968) results also suggest atelectasis when oxygen is breathed at volumes close to residual volume. Gas trapping has been found in man breathing at normal volumes, particularly when closing volume is high (Don et al, 1971). It is hard to see how changes in surfactant or in the properties of the chest wall could account for the increase in closing volume with age. Leith and Mead (1967) concluded that the larger residual volumes in elderly subjects were due to dynamic collapse of airways.

What are the factors determining the patency of intrapulmonary airways? The airway lumen is maintained by a balance of forces — the distending force of lung tissue elasticity being opposed by airway smooth muscle tone and the intrinsic elastic recoil of the airway itself. At low lung volumes the elastic recoil of the dependent parts of the lung is low, probably less than 1cm H_2O and a slight imbalance between lung recoil and bronchomotor tone could in theory lead to airway collapse. With increasing age, the lung recoil pressure for a given volume decreases and the volume at which the dependent airways close increases. These notions receive support from the measurements of Holland et al (1968). They found that the lung distending pressure (measured with the oesophageal balloon) at which phase IV appeared was lower in elderly people than at an equivalent lung **volume** in a younger group, suggesting a loss of elasticity. An increase in closing volume associated with normal lung elasticity suggests intrinsic changes in small bronchi rather than loss of tissue support. Do those who have an abnormal closing volume for their age have a disorder of lung elasticity or of bronchial structure? Closing volume is put forward as the simple test of choice for small airways disease but measurements of lung static recoil are required to distinguish primary airway abnormalities from bronchial closure secondary to loss of tissue support.

CLOSING VOLUME IN CHILDREN

Mansell et al (1972) have recently shown that closing volume is at a minimum in late adolescence and increases with decreasing age. At 16 years of age phase IV/VC% was about 2% increasing to 20% at 7 years of age. There is also a decline in arterialized capillary oxygen tension (Mansell et al, 1972) and lung elastic recoil (Zapletal et al, 1971) in young children. Thus at the beginning and end of man's life-span a reduction in lung elasticity leaves the lower zone airways more liable to collapse and the lungs more prone to respiratory infection.

CONCLUSIONS

1. In normal subjects closing volume is a sensitive, reproducible and easily measured index of uneven ventilation.

2. The range of values in a normal population needs further study.

3. In normal subjects the change of CV with age probably reflects the effects of changes in lung elasticity on the patency of small airways.

4. Closing volume is abnormally high in some cigarette smokers who have a normal FEV_1.

5. In cases where closing volume is abnormal, the simultaneous measurement of lung elastic recoil may help to distinguish the part played by a reduction in tissue elasticity from intrinsic bronchial changes.

REFERENCES

Anthonisen, N. R., Danson, J., Robertson, P. C. and Ross, W. R. D. (1969/70) Respiration Physiology, **8**, 58

Bates, D. V., Gordon, C. A. and Paul, G. I. (1966) Medical Services Journal, Canada, **22**, 5

Bjurstedt, H., Hesser, C. M., Liljestrand, G. and Matell, G. (1962) Acta physiologica Scandinavica, **54**, 65

Burger, E. J. and Macklem, P. T. (1968) Journal of Applied Physiology, **25**, 139

Collins, J. V., Clark, T. J. H., McHardy-Young, S., Cochrane, G. M. and Crawley, J. (1972) British Journal of Diseases of the Chest, **67**, 19

Craig, D. B., Wahba, W. M., Don, H. F., Couture, J. G. and Becklake, M. R. (1971) Journal of Applied Physiology, **31**, 717

Daly, W. J. and Donduraut, 0. (1969) Journal of Applied Physiology, **18**, 513

Dollfuss, R. E., Milic-Emili, J. and Bates, D. V. (1967) Respiration Physiology, **2**, 234

Don, H. F., Craig, D. B., Wahba, W. M. and Couture, J. G. (1971) Anaesthesiology, **35**, 582

Farebrother, M. J. B., Paredes Martinez, R., Soejima, R. and McHardy, G. J. R. (1973) Clinical Science, **44**, 181

Fowler, W. S. (1949) Journal of Applied Physiology, **2**, 283
Freedman, S. and Maberly, D. J. (1972) Lancet, **ii**, 1321
Greene, M., Travis, D. M. and Mead, J. (1972) Journal of Applied Physiology, **33**, 827
Greene, M. and Travis, D. M. (1973) Lancet, **i**, 158
Holland, J., Milic-Emili, J., Macklem, P. T. and Bates, D. V. (1968) Journal of Clinical Investigation, **47**, 81
Hughes, J. M. B., Rosenweig, D. Y. and Kivitz, P. B. (1970) Journal of Applied Physiology, **29**, 340
Hyatt, R. E. and Okeson, G. C. (1971) Physiologist, **14**, 166
Jones, J. G. and Clarke, S. W. (1969) Clinical Science, **37**, 343
Leblanc, P., Ruff, F. and Milic-Emili, J. (1970) Journal of Applied Physiology, **28**, 448
Leith, D. and Mead, J. (1967) Journal of Applied Physiology, **23**, 221
Mansell, A., Bryan, C. and Levison, H. (1972) Journal of Applied Physiology, **33**, 711
McCarthy, D. S. and Craig, D. B. (1972) Lancet, **ii**, 1321
McCarthy, D. S., Spencer, R., Greene, R. and Milic-Emili, J. (1972) American Journal of Medicine, **52**, 747
Mead, J. and Collier, C. (1959) Journal of Applied Physiology, **14**, 669
Mellemgaard, K. (1966) Acta physiologica Scandinavica, **67**, 10
Milic-Emili, J., Henderson, J. A. M., Dolovich, M. B., Trop, D. and Kaneko, K. (1966) Journal of Applied Physiology, **21**, 749
Needham, C. D., Rogan, M. C. and McDonald, I. (1954) Thorax, **9**, 313
Newberg, L., Jones, J. G. and Nadel, J. A. (1972) Lancet, **ii**, 1418
Nunn, J. F., Coleman, A. J., Sachihanandan, R., Bergman, N. A. and Laws, J. W. (1965) British Journal of Anaesthesia, **37**, 3
Robertson, P. C., Anthonisen, N. R. and Ross, D. (1969) Journal of Applied Physiology, **26**, 438
Sorbini, C. A., Grassi, V., Solinas, E. and Muiesan, G. (1968) Respiration, **25**, 3
Streider, D. J. and Kazemi, H. (1967) Annals of Thoracic Surgery, **4**, 523
Travis, D. M., Greene, M. and Don, H. F. (1972) Physiologist, **15**, 288
Ward, R. J., Tolas, A. G., Benveniste, R. J., Hansen, J. M. and Bonica, J. J. (1966) Geriatrics, **21**, 139
Zapletal, A., Misur, M. and Samanek, M. (1971) Bulletin Physio-pathologie respiratoire, **7**, 139

Clinical Aspects of Closing Volume Measurement

T J H CLARK, J V COLLINS

The insight into closing volume measurement provided by Dr Hughes in his review of its physiology may prompt the perspicacious to doubt its clinical value. To demonstrate closing volume demands lungs which allow an orderly sequential filling during inspiration in such a way as to produce an alveolar concentration gradient of a marker gas which empties out of alveoli in reverse order with the movement of gas remaining influenced by the usual gravitational forces acting on the lungs. This delicate physiological edifice is likely to be easily damaged by disease and the measurement of closing volume may not be possible in most patients now seen with respiratory symptoms. To date, these gloomy prognostications have proved partially correct and it has been found to be impossible to make sense of closing volume measurements in patients with much in the way of airways obstruction. This would be expected as airways obstruction is associated with errors of gas mixing which will produce unpredictable and inconstant gradients of marker gas within the alveolar gas phase. Such inefficiency of gas mixing makes it impossible to sample representative alveolar gas and in the closing volume trace produces a sloping alveolar plateau with no clear junction between phases III and IV as seen in normal subjects (Figure 1). In addition to the difficulties obtaining a closing volume in patients with airways obstruction there are two other reasons for questioning the clinical value of this new test. The first is strictly utilitarian and stems from the possibility that closing volume reflects regional residual volume. One might therefore expect closing volume to provide no more information than that given by measurements of residual volume. This now appears to be incorrect and closing volume is found to be more sensitive than residual volume and I will provide some evidence for this later.

The other more general reason for doubting the clinical usefulness of measurements of closing volume rests upon doubts about its origin. If the closing volume is abnormally large it will be difficult to draw conclusions

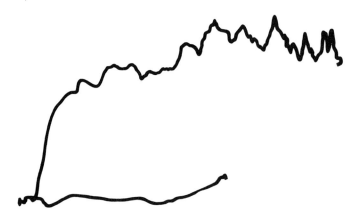

Figure 1. Closing volume result in young man with asthma. 133 Xe bolus technique. Note failure to show terminal rise in 133 Xe concentration close to residual volume. Expiration begins at TLC on left and ends at RV on right. Expired 133 Xe concentration shown on ordinate

about the nature of the increase either in terms of physiological mechanisms or pathology. This limitation is, however, common to all tests of lung function which need to be handled by clinicians in the same way as blood pressure or haemoglobin values and I hope you will resist the temptation to regard closing volume solely as a test of airways of a specific size from certain parts of the lungs.

At this stage it is worth stressing that closing volume abnormalities may be present when conventional tests of airway resistance are normal. This is because small airways normally contribute little to total airways resistance and airway diseases may largely occur in small airways with consequently a normal airways resistance and FEV_1. It is likely that the major site of airways obstruction in chronic obstructive bronchitis is in airways smaller than 2mm (Hogg et al, 1968) and the early stages of this disease can therefore only be revealed by tests of small airways behaviour. This accounts for the increasing interest in closing volume which reflects the performance of this part of the bronchial tree. Work with closing volume has only just passed from the physiologist to the clinician and this I hope will account for some of my caution about its clinical value.

In summary, the closing volume measurement reflects small airway behaviour and is unlikely to be helpful in advanced respiratory disease and where it can be measured validly its interpretation must remain in terms of small airway function rather than specific diagnosis. With these reservations in mind I will now turn to two problems where there is likely to be a significant clinical benefit from measurement of closing volume.

DETECTION OF FLUID OVERLOAD

When fluid accumulates within the pulmonary circulation one of the earlier consequences is extravasation of fluid around the vessels and small airways and this might be expected to alter airway calibre. Patients with hepatic cirrhosis have been shown to have abnormal distribution of ventilation which can be explained in terms of basal airway narrowing secondary to excess

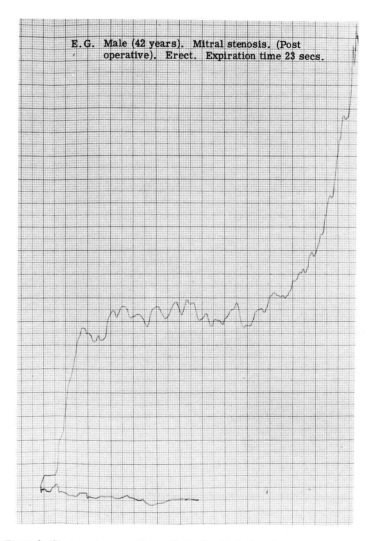

Figure 2. Closing volume result in patient with mitral stenosis. Volume on abscissa and expired 133 Xe concentration on ordinate. Note clear junction between phase III and phase IV as expiration approaches RV. Phase IV/VC% is abnormally large in this patient

lung fluid (Milic-Emili et al, 1971). We have previously shown (Collins et al, 1972) that closing volume is often increased in patients with mitral or aortic valve disease and this would support the idea that closing volume reflects pulmonary fluid overload (Figure 2).

This simple explanation for an increased closing volume in left heart failure may require some modification as the mechanical abnormalities of

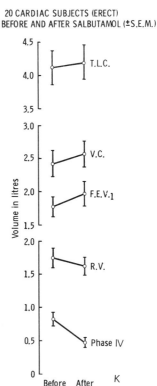

20 CARDIAC SUBJECTS (ERECT)
BEFORE AND AFTER SALBUTAMOL (±S.E.M.)

Figure 3. Changes in lung volumes in patients with chronic heart failure following salbutamol inhalation. The only significant change is in phase IV volume

lungs associated with mitral stenosis are known to be more than can be explained by simply displacing air in alveoli with blood and fluid within the lung (Wood et al, 1971). We have also shown that the closing volume in many of these patients is markedly affected by salbutamol and also by atropine in a somewhat smaller proportion of patients (Figure 3).

This suggests that part of the explanation for the increased closing volume in patients with left heart failure lies in bronchoconstriction and this may subserve the florid clinical extreme of cardiac asthma although this is likely to be too simple a view. It is of more than passing interest to be able to obtain a satisfactory closing volume trace in patients with severe and chronic left heart failure which is to be contrasted with the findings in patients with bronchial asthma and a comparable vital capacity. This implies well preserved gas mixing and a normal distribution of inspired air in patients with left heart failure and this may provide a useful basis for distinguishing cardiac and bronchial asthma, particularly when combined with the divergent effects these two conditions have on static lung volumes.

These studies on patients with left heart failure support the notion that closing volume may prove a valuable method for assessing pulmonary fluid volume and this would have particular clinical benefit in patients undergoing dialysis. To examine this idea we have also looked at the effect of acute intravenous saline load on closing volume in normal subjects. One or two litres of normal saline have been rapidly infused over 20 minutes into healthy subjects sitting upright and this produced no adverse clinical effects. Lung volumes were only slightly reduced but in three out of the four subjects given 2 litres, closing volume was increased and in the fourth subject the closing volume trace became abnormal with the slope of the alveolar plateau increasing as lung volume decreased during expiration. The increase in closing

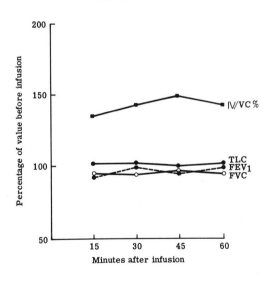

Figure 4. Percentage change in closing volume (expressed as IV/VC%) compared with changes in other lung volumes following rapid intravenous infusion of 1 litre of normal saline

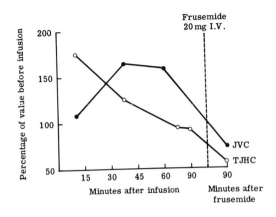

Figure 5. Changes in phase IV /VC% in two subjects rapidly infused with 2 litres normal saline

volume was more in percentage terms than the change in static lung volumes (Figures 4 and 5) and this supports the view that it is a more sensitive test than measurement of residual volume.

Although the exact mode of action of saline infusion is not known these preliminary studies also support the idea that closing volume is especially influenced by the calibre of small airways as it is known that pulmonary oedema mainly involves smaller intrapulmonary airways.

These observations have raised the possibility that closing volume measurements may provide useful clinical information about pulmonary oedema and might be of particular value monitoring response to treatment in patients with left heart failure and in patients with renal failure on haemodialysis.

EARLY DETECTION OF AIRWAY DISEASE

Doubts about the clinical value of closing volume measurement in part stem from the fact that it is critically affected by abnormal gas mixing and un-homogenous gas distribution and will thus be difficult to use in patients with advanced airway disease. This sensitivity to airway abnormalities can be used to clinical advantage if the test is used to detect early disease. This would be especially likely if the disease begins in small airways as this is the probable site of airway closure in the production of closing volume in healthy subjects. Other tests of small airway behaviour have also shown that abnormalities occur in the presence of otherwise normal lung function (McFadden & Linden, 1972; Ingram & O'Cain, 1971) and closing volume needs to be seen as one of a number of means of assessing small airway behaviour.

Of the other tests, frequency dependent compliance is technically very difficult and is too variable and tests of maximum mid-expiratory flow rate appear to be less sensitive than closing volume. Closing volume, therefore, seems to be the most suitable test of small airway function for clinical application.

Use of closing volume to detect early airway disease could be of profound clinical significance (Macklem, 1972). At present patients with airways obstruction are usually seen late in the natural history of their illness. The remorseless and accelerated decline in ventilatory capacity does not usually make its presence felt clinically until the patient has relatively advanced and irreversible airways obstruction and our puny efforts are directed towards wrestling with the final stages of a process that probably began a generation earlier and may have been reversible in the formative years. The opportunity to identify patients at risk in their twenties rather than palliating the ravages of airways obstruction later in life is one that may be within our grasp.

The close relationship between airways obstruction, bronchitis and cigarette smoking is of relevance in this context. Smokers are clearly at risk even at the outset and they demand special attention. It is possible that to demonstrate to a young man of 25 years that his airways are affected and are equivalent to, say, a man twice his years, might provide that necessary persuasion to stop smoking that current health education fails to achieve. All this may be possible if a method could be found which is capable of large scale use and could clearly identify early airway abnormalities.

Closing Volume and Age

It has been established that closing volume expressed either as phase IV %vital capacity or as %TLC increases linearly with age and a number of

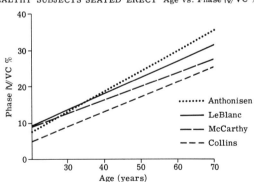

Figure 6. Phase IV/VC% and age in healthy subjects. Results of four studies. For further details see Collins et al (1973)

reports have given broadly similar results (Figure 6). There is some doubt about the confidence limits so far used to define normality and this is of crucial importance for a test which aims to pick out individuals with early airway disease. It seems likely that the existing confidence limits may not be sufficiently close to the mean to enable the test to be as useful as a screening test as first hoped (Collins et al, 1973).

It may also prove valuable to look more closely at the slope of phase III (the alveolar plateau) which bears a close relation to the phase IV volume but as yet the confidence limits for this slope have not been fully explored.

Technical Aspects

For a test to be of real value it must be capable of widespread use and therefore be simple to perform, safe, cheap and easy to use. On all counts closing volume offers great promise. The patient need only be able to make a couple of vital capacity manoeuvres and should only be taxed by the need for the definitive inspiration and expiration to be made slowly and evenly. At present a large body of experience has been gained using radio-Xenon and this is not suitable for large population surveys. This should not provide an intractable problem as other foreign gases can be used and at present great interest is being expressed in helium using a critical orifice helium analyser which looks very promising (Green & Travis, 1972).

The technique is easy to commission and compares favourably with mass X-ray techniques in terms of cost and acceptibility and would serve a similar function but looking for an early functional defect rather than a structural lesion shown up by X-ray.

Smoking

The earlier studies on closing volume in normals include studies made on smokers and this contributed to some of the large scatter of normal values for it is now realised (McCarthy et al, 1972) that smokers commonly have abnormal closing volumes (Figure 7). Studies are being made of the progress of closing volume in those who continue to smoke and in those who are persuaded to stop smoking. Two important facts need to be established: firstly it must be shown that the closing volume changes are reversible in young smokers who stop and the physiological factors responsible for the increased airway closure should be unravelled. McFadden and Linden (1972) have already shown maximum mid-expiratory flow rates may return to normal if the subject stops smoking and similar reversibility of frequency dependent compliance has been shown by Ingram and O'Cain (1971) and it is therefore likely that closing volume measurements will also support the idea that airway obstruction is reversible in its early stages.

The other enigma requiring explanation is the finding that abnormal lung

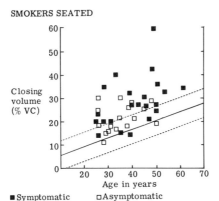

SMOKERS SEATED

Figure 7. Closing volume expressed as phase IV /VC% and age in smokers.
Average regression + 2 SD for 66 non-smokers is also shown. Argon bolus
method. From McCarthy et al (1972). Published by kind permission of the
Editor "American Journal of Medicine"

function in young smokers is much more common than the development of
chronic obstructive bronchitis in older smokers. To this problem can be
added the lack of correlation between closing volume and clinical features
of cough and sputum. One cannot use symptoms of bronchitis as a sign of
small airway involvement and in particular absence of symptoms does not
exclude abnormal closing volume (McCarthy et al, 1972). This draws attention to the need to concentrate more closely upon the relationships between
clinical features, the sites of airway disease and the pathological changes
occurring in different parts of the bronchial tree.

The ability to identify smokers at risk and to look at their natural history
using closing volume measurements is clearly a development of great potential but much work is still required to make the method cheaper and simpler
to use in mass surveys. Further work is also required to define the limits
of normal and the physiological basis of closing volume before its value can
be fully realised.

REFERENCES

Collins, J. V., Clark, T. J. H. and McHardy-Young, S. (1972) Thorax,
    27, 260
Collins, J. V., Clark, T. J. H., McHardy-Young, S., Cochrane, G. M.
    and Crawley, J. (1973) British Journal of Diseases of the Chest, 67, 19
Green, M. and Travis, D. M. (1972) Lancet, 11, 905
Hogg, J. C., Macklem, P. T. and Thurlbeck, W. M. (1968) New England
    Journal of Medicine, 278, 1355
Ingram, R. H. Jr. and O'Cain, C. F. (1971) Entretiens de Physio-
    pathologie Respiratoire, Nancy, 8e series (Ed) R. Peslin.
    Masson & Cie, Paris
Macklem, P. T. (1972) American Journal of Medicine, 52, 721
McCarthy, D. S., Spencer, R., Greene, R. and Milic-Emili, J. (1972)

American Journal of Medicine, **52**, 747
McFadden, E. R. Jr. and Linden, D. A. (1972) American Journal of Medi-
cine, **52**, 725
Milic-Emili, J., Ruff, F., McCarthy, D. S., Stanley, N., Iliff, N. D. and
Hughes, J. M. B. (1971) in 'Central Haemodynamics and Gas Exchange'.
(Ed) C. Giuntini. Minerva Medicine
Wood, T. E., McLeod, P., Anthonisen, N. R. and Macklem, P. T. (1971)
American Review of Respiratory Diseases, **104**, 52

Current Status of Radioisotope Investigations of the Lungs: Basic Techniques

D MELVILLE ACKERY

Radioisotope investigations of lung function require the administration of radioactivity to the patient and subsequent detection of radiation emitted from the body to external, usually scintillation, detectors. Measurements can be made to determine the relative or absolute pulmonary artery blood perfusion, or the ventilatory function of the lungs. The major contribution of radioisotopes is that regional measurements of pulmonary function are possible. Hitherto only the effectiveness of total gaseous exchange could be determined routinely by non-radioactive lung function tests or by blood gas analysis.

The use of radioactive tracer techniques is now firmly established in clinical practice and can provide valuable evidence of lung dysfunction. In particular, they may be of assistance in the diagnosis of pulmonary thrombo-embolism (Poulose et al, 1970), they provide a useful preoperative assessment of those patients selected for lung resection (Fraser et al, 1970) and serial measurements can demonstrate response to therapy (Winebright et al, 1970). The more commonly used radionuclides are shown in Figure 1.

RADIONUCLIDE	PHYSICAL HALF LIFE	USEFUL PHOTON ENERGY (kev)	CHEMICAL FORM	USE
NITROGEN – 13	10 mins	510	N₂	VENTILATION
OXYGEN – 15	2 mins	510	O₂ or CO₂	VENTILATION / PERFUSION
KRYPTON – 81m	13 secs	190	Kr gas	VENTILATION / PERFUSION
XENON – 133	5·3 days	81	Xe gas	VENTILATION / PERFUSION
XENON – 127	36·4 days	−200	Xe gas	VENTILATION / PERFUSION
TECHNETIUM – 99m	6 hours	140	macroaggregated albumin / albumin aerosol	PERFUSION / VENTILATION
INDIUM – 113m	100 mins	393	ferric hydroxide	PERFUSION
IODINE – 131	8 days	364	macroaggregated albumin	PERFUSION

Figure 1. Radionuclides for pulmonary function

RADIOACTIVE GAS STUDIES
OF REGIONAL PERFUSION AND VENTILATION

The measurement of regional lung function with radioactive gases is a simple and safe alternative to previous methods of gas analysis requiring selective catherisation of lobar bronchi. Xenon-133 was first used for this purpose (Knipping et al, 1957) and has remained the most popular radioactive gas for these measurements.

Radioisotopes of elements of the principal respiratory gases — carbon dioxide, oxygen, and nitrogen may also be used, and are made by cyclotron bombardment, but all are short-lived and therefore not available for clinical work except in special centres. Oxygen-15 labelled oxygen (Dyson et al, 1960) and carbon dioxide (West & Dollery, 1960) have been used to measure regional ventilation and blood flow at the Hammersmith Hospital where vicinity to the Medical Research Council cyclotron makes this possible.

Xenon-133 is reactor-produced with a half life of 5.3 days. Its primary energy emission is at 81 KeV, which is too low to be ideal for patient measurements, since many gamma photons are scattered out of the direct path to the detector. It is a poorly soluble gas, but with a partition co-efficient sufficiently high between saline and air to allow intravenous injection of several millicuries for blood flow studies. When xenon in saline is injected it is carried in solution to the lung and because of its low solubility most of the radioactive gas passes into the alveolar space. Diffusion of gas within the lung is minimised if the patient holds his breath during the procedure, and distribution of activity within alveolar gas can be measured. This regional distribution is proportional to the relative blood flow to each part of the lung.

Measurement of regional ventilation can also be determined with xenon-133. For this the patient breathes from a closed circuit spirometer which contains 1 millicurie of xenon-133 per litre of oxygen. The circuit contains carbon dioxide absorbent and a mixing pump. Distribution of activity is measured at breathhold following a single breath to total lung capacity. The patient is then instructed to breath quietly at tidal volume from the circuit and the wash-in of xenon is measured over a period of several minutes, during which poorly ventilated spaces of the lung should largely equilibrate with the spirometer concentration. To complete the procedure, the patient is switched out of the circuit and allowed to breathe room air, and the wash-out rate of xenon from the lung is measured.

Solubility of xenon in blood can cause error in the wash-in and wash-out measurement (Matthews & Dollery, 1965). Increasing activity in the blood gives a count rate from vascular tissues within the thorax and from the chest wall. Consequently, activity levels measured over the chest are higher than those which would be obtained from intra-pulmonary gas alone.

Methods to correct for this are difficult and seldom applied; instead the error is kept small by restricting the rebreathing period.

DETECTION EQUIPMENT

Three methods can be used to detect gaseous activity within the lungs. All must have a fast response to enable measurements to be completed within the period of a breathhold.

Multiple fixed detectors

Scintillation probe detectors are directed at the anterior and posterior aspects of the chest. These may view two areas of each lung (8 counters in total) or three areas (12 counters). The output from the front and back probe is added and fed to a chart recorder, displaying traces of activity for each pulmonary region. This technique, which has been termed 'radiospirometry', has been shown to give very similar results to those obtained by differential spiro-metry (Miörner, 1968) and is in routine clinical use in some centres.

Moving detectors

An alternative to a number of fixed probes is to have just four counters, one pair over each lung (Dollery & Gillam, 1963). These are designed so that the activity in a 'slice' of lung is measured. The probes are attached to a vertical stand and can be moved from base to apex during breathhold. A trace of activity is obtained for each lung proportional to the positional count rate detected by the paired probes as they move up the chest. This vertical profile of activity is then related to the regional perfusion or ventilation.

Scintillation camera

This is a recent advance in the development of radiation detection equipment. It consists of a single large scintillation crystal which remains static in rela-tion to the patient during the measurement period. Between the face of the crystal and the patient is a lead multi-hole collimator which permits radiation to enter the detector only perpendicular to the crystal face. Thus gamma radiation emitted from a region of the chest will only interact with that part of the crystal overlying that particular region.

Thousands of interactions take place in the crystal every second, and the spatial position of each is determined by the electronic circuits attached to the crystal. Thus an interaction taking place in the crystal in a particular position will be given that same co-ordinate on a display oscilloscope or polaroid film. During this period of measurement a two-dimensional image of activity within the chest is accumulated on the display. An image of suffi-cient accuracy can be obtained in about thirty seconds, which permits the scintillation camera to be used for breathhold gas studies of perfusion and ventilation. A quantitative output, which will be discussed later, enables successive images to be stored on magnetic tape for subsequent mathematical analysis.

A scintillation camera is the instrument of choice for radioisotope pulmonary investigations, but it is expensive. It has the great advantage that the physician can be given a two dimensional display of function which can be more easily related to the patient and the chest X-ray than can the traces obtained from probe systems.

Not unexpectedly errors are encountered in scintillation camera measurements. Limitations of present day instruments restrict the spatial resolution of detection to about four centimetres, meaning that regions of diminished activity of less than this size cannot be distinguished from surrounding regions of normal activity. The response of the scintillation camera is less good for activity measured at a distance from its surface, so that a count rate from a part of the lung furthest from the camera may be much less than that for the same activity in a region near to the detector. This difficulty is not encountered when probe systems are used, as detectors are placed both front and back of the chest and their outputs added, which gives a uniform response through the chest.

Currently available commercial scintillation cameras are unable to include the image of activity from the whole of both lungs in the field of view of the crystal. To overcome this draw-back, and to enable the relative function of all regions of both right and left lungs to be compared in one image, a diverging collimator is fitted which effectively increases the useful detection area of the crystal at the expense of some acceptable distortion of the image.

Xenon-133 is commonly used for pulmonary function studies with the scintillation camera although its low energy photon emission limits both sensitivity (number of counts accumulated in unit time) and spatial resolution. Recent investigations carried out by us with xenon-127 suggest that this radionuclide may be better. Xenon-127 has a principal energy of about 200 KeV, which is ideally suited to the scintillation camera, and gives a higher count rate than that of xenon-133, for a comparable patient radiation dose. At present xenon-127 is not commercially supplied, but its promise of improved images for lung function studies with a scintillation camera should create sufficient demand for its availability.

RADIOACTIVE PARTICLES FOR PULMONARY PERFUSION AND VENTILATION STUDIES

An alternative to using radioactive gases for studying regional perfusion or ventilation is to use labelled particles. Particles have the advantage of remaining for some time in the capillary bed, or on the pulmonary mucosal surface, and radiation detectors with a slower time response than the scintillation camera can be used. Measurements are usually made with a rectilinear scanner, although other detectors, already described, can be used.

BLOOD FLOW STUDIES

Flow of blood through the pulmonary microcirculation is demonstrated by the intravenous injection of aggregated particles of a size range 10 to 50 microns (Taplin et al, 1966a). These are injected into an antecubital vein and are randomly mixed in blood in its passage through the right side of the heart. It is assumed that the particles respond to haemodynamic forces in a similar way to blood cells. The particles are ejected into the pulmonary arterial circulation and become lodged in small vessels of the pulmonary capillary bed, the small cross-sections of which prevent further passage. Particles are labelled before injection with a suitable radioisotope, and scanning of the chest after injection demonstrates the functional state of the pulmonary circulation. Regions in which pulmonary arterial blood flow is low or absent will show on the scan as areas of reduced activity.

Most injected particles should become trapped in the pulmonary capillaries at the first passage through the lung if care has been taken at preparation to ensure the correct particle size. This gives a high concentration of activity in the lungs, and effectively 'fixes' in time the perfusion pattern soon after injection. Subsequent scanning displays a two dimensional image of the blood flow at the time of injection, not at the time of the scan.

In spite of the potential risk the procedure has been shown to be safe. Animal experiments have indicated a wide margin of safety for the injection, even when the pulmonary circulation is severely impaired. A very low mortality in humans is reported for the procedure, which has been used widely over a number of years for the investigation of pulmonary vascular disorders. A typical injection contains less than one million particles, which enter a pulmonary circulation of approximately 280 billion capillaries.

Particles of macroaggregated human serum albumin are commonly used for the investigation. Recently commercial supplies of microspheres of human serum albumin have become available, which have the advantage of a more predictable size than laboratory prepared macroaggregates. Technetium-99m is the usual radioactive label. It has the advantage over iodine-131, which was previously used, that higher activities can be given to the patient with increased regional count rates, giving technically superior results.

Alternatively, an inorganic particle can be injected for lung scanning. Ferric hydroxide is the commonest of these, and is labelled with indium-113m. Precipitation of the hydroxide at pH 9 ensures a fairly uniform particle size, and gives technically good scans. Minor reactions have been reported following the intravenous injection of this compound, and for this reason some departments have given up using it in favour of macroaggregated albumin.

Lung scanning following particle injection is a simple procedure, and is now widely used as a clinical investigation. It requires less cooperation on the part of the patient than do gas perfusion studies, which necessitate breathhold procedures, and scanning has the advantage that views from all sides of the chest can be made following a single injection. Lateral perfusion scans are particularly useful in suspected pulmonary embolism, as losses of perfusion can be related more easily in this view to regional segmental anatomy.

Most rectilinear scanners operate only in the horizontal plane, and may be limited when the patient is distressed and cannot lie flat or still for long periods. The scintillation camera is better in this situation.

RADIOACTIVE AEROSOLS FOR VENTILATION STUDIES

A good deal is known about the behaviour of particles which are inhaled into the lungs. Much investigation has been undertaken into the hazards of inhaled dusts, particularly those that are radioactive, and mathematical models have been proposed. It has been shown that distribution of inhaled particles on mucosal surfaces, and their subsequent removal, depends largely on the size of the particles. Particle density and inspiration flow rate are also important factors.

Methods have been described (Taplin et al, 1966b) for determining ventilatory function by the administration of radioactive aerosols into the inspired air. Technetium-99m albumin solution is used, and particles of about 1 to 5 microns are produced by an intermittent positive-pressure nebuliser. These are inhaled over a ten minute tidal breathing period. Particles adhere to mucosal surfaces of the airways and alveoli, and remain in situ sufficiently long for rectilinear scans of four views (anterior, posterior, right and left lateral) to be completed.

Aerosol is accumulated at sites of partial airway obstruction where airflow is excessively turbulent. Activity is not seen distal to obstructed airways, or in those regions where airways remain patent but air has ceased to flow, eg when alveoli are collapsed or filled with fluid.

Aerosols are less commonly used for clinical ventilation measurements than radioactive gases. Distribution of particles in the lungs gives only a qualitative impression of regional ventilation and the underlying physiological principles are better understood for gases than for aerosols.

The aerosol technique does allow a study of regional airflow at those hospitals where a scintillation camera is not available, and the distribution of aerosol in the lateral view may have value when exact anatomical localisation of activity is required. Lateral views are less easy to obtain with gases.

DOSIMETRY

All radioisotope procedures are limited by the radiation dose which can be received by the patient. The radiation dose is the accumulated energy which is deposited per gram of tissue over the period during which the radioisotope resides in the body and remains active.

Generally radioisotopes with a short physical half life are chosen for clinical studies so that activity decays to insignificant levels as soon as possible after the completion of an investigation. In the case of radioactive gas studies, physical half life is less important since the residence time of the gas within the body is short.

For the procedures described, radiation doses vary from a few hundred millirad for gas studies to nearly two rad for perfusion studies with particles (ICRP, 1971). Chest radiography gives about twenty millirad for straight films, and about six rad for pulmonary angiography.

QUANTITATIVE STUDIES WITH A SCINTILLATION CAMERA

The image of activity obtained from a scintillation camera is usually displayed on an oscilloscope or polaroid film. This display of regional perfusion or ventilation may assist in the diagnosis or management of a patient, but is limited in that it is qualitative. The next step is to quantify the functional image using digital electronics, enabling it to be stored and used subsequently for analysis of gas flow in and out of the lung, and for other parameters of pulmonary function.

This is done in the following way (Figure 2). Data from the scintillation camera is fed to an analogue-to-digital converter. The purpose of this is to place a grid, or matrix of lines, over the image. The matrix usually consists of 64 by 64 lines, so that the image is transposed into 4096 points, each of which has a value proportional to the count rate at that point in the image. In terms of the patient each point in the 64 by 64 matrix corresponds to an 'element' of activity through the chest with a 0.5 cm by 0.5 cm cross-section.

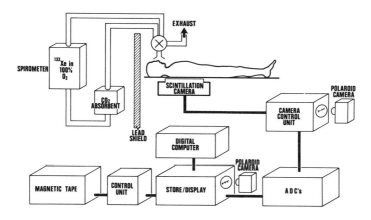

Figure 2. Schematic view of scintillation camera system

A numerical value is obtained for the activity in each element of lung.

The element of lung is chosen intentially to have a cross-sectional area less than the smallest area of the lung which can be resolved by the scintillation camera, for it is necessary that any mathematical treatment of data should carry less spatial error than the original data.

Once the image is in quantitative terms, it is stored as 4096 numbers on either magnetic tape or disc. A number of successive images, or matrices, at selected time intervals may be stored for an investigation.

When the investigation is completed matrices are played back from the tape to give an image on the oscilloscope of the cumulative counts throughout the total procedure. From this are selected regions of interest. The tape is then replayed, this time to give the total activity within each chosen region of interest for each matrix plotted against time. This trace is a histogram display of the dynamic flow of radioactivity through that part of the organ selected by the region of interest. During the radioxenon rebreathing procedure a rising trace is obtained as the lungs attain the specific activity of the spirometer. On switching to air, the ash-out of xenon in time from each region of the lung can be measured.

With a digital computer, semilogarithmic curve fitting to the xenon curves gives rate constants for regional wash-in and wash-out of gas, and diversion of the ventilation matrix by that of perfusion gives a display of regional ventilation - perfusion ratios.

These data handling and computing facilities have recently been made available to our department, and we are at present evaluating the clinical advantages of presenting images of regional lung function in quantitative terms.

ERRORS DUE TO PHYSIOLOGICAL AND OTHER FACTORS

Once quantitative analysis and comparison of radioactive pulmonary function tests become possible, it is necessary that the factors which may give rise to error in the technique are properly understood and minimised.

a) Gravitational effects

In the normal upright lung both blood flow and ventilation per unit volume of lung are relatively increased at the lung bases compared to the apical regions (West, 1967). This gravitational effect is greater for perfusion than ventilation. If studies are done with the patient upright interpretation of the result must allow for this gradient. Both blood flow and ventilation become more uniform in the lung with the patient supine, but some gravitational gradient can still be observed across the chest from anterior to posterior.

b) Lung volume

Quantitative comparisons of pulmonary activity should take account of the volume of the lung at the time of measurement. The lung alters considerably in size from inflation to deflation, and measurements made at fixed positions on the chest wall may not relate to specific lung regions unless they are made at the same volume.

c) Closing volumes

The volume to which inspiration of xenon is taken is important, as, at higher volumes, airways normally closed will open and distribution of activity will be different to that at lower volumes.

d) Rate of inspiration

It has been shown in normal subjects that the inspiratory flow rate will affect distribution of xenon in the lung (Hughes et al, 1972). The different distributions for fast and slow inspirations are thought to reflect the relative importance of airways resistance and lung compliance. Either resistance or compliance may be altered by disease.

e) Radioisotope photon energy differences

Differences in the response of the scintillation camera to gamma photons of different energies may lead to error in the computation of regional ventilation-perfusion relationships, particularly so when attenuation of the radiation is increased by pleural effusion or thickening. If possible radioisotopes should have similar energies for both measurements.

SUMMARY

Radioisotopes are valuable for investigating regional function in the normal and abnormal lung. The procedures are usually simple and safe. Detailed quantitative studies of ventilation and blood flow are probably best done with radioactive gases and a scintillation camera with associated data processing, but techniques using particles and a rectilinear scanner are of great assistance for routine clinical investigation, particularly when pulmonary vascular disorders are suspected.

REFERENCES

Dollery, C. T. and Gillam, P. M. S. (1963) Thorax, 18, 316
Dyson, N. A., Hugh-Jones, P., Newbery, G. R., Sinclair, J. D. and
    West, J. B. (1960) British Medical Journal, 1, 231
Fraser, H. S., Macleod, W. M., Garnett, E. S.and Goddard, B. A. (1970)
    American Review of Respiratory Disease, 101, 349
Hughes, J. M. B., Grant, B. J. B., Greene, R. E., Iliff, L. D. and
    Milic-Emili, J. (1972) Clinical Science, 43, 583
ICRP Publication 17, Protection of the Patient in Radionuclide Investigations
    (1971). Pergamon Press, Oxford
Knipping, H. W., Bolt, W., Valentin, H., Venrath, H. and Endler, P. (1957)
    Münchener medizinische Wochenschrift, 99, 1
Matthews, C. M. E. and Dollery, C. T. (1965) Clinical Science, 28, 573

Miörner, G. (1968) Scandinavian Journal of Respiratory Diseases, Supplementum No. 64

Poulose, K. P., Reba, R. C., Gilday, D. L., Deland, F. H. and Wagner, H. N. (1970) British Medical Journal, **3**, 67

Taplin, G. V., Johnson, D. E., Kennady, J. C., Dore, E. K., Poe, N. D., Swanson, L. A. and Greenberg, A. (1966a) in 'Radioactive Pharmaceuticals', AEC Symposium. (Ed) G. A. Andrews, R. M. Kniseley and H. N. Wagner. US Atomic Energy Commission, Division of Technical Information. Page 525

Taplin, G. V., Poe, N. D. and Greenberg, A. (1966b) Journal of Nuclear Medicine, **7**, 77

West, J. B. and Dollery, C. T. (1960) Journal of Applied Physiology, **15**, 405

West, J. B. (1967) Annual Review of Medicine, **18**, 459

Winebright, J. W., Gerdes, A. J. and Nelp, W. B. (1970) Archives of Internal Medicine, **125**, 241

Current Status of Radioisotope Investigations of the Lungs: Clinical Aspects

G M STERLING

Although radioisotopes have been used for over ten years for examination of pulmonary physiology and pathology, there is still some doubt about their place in clinical investigation. The techniques are relatively easy to apply and by the use of suitable materials it is possible to assess perfusion and ventilation of the lungs both separately and in relation to one another. The difficulties arise in the interpretation and as with other forms of pulmonary testing, radioisotopes frequently give pathologically non-specific results, though they may be useful in the study of regional lung function. It is convenient to consider radioisotope investigation of the lungs under the broad headings of: (a) Perfusion and (b) Ventilation, but there is a degree of overlap and, for instance, some of the problems of perfusion scanning have only been revealed by the more widespread use of simultaneous ventilation scans. The actual techniques used depend on local facilities and the available range has already been described: our own experience involves a conventional rectilinear scanner for perfusion studies and a gamma camera for ventilation studies. For a fuller account of clinical techniques see Blahd (1971) and Gilson and Smoak (1970).

PERFUSION SCANNING

This is the most familiar routine use of radioisotopes in the lung and usually involves intravenous injection of a labelled particulate (eg I^{131} labelled macroaggregated human albumin or Indium) the majority of which is retained in the lung capillary bed and remains there long enough for anterior, posterior and lateral scans to be made. Alternatively an almost insoluble gas such as Xenon can be injected in saline and is evolved into the alveoli during one passage through the pulmonary circulation and can be counted during a period of breath holding using moving or fixed counters or a gamma camera. This technique gives slightly different information since the labelled particulates will be held in any part of the pulmonary circulation which is being perfused, whereas the gas will not be able to leave the circulation unless it comes into contact with aerated alveoli. Anatomically, therefore, it may give a false appearance of avascularity in areas of atelectasis which are in fact perfused but not ventilated. Functionally, though, this information is useful in determining the site and extent of non-gas-exchanging lung, which would not be demonstrated by the conventional particle techniques.

i) PHYSIOLOGICAL STUDIES

One of the early uses of the perfusion scan was in the investigation of the influence of gravity on the distribution of pulmonary blood flow in the upright posture, and it is now established that in normal subjects there is preferential perfusion of the dependent parts of the lungs with a gradient of increasing perfusion from apex to base at lung volumes above Functional Residual Capacity (Dollery & Gillam, 1963; Dollery & Hugh-Jones, 1963). In accordance with the radiographic appearances, this gradient is lost or even reversed in patients with high pulmonary venous pressure due to mitral valve disease (Dawson et al, 1965), and may also be diminished in pulmonary arterial hypertension (Secker-Walker, 1968). Some attempts have been made (Friedman & Braunwald, 1966; Hughes et al, 1969) to use this technique as a simple indirect index of left atrial pressure but the correlation is imperfect and it is more satisfactory to make direct measurements of pulmonary arterial wedge pressure at right heart catheter. However, the technique may be helpful in assessment of post-operative improvement, since it can be repeated more readily than cardiac catheterisation (Krishnamurthy et al, 1972). Although there has been little further clinical application of changes in the normal gravitational distribution of pulmonary perfusion, these findings have been important in demonstrating one of the major physiological factors that may interfere with the interpretation of of perfusion scans.

The second major physiological application of perfusion scanning in conjunction with ventilation studies (see below) has been in the attempted calculation of regional ventilation/perfusion ratios, using dissolved Xenon[133]. After intravenous injection, relative regional perfusion is estimated during a period of breath holding. Regional ventilation is then assessed during washout of the Xenon evolved into the alveoli or after inhalation of Xenon gas and rebreathing to equilibrium, though error may be introduced by the slight but significant solubility of Xenon in plasma and tissue fluids. Using this combined technique relative ventilation/perfusion ratios can be derived for different lung regions (Newhouse et al, 1968), but quantitative results can only be obtained during continuous infusion of Xenon and require a 'steady state' and complex assumptions and calculations (Anthonisen et al, 1966). Moreover, in some diffuse lung diseases, local ventilation/perfusion abnormalities may be occurring in volumes of lung too small to be discriminated by isotope counting, so the technique is not yet of routine clinical use and is bound always to be of limited application.

ii) CLINICAL USES

Pulmonary embolism

The major clinical application of perfusion scanning is in the diagnosis and assessment of pulmonary embolism. Following the initial demonstration of the value of the technique in detecting large experimental and clinical pulmonary emboli (Sabiston & Wagner, 1964; Wagner et al, 1964) many reports of the characteristic wedge-shaped or irregular perfusion defects have appeared (Secker-Walker, 1968 – Figure 1). Some of these clinical descriptions have lacked angiographic or pathological confirmation of the

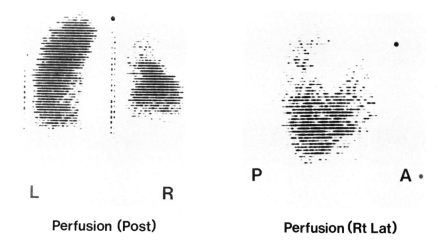

L   R

Perfusion (Post)   **Perfusion (Rt Lat)**

Figure 1. Pulmonary embolism: characteristic large perfusion defect, but in an unusual situation in the right upper lobe

scan findings, but other fuller studies have generally shown a good correlation between the scan and the angiogram. In one series of 27 arteriographically proven pulmonary emboli, 22 were detected in the appropriate sites by scanning while 4 showed less evenly widespread defects than indicated by the angiogram: in only 1 case was the scan reported as normal, and this patient had a block in one of the right basal segmental arteries close to the diaphragm, where the scan interpretation is bound to be difficult (Fred et al, 1966).

Thus scanning gives essentially similar geographical evidence about the site of perfusion defects to angiography, but should be regarded as complementary to rather than a routine substitute for the latter technique, since the scan gives less precise anatomical information about the mechanism of any defects found. For example, perfusion defects due to arterial compression resulting from primary lung disease can be distinguished from pulmonary emboli by angiography, but not by scanning which will show simply a region of relative avascularity. It should therefore be emphasised that the scan is of little diagnostic value in the presence of a local radiographic abnormality, since almost any disease process, such as pneumonia or pulmonary fibrosis, which shows up radiographically is likely to cause a local reduction in perfusion.

The particular advantages and uses of scanning in pulmonary embolism are:

1. Ease of performance: all that is required is a single intravenous injection as opposed to cardiac catheterisation.

2. For screening purposes: perfusion defects may be located prior to selective angiography, which especially with primary magnification techniques allows more accurate detection of emboli in small arteries.

3. Safety: there is some doubt about the danger, if any, of pulmonary angiography in seriously ill patients with pulmonary hypertension, but some serious arrhythmias and even deaths have been described in association with the procedure (Fred et al, 1966) whereas scanning seems almost completely safe. Moreover, the particles injected for scanning do not appear to affect any of a wide variety of pulmonary tests including those of mechanics, distribution of ventilation and gas exchange (Gold & McCormack, 1966).

4. Repeatability: within the limits of radiation dosage it is easy to repeat perfusion scans and follow the progress and resolution of perfusion defects due to pulmonary emboli. In this way it has been shown that many such defects improve over a few days or weeks and may disappear entirely (Wagner et al, 1964; Tow & Wagner, 1967) and the method has also proved useful in assessment of the effectiveness of thrombolytic therapy in experimental pulmonary embolism (Wagner et al, 1964). An unchanging scan following an acute episode makes pulmonary embolism an unlikely cause, and the appearance of new defects in a patient already on anticoagulants suggests failure of the treatment and the need for more radical measures such as vena caval ligation.

The main disadvantage of lung perfusion scanning in the diagnosis of pulmonary embolism is that the results are non-specific in terms of pathology. Local perfusion defects may occur not only with radiologically apparent lung lesions but are also common in patients with airway obstruction due to asthma, bronchitis or emphysema without any local abnormality on X-ray. These patients can usually be differentiated by means of pulmonary function tests especially if they have generalised disease, but they may show only slight disturbance of function in, for instance, localised bullous emphysema. Attempts to improve the accuracy of differential diagnosis of localised perfusion defects have led to the more widespread use of radioactive gases, usually Xenon[133], to investigate regional ventilation in relation to perfusion.

VENTILATION 'SCANNING'

Several techniques have been developed for counting the emission from inhaled isotopes in order to study regional ventilation or droplet deposition. Because of the limited duration of breath holding and rapid changes in count rate as gas is 'washed in' or 'washed out', it is impossible to use a rectilinear scanner for counting, and the most detailed information is obtained from a gamma camera image, though banks of separate static counters or pairs of moving counters are more widely available and generally give an adequate picture of the distribution of inhaled radioactive particles. It is, therefore, strictly inaccurate to speak of ventilation 'scanning' though the term is frequently used for convenience as a synonym for 'counting' or 'imaging' and will be used in this way at times in the present account.

The two main methods employed for the study of distribution of ventilation are the inhalation of radioactive aerosol particles and the inhalation of a labelled gas, usually an isotope of Xenon. Early studies involved the use of isotopes of oxygen and gave particularly useful physiological results, but the short half-life of O_2 makes it impracticable for routine use unless the department of nuclear medicine happens to be adjacent to a cyclotron (Dollery et al, 1962).

a) Radio-aerosols

Inhalation of radioactive-labelled aerosol droplets has been used to study distribution of inhaled particles, their pattern of deposition and their rate of removal from the lung. The technique also gives information about the distribution of inhaled gas, though for the latter purpose radioactive gases themselves are more satisfactory. The aerosol method has been quite widely used in America and has been claimed to help differentiate chronic bronchitis from emphysema in patients with chronic airway obstruction but this has not yet been confirmed and aerosols are not generally in routine use for investigation of lung disorders in this country.

b) Inhaled gases: physiological studies

These have shown that at normal lung volumes there is a slight gradient of increasing ventilation from the apex down the lung, but that the difference between ventilation of apices and bases is much less than the difference in

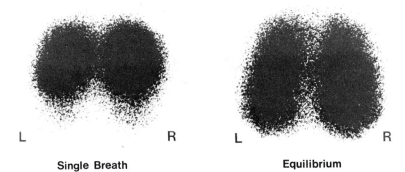

Single Breath   Equilibrium

Figure 2. Distribution of inspired gas in normal erect subject: a small bolus of Xenon[133] was inhaled at Residual Volume followed by slow inspiration to Total Lung Capacity, at which volume counts were made during breath-holding. Gas is mainly in the upper zones compared with more even distribution after rebreathing to equilibrium

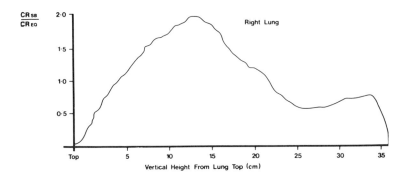

Figure 3. Distribution of inspired gas (data taken from Figure 2): Ratio of counts after a single breath (from Residual Volume) to counts after equilibrium, down a sagittal slice of the lung. This allows a more quantitative assessment of the preferential distribution of gas to the upper zones at the start of inspiration shown in Figure 2

perfusion (Ball et al, 1962; Anthonisen et al, 1966). Radioactive gases have also been used for the measurement of closing volume and were essential in establishing that during slow inspiration from low lung volume gas is initially distributed to the upper parts of the lungs (Milic-Emili et al, 1966 – Figures 2 & 3), probably due to the closure of small airways in the dependent lung regions. However, radioactive gases are limited in this use for reasons of dosage and for clinical purposes closing volume is now usually measured with an inert tracer gas such as helium, argon or nitrogen, which can be given repeatedly to the same subject.

CLINICAL USES

The main clinical application of the ventilation image is as an adjunct to perfusion scanning, particularly in the investigation and differential diagnosis

352

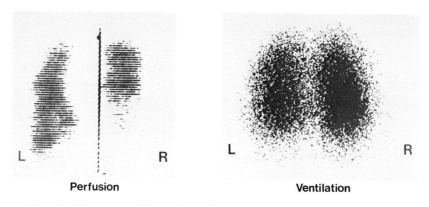

L   R   L   R

Perfusion   **Ventilation**

Figure 4. Pulmonary embolism: the perfusion scan, made with a rectilinear scanner, shows a large defect in the right lower lobe but there is no corresponding loss of ventilation on the gamma camera image. The patient was supine for both procedures

of pulmonary embolism. Generally in this condition, regional ventilation is normal (Figure 4), at least if the tests are not done until 24-48 hours after the time of the embolus (Medina et al, 1969; DeNardo et al, 1970). Experimentally, occlusion of one pulmonary artery in the dog and in man leads to diminution of ventilation as well as perfusion in the affected area, probably due to local hypocapnia (Allgood et al, 1968; Swenson et al, 1961), but this compensating response is apparently short-lived and is rarely seen in clinical pulmonary embolism (Bass et al, 1967) although there are occasional exceptions. In airway obstruction, on the other hand, local perfusion defects are common and the ventilation image is of particular value in differentiating patients with local bullous emphysema from those with pulmonary embolism.

COMBINED PERFUSION AND VENTILATION 'SCANS'

As indicated in the preceding section, the combination of perfusion and ventilation scanning gives more useful information than either technique alone and numerous attempts have been made to derive absolute ventilation/perfusion ratios from radioactive studies. In physiological conditions this is possible, but the quantitative methods have had only disappointingly limited application in clinical investigation. For one thing, the discrimination of any current counting system is limited to areas of lung 2-4 cms square, and therefore only relatively large areas of abnormal ventilation/perfusion balance can be detected. Moreover, the methods depend upon equilibrium being attained (Anthonisen et al, 1966), or upon measurement of total cardiac output (Heckscher et al, 1968), which may not be possible in pathological conditions of the lung. Clinically, combined perfusion and ventilation scanning has been confined largely to qualitative description and localisation of regional abnormalities of function, but even at this level is often of some practical help in diagnosis and management.

353

i) AIRWAYS OBSTRUCTION: ASTHMA, BRONCHITIS, EMPHYSEMA

In all the clinical varieties of airways obstruction patchy defects in both perfusion and ventilation are common, and the areas involved usually coincide anatomically (Figures 5 & 6). The main use of the combined technique in emphysema is in the determination of the extent of known defects and in the detection of unexpected ones. The latter information may be valuable when surgical removal of an area of bullous emphysema is being considered, and

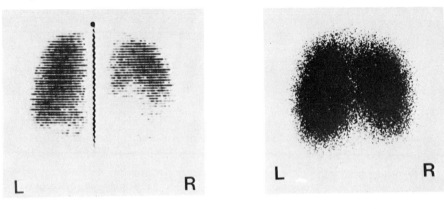

Perfusion   **Ventilation**

Figure 5. Obstructive emphysema: the perfusion scan (made with the rectilinear scanner) shows a large defect at the right base and there is also a reduction in counts at the right base in the ventilation image (made with the gamma camera)

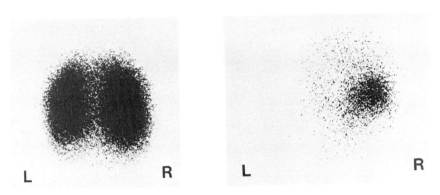

Xe Washout 1 min   **Xe washout 7mins**

Figure 6. Obstructive emphysema (same patient as Figure 5): The 'equilibrium' ventilation image after only 1 min of wash-out shows relatively increased counts at the right base compared with the single-breath image in Figure 5. The size of the ventilation defect is better shown by the area of retention of Xenon at the right base after 7 mins wash-out.

the state of the remainder of the lung needs assessment, but in general the technique gives only an approximate guide to the function of the remaining lung. In asthma, as might be expected, ventilation is characteristically more widely affected than perfusion, in contrast to the findings in pulmonary embolism, and defects become worse as symptoms increase but are reversible with treatment (Heckscher et al, 1968). Interpretation of these results is often difficult because the different techniques of inhalation of radioactive gas used may affect the distribution of that gas (Robertson et al, 1969) and because the effects of gravity have not always been considered carefully. However, in one study in which these factors were taken into account there was found to be good correlation between regions of reduced perfusion and ventilation in 17 out of 18 asthmatic subjects (Wilson et al, 1970). The extent of ventilation involvement was greater than that of perfusion, and ventilation wash-out studies performed after injection of radioactive Xenon showed areas of slow gaseous wash-out in which perfusion was apparently normal, indicating evolution of gas into aerated but poorly ventilated alveoli. Although regional abnormalities of lung function in asthma usually improve with treatment, some may persist when the patients are in symptomatic remission.

The value of radioisotopes in separating the bronchitic from the emphy-sematous type of chronic airway obstruction has not yet been substantiated, although this seems a promising field for further investigation. In theory one would expect to find more severe regional perfusion defects in emphysema than in bronchitis (Lopez-Majano et al, 1966) but the difficulty comes in differentiating the two types reliably by physiological tests in life in order to test the correlation with the scan findings, and confirmatory pathological comparisons may take years to complete.

ii) CARCINOMA OF BRONCHUS

The effects of bronchial carcinoma on regional blood flow and ventilation have been quite extensively studied by radioactive techniques which have yielded some interesting results. Usually a carcinoma is accompanied by a reduction in both perfusion and ventilation often over an area larger than that suggested by the size of the neoplasm itself or by associated lung collapse or consolidation (Maynard et al, 1969). The mechanism of the reduced perfusion is thought to be mainly compression of the pulmonary arteries by tumour, or rarely direct invasion, although the extent of involvement of the pulmonary vasculature has not often been assessed by detailed pathological studies and local hypoxia has been suggested as an alternative mechanism (Wagner et al, 1965) as has pulmonary venous occlusion and local obstructive emphysema (Fraser et al, 1970). Centrally situated growths may affect surprisingly large areas of pulmonary perfusion through involvement of the larger pul-monary arteries (Figure 7), and the extent of perfusion loss has been used

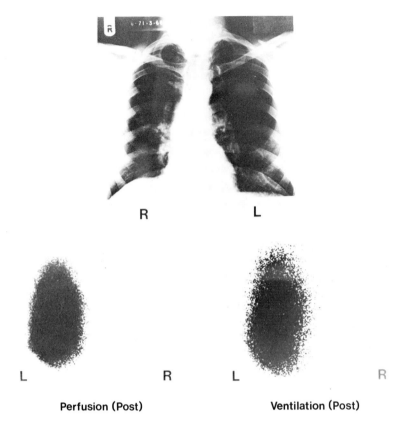

Perfusion (Post) **Ventilation (Post)**

Figure 7. Carcinoma of bronchus: CXR shows only slight right hilar enlargement, but perfusion and ventilation images (both obtained with the gamma camera) show almost absent function on the right side.

by some authors as a guide to resectability. It has been suggested that the relative reduction of perfusion on one side to less than one third of the total indicates an inoperable growth (Secker-Walker et al, 1971), but the correlation is not perfect and the method cannot at present be regarded as giving more than an approximate idea of whether resection of a tumour is possible. The hope that perfusion scanning might be useful in early detection of bronchial carcinoma (Wagner et al, 1965) has not been fulfilled, largely because most patients already have X-ray abnormalities when first seen. The mechanism of the reduction in ventilation is not entirely clear, since areas involved are often larger than predicted from the extent and degree of bronchial obstruction. Radioactive ventilation studies have already proved a useful adjunct to clinical examination and conventional radiology in revealing unexpected defects which may be of functional importance. Another important and increasing use of radioisotopes in carcinoma of the bronchus is in predicting whether residual lung function will be adequate after lobectomy or pneumonectomy. At present, routine lung scanning gives only qualitative information about regional lung function, but it is helpful to know whether the opposite lung has evenly distributed perfusion and ventilation prior to operation. Although interpretation is still subjective and rather crude, the presence of marked abnormalities in the lung to be left behind would weigh against operation in a patient with impaired overall lung function. Conversely, resection would be more readily attempted in the presence of poor function if the scan showed severe abnormalities confined mainly to the side to be resected (see Figure 7), although against this must be considered the suggestion that a gross perfusion defect indicates a central growth unlikely to be technically removable. This application of radioisotope investigation of the lungs is already proving of some practical value but needs to be put on a more exact quantitative basis before it is widely used.

iii) MISCELLANEOUS CONDITIONS

Old age: This is an important factor, like posture, which can alter the normal distribution of perfusion and ventilation. In the upright posture, perfusion to the upper lung zones is increased, although remaining less than to the lower zones, while the normal preferential distribution of ventilation to the lower zones at resting tidal volume is lost with increasing age (Holland et al, 1968). In theory these changes could contribute to the increased alveolar-arterial oxygen difference in old age, but more quantitative studies are needed to confirm this. However, age should clearly be taken into account in interpreting radioisotope tests done in the upright posture.

Obesity: Another potential cause of perfusion/ventilation abnormalities is obesity, particularly since there is often evidence of increased physiological 'shunting' of pulmonary blood flow in the Pickwickian syndrome. In one study it was found that perfusion was distributed slightly more evenly than usual in the upright posture in obese subjects. Ventilation of the lower zones tended to be decreased in the more severely affected subjects, whose expiratory reserve volume was less than 0.41 and averaged only 21% of predicted (Holley et al, 1967). Only a small number of subjects was investigated and the effects of moderate obesity seemed to be negligible, but weight is yet another factor to be considered in the interpretation of scans done in the upright posture.

Lung infiltration: There has been little systematic work on the distribution of injected and inhaled isotopes in lung infiltration apart from pulmonary congestion and oedema. Individual results suggest patchy defects in perfusion and ventilation, but there are usually X-ray abnormalities visible and it is not yet known whether isotope studies can detect altered function

357

in the absence of radiological findings.

Hepatic Cirrhosis: The mechanism of the hypoxaemia sometimes seen in patients with cirrhosis but grossly normal pulmonary function has been investigated with inhaled and injected Xenon. There is increased air-trapping and closing volume, attributed to premature closure of airways in dependent lung regions (Ruff et al, 1971) and the authors suggest that this leads to sufficient lowering of basal ventilation/perfusion ratios to cause arterial hypoxaemia by means of increased 'venous admixture'.

SUMMARY AND CONCLUSIONS

Radioisotope studies of the lung give useful physiological and clinical information and are already established as a vital adjunct to other forms of pulmonary investigation since, apart from bronchospirometry, there is no other way of examining regional lung function. However, it is important to remember that these techniques rarely give a specific pathological answer and that they must be interpreted with care, in the light of the clinical and physiological findings in any particular patient.

In making the differential diagnosis of pulmonary thromboembolism from other forms of local lung disease, ventilation as well as perfusion needs to be assessed but, given a firm clinical diagnosis, conventional perfusion scanning alone may be helpful in demonstrating the extent of embolic obstruction and the rate of resolution. In carcinoma of the bronchus, combined ventilation and perfusion studies may give a guide to likely residual lung function after resection but more quantitative work is needed before this kind of information can be used widely for prediction. Some quantitative data on ventilation/perfusion relationships are already available from physiological studies but their application to patients with severely diseased lungs is not yet established, and the role of isotope investigation particularly in chronic airway obstruction needs to be more clearly defined.

REFERENCES

Allgood, R. J., Wolfe, W. G., Ebert, P. A. and Sabiston, D. C. Jnr. (1968) American Journal of Physiology, **214**, 772

Anthonisen, N. R., Dolovich, M. B. and Bates, D. V. (1966) Journal of Clinical Investigation, **45**, 1349

Ball, W. C. Jnr., Stewart, P. B., Newsham, L. G. S. and Bates, D. V. (1962) Journal of Clinical Investigation, **41**, 519

Bass, H., Heckscher, T. and Anthonisen, N. R. (1967) Clinical Science, **33**, 355

Blahd, W. H. (1971) 'Nuclear Medicine', 2nd Edition. McGraw Hill, N Y

Dawson, A., Kaneko, K. and McGregor, M. (1965) Journal of Clinical Investigation, **44**, 999

DeNardo, G. L., Goodwin, D. A., Ravasini, R. and Dietrich, P. (1970) New England Journal of Medicine, **282**, 1334

Dollery, C. T. and Gillam, P. M. S. (1963) Thorax, **18**, 316

Dollery, C. T. and Hugh-Jones, P. (1963) British Medical Bulletin, **19**, 59

Dollery, C. T., Hugh-Jones, P. and Matthews, C. M. E. (1962) British Medical Journal, **1**, 1006

Fraser, H. S., Macleod, W. M., Garnett, E. S. and Goddard, B. A. (1970) American Review of Respiratory Disease, **101**, 349

Fred, H. L., Burdine, J. A. Jnr., Gonzalez, D. A., Lockhart, R. W., Peabody, C. A. and Alexander, J. K. (1966) New England Journal of Medicine, **275**, 1025

Friedman, W. F. and Braunwald, E. (1966) Circulation, **34**, 363

Gilson, A. J. and Smoak, W. M. (1970) 'Pulmonary Investigation with Radionuclides', C. T. Thomas, Springfield, Illinois

Gold, W. M. and McCormack, K. R. (1966) Journal of the American Medical Association, **197**, 146

Heckscher, T., Bass, H., Oriol, A., Rose, B., Anthonisen, N. R. and Bates, D. V. (1968) Journal of Clinical Investigation, **47**, 1063

Holland, J., Milic-Emili, J., Macklem, P. T. and Bates, D. V. (1968) Journal of Clinical Investigation, **47**, 81

Holley, H. S., Milic-Emili, J., Becklake, M. R. and Bates, D. V. (1967) Journal of Clinical Investigation, **46**, 475

Hughes, J. M. B., Glazier, J. B., Rosenzweig, D. M. and West, J. B. (1969) Clinical Science, **37**, 847

Krishnamurthy, G. T., Srinivasan, N. V. and Blahd, W. M. (1972) Journal of Nuclear Medicine, **13**, 604

Lopez-Majano, V., Tow, D. E. and Wagner, H. N. (1966) Journal of the American Medical Association, **197**, 121

Maynard, C. D., Miller, R. P., Heaphy, L. J. and Whitley, J. E. (1969) Radiology, **92**, 903

Medina, J. R., L'Heureux, P., Lillehei, J. P. and Loken, M. K. (1969) Circulation, **39**, 831

Milic-Emili, J., Henderson, J. A. M., Dolovich, M. B., Trop, D. and Kaneko, K. (1966) Journal of Applied Physiology, **21**, 749

Newhouse, M. T., Wright, F. J., Ingham, J. K., Archer, N. P., Hughes, L. B. and Hopkins, O. L. (1968) Respiration Physiology, **4**, 141

Robertson, P. C., Anthonisen, N. R. and Ross, D. (1969) Journal of Applied Physiology, **26**, 438

Ruff, F., Hughes, J. M. B., Stanley, N., McCarthy, D., Greene, R., Aronoff, A., Clayton, L. and Milic-Emili, J. (1971) Journal of Clinical Investigation, **50**, 2403

Sabiston, D. C. and Wagner, H. N. Jnr. (1964) Annals of Surgery, **160**, 575

Secker-Walker, R. H. (1968) British Medical Journal, **2**, 206

Secker-Walker, R. H., Provan, J. L., Jackson, J. A. and Goodwin, J. (1971) Thorax, **26**, 23

Swenson, E. W., Finley, T. N. and Guzman, S. V. (1961) Journal of Clinical Investigation, **40**, 828

Tow, D. E. and Wagner, H. N. Jnr. (1967) New England Journal of Medicine, **276**, 1053

Wagner, H. N. Jnr., Lopez-Majano, V., Tow, D. E. and Langan, J. K. (1965) Lancet, i, 344

Wagner, H. N. Jnr., Sabiston, D. C. Jnr., McAfee, J. G., Tow, D. and Stern, H. S. (1964) New England Journal of Medicine, **271**, 377

Wilson, A. F., Surprenant, E. L., Beall, G. N., Siegel, S. C., Simmons, D. H. and Bennett, L. R. (1970) American Journal of Medicine, **48**, 416

Gallstone Formation

K W HEATON

Cholelithiasis is a metabolic disease, but it is only very recently that physicians have regained their old interest in it. I believe there are three reasons for this re-awakening.

(1) The possibility of effective medical treatment is appearing as a result of experiments which Dr Dowling will describe.

(2) Our understanding of the physiology and biochemistry of bile has increased enormously in the last 15 years and we now have a reasonably clear idea of how cholesterol gallstones arise; that is their pathogenesis.

(3) The epidemiology of gallstones has at last begun to attract the interest which it deserves, and many of us have been astonished to find that whereas gallstones are extremely common in Western society they are rare or non-existent in some communities. This has led us to question why gallstones arise, that is their aetiology, and in doing so to look seriously at a revolutionary new hypothesis about 'civilised' eating habits.

In this paper I shall discuss briefly the second and third of these reasons. The subject is discussed more fully elsewhere (Small, 1970; Heaton, 1972; Redinger & Small, 1972; Heaton, 1973).

THE NATURE OF THE PROBLEM

In most countries gallstones form within the gallbladder and are composed mainly of crystalline cholesterol. A random sample of 47 English stones contained nearly 60% of cholesterol (Sutor & Wooley, 1971). There is probably no value in separating mixed stones from cholesterol stones since the cholesterol content of gallstones varies continuously from nearly 100% to very low levels (Lancet, 1968). The second most abundant component is calcium salts, and English stones are unusually rich in calcium carbonate (33%), but the significance of calcium precipitation is obscure. Except for the uncommon pure pigment stone, bile pigments are minor components, usually present as calcium bilirubinate. The main interest of bile pigment is that it is regularly found in the centre of a gallstone. This has excited much interest but again its significance is unclear.

The major developments in our understanding revolve round cholesterol and the factors determining its solubility or insolubility in bile.

The cholesterol in gallstones comes from the bile. We do not know why bile contains cholesterol – it has no obvious function. It may just be an accidental passenger, leaked out of the liver cell membrane as bile is secreted into the canaliculus. However, it is there in a concentration of about 130 mg per 100 ml, which is around 5% of the total organic solids in freshly secreted hepatic bile. Cholesterol is a lipid which is completely insoluble in water, so special mechanisms are necessary to keep it in solution. In the blood this mechanism is minute negatively charged particles – the lipoproteins. In the bile it is also minute negatively charged particles, the micelles. The structure of these micelles is considered in the next paper by Dr Hermon Dowling. Suffice it now to say that a solution containing micelles is water-clear and completely stable. Normal bile is a micellar solution. It is also a one-phase system, that is to say it is all in one physical state – liquid. Bile containing a gallstone is a two-phase system; it contains cholesterol in two physical states, solid and liquid, which are more or less in equilibrium with one another. The gallstone is present because at some time the bile has been unable to hold in solution all the cholesterol within it.

FACTORS DETERMINING THE SOLUBILITY OF CHOLESTEROL IN BILE

The formation of micelles is a property of detergents. Bile owes its detergent properties to the combined action of two substances, bile salts and lecithin, which is a phospholipid. Neither substance can do the job by itself, but bile salts are the key material for two reasons:

(1) They are largely responsible for the fact that bile is secreted at all. The liver cells secrete bile salts into the canaliculi by an active transport process. In doing so, they create an osmotic gradient across the canalicular membrane which drags water through the membrane. This mechanism accounts for most of the water in bile.

(2) Bile salts exert a profound influence over the secretion of lecithin. If the bile salt secretion rate is artificially lowered, for example by draining off the bile salt pool through a T-tube in the common bile duct so that the only bile salts available to be secreted are newly synthesised ones, then the secretion of lecithin falls dramatically. If bile salt secretion is then artificially boosted by feeding a bile salt mixture by mouth, there is a parallel increase in lecithin secretion, which falls and rises as bile salt feeding is stopped and then started again (Figure 1). Notice, however, that cholesterol secretion varies much less than the other two. This implies that the relative proportions of these three substances, cholesterol, lecithin and bile salts, are likely to be very variable, since they depend on changes in

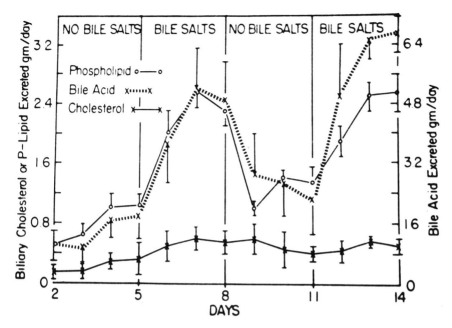

Figure 1. Excretion through a T-tube of bile salt, phospholipid and cholesterol during 3 day periods without and with the oral administration of bile salt (1.8 - 2.2 g per day in 3 divided doses). Each point represents the average value from 5 patients. From Bell et al, 1971

the secretion rates of three materials. Two of these materials seem to change together but the third is largely independent.

It is essential that we have a way of expressing the relative proportions of cholesterol, lecithin and bile salts, because in them lies the answer to the question, 'When is cholesterol soluble in bile, and when is it insoluble?' Fortunately, a simple technique is at hand to do this, a technique known as triangular co-ordinates. This was introduced five years ago by Donald Small of Boston, and it has done much to stimulate thought and work in this field. There are three stages in its use. First, measure the concentrations of the three materials in moles and add them together. Second, express the amount of each material as a percentage of the sum. For example, in a sample of hepatic bile, the measured concentration of bile salts may well be 40 mmol/l, that of lecithin 7.5 mmol/l and that of cholesterol 2.5 mmol/l. The sum of these is 50 mmol/l, so that amounts of each are 80%, 15% and 5% respectively. (Obviously, the amounts of the three materials always add up to 100 percent). Thirdly, plot the percentages in an equilateral triangle, each side of which represents the percentage of one component. The results of the foregoing example have been plotted in this way in Figure 2.

The importance of this technique in relation to gallstone formation is

365

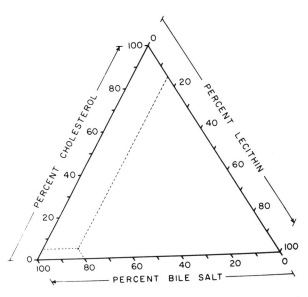

Figure 2. Triangular co-ordinates used to represent by a single point a mixture of
three components, namely 80% bile salt, 15% lecithin and 5% cholesterol. A mixture
of equal parts of all three components would be represented by a point in the centre
of the triangle

that it enables us to define precisely the limits within which the composition
of bile can vary without jeopardising the solubility of cholesterol. These
limits were defined by Small et al (1966) in a series of in vitro experiments
using a large number of artificial biles. They mixed together cholesterol,
lecithin and bile salts in all possible proportions and then examined the
mixtures for the presence of crystals and liquid crystals. Their findings
are summarised in Figure 3. This shows that most of the mixtures contained crystals and/or liquid crystals. Only mixtures in the small area
under the curved line were wholly liquid. We may regard this as the zone
of guaranteed cholesterol solubility, and the line as the line of cholesterol
saturation. Below it the mixture is unsaturated, above it it either contains
solid cholesterol or is supersaturated and liable to precipitate cholesterol
at any time.

If bile behaves like these in vitro mixtures, then the composition of
normal bile should lie within the liquid or micellar zone, whereas gallstone-
forming bile should lie on the boundary line if it is saturated with cholesterol,
and over the line if it is supersaturated. Broadly speaking this is true. The
original work of Admirand and Small (1968) suggested a sharp distinction
between gallstone patients and controls (Figure 4). Subsequently, it has
become clear that there is some overlap, but all workers find that, on

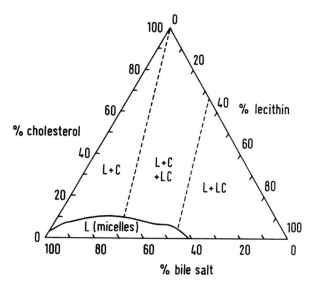

Figure 3. The physical state of all possible mixtures of cholesterol, lecithin and bile salt at 37°C and with 10% water content. L = liquid, C = crystals, LC = liquid crystals. Modified from Admirand and Small, 1968

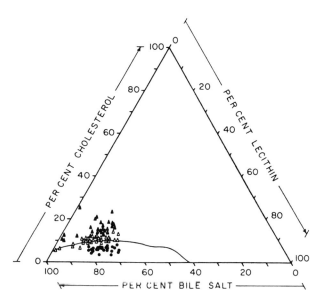

Figure 4. The composition of gallbladder bile, expressed by triangular co-ordinates, from patients with cholesterol or mixed gallstones (triangles) and from controls (circles). The limits of cholesterol solubility, as determined from artificial bile salt-lecithin-cholesterol mixtures, are shown by the curved line. The black triangles represent biles which contained microcrystals of cholesterol, the white triangles those without microcrystals. From Admirand and Small, 1968

average, gallstone-bearing bile is significantly more saturated with cholesterol than control patients' bile.

The existence of this overlap has caused some confusion and misunderstanding. There are probably two reasons for it. The first is that in a community where gallstones are very common, many ostensibly normal people are in a pre-gallstone state. For example, in Sweden, no less than 70 percent of women develop gallstones by the age of 70, and about half as many men (Sternby, 1968). It is therefore not surprising that when 19 normal Swedes were studied, 12 were found to have supersaturated gallbladder bile, even though they were at the time free of biliary disease (Figure 5). Why did these 12 Swedes not actually have cholelithiasis? Probably because at the time they lacked a nucleating or seeding agent to initiate stone growth or because they were emptying their gallbladders to effectively that microstones were continually being washed out.

The second reason for the overlap is that the gallstone-forming diathesis like the duodenal ulcer diathesis is intermittent. On repeated cholecystography many patients show no change in the size of their stones. Very probably the secretion of stone-forming or lithogenic bile is also intermittent. This would explain why several groups of workers have recently found normal, undersaturated bile in some patients with gallstones. Gallstone-bearing bile is not always gallstone-forming bile, nor is gallstone-forming bile always gallstone-bearing bile. Nevertheless, the fundamental fact remains that cholesterol-rich stones can form and grow only when bile is supersaturated with cholesterol.

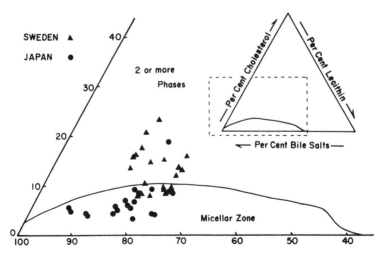

Figure 5. The composition of gallbladder bile samples from control subjects free of biliary disease in Sweden and Japan. Only one of the Japanese biles, but most of the Swedish ones are supersaturated. From Nakayama and van der Linden, 1971

THE ORIGIN OF LITHOGENIC BILE

After it enters the gallbladder, bile is not changed in any way except by being concentrated, that is by having water and electrolytes extracted. The act of concentration does not make bile any more liable to precipitate out cholesterol. Bile which is supersaturated in the gallbladder was already supersaturated when it was secreted by the liver cell. This is illustrated by Figure 6, which shows that bile aspirated through a needle from the common hepatic duct was supersaturated in gallstone patients, saturated in control subjects with no biliary tract disease, and under-saturated in patients with pigment stones. Incidentally, the latter finding is important since it validates the present approach. A pigment stone provides a perfect nucleus for the precipitation of cholesterol. By remaining a pure pigment stone it demonstrates that there is no surplus cholesterol available in the bile bathing it.

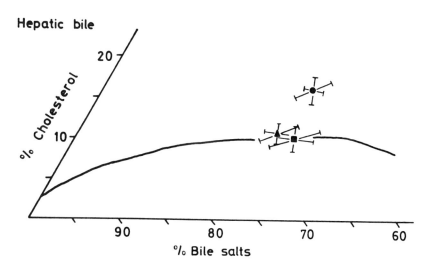

Figure 6. The composition of hepatic bile from patients with cholesterol stones (circles), control subjects (triangles) and patients with pigment stones (squares). From Schaffer et al, 1972

The fact that bile is already lithogenic when secreted by the liver means that we may legitimately regard cholesterol gallstone disease as a liver disease. The gallbladder is the innocent victim of a delinquent liver. It suffers simply because it is a cul-de-sac in which stones can grow and out of which they can have great difficulty in escaping.

The question 'Why do people form gallstones?' may now be re-phrased as 'Why do people secrete bile which is supersaturated with cholesterol?'

There are two possible mechanisms: (1) The liver secretes excess cholesterol. (2) The liver secretes too little bile salts. A theoretical third possibility, too little lecithin, need not be discussed separately since lecithin secretion is almost totally dependent on bile salt secretion. At the present time it seems likely that both mechanisms are at play: (1) Bile cholesterol secretion is increased, probably as a result of excessive cholesterol synthesis (2) Bile salt secretion is reduced, probably because the size of the circulating bile salt pool is only half the normal, which in turn is due to impaired bile salt synthesis. Let us consider each of these metabolic abnormalities in turn.

CHOLESTEROL EXCESS

In 1954, Isaksson showed that although gallbladder bile from stone patients is considerably more dilute than normal bile, it contains more cholesterol. Expressed as a percentage of total solids, the cholesterol was increased by 40%. Obviously this suggests that the liver is secreting too much cholesterol into the bile, but it is only very recently that advances in experimental technique have enabled research workers to check this by measuring bile secretion in intact subjects. Grundy et al (1972) have investigated a group of American Indian women with gallstones and have shown that they do indeed secrete excessive amounts of cholesterol – on average 47 mg per hour, compared with 29 mg per hour in white controls without gallstones. It remains to be seen whether this oversecretion of cholesterol is also present in white subjects with gallstones, but it is hard to see why it should not be.

BILE SALT DEFICIENCY

The human body contains about 3 grams of bile salts. This 'pool' of bile salts spends part of its time resting in the gallbladder (that is during fasting), but most of the time it is on the move, going round the enterohepatic circulation – liver, biliary tract, duodenum, jejunum, ileum, portal blood, liver again, and so on. In normal subjects, the bile salt pool circulates about six times in each 24 hour period. Therefore the total amount of bile salts secreted each day is six times 3 grams, or 18 grams. Only a very small fraction of this is lost in the faeces, about half a gram a day, or 3% of what enters the gut. This $\frac{1}{2}$ g is of course replaced by $\frac{1}{2}$ g of newly synthesised bile salt, made in the liver from cholesterol. Liver synthesis is homeostatically controlled by the amount of bile salt returning to the liver in the portal vein, in other words by a negative feedback system.

In patients with cholesterol-rich gallstones the size of the circulating bile salt pool is markedly reduced. The first time it was measured, in male patients in Boston, it was half the normal size (Vlahcevic et al, 1970). In Bristol, we have studied middle-aged women with gallstones and have found them to have an average bile salt pool of 1.8 grams, compared with 2.8 grams in matched controls (Figure 7). Obviously these findings make

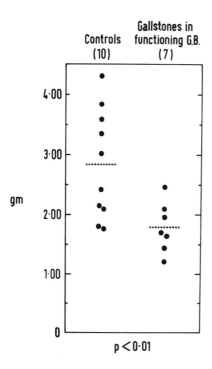

Figure 7. The size of the bile salt pool in middle-aged women with gallstones and in matched controls (Pomare & Heaton, 1972)

it likely that bile salt secretion is diminished. Indeed, American Indian girls, most of whom will develop gallstones by the age of 25, have very small bile salt pools (Vlahcevic et al, 1972) and we now know from the work of Grundy et al (1972) that they have very low bile salt secretion rates. It is just possible that a small bile salt pool is compensated by more frequent cycling of the pool. Nevertheless, at the present time it is generally accepted that shrinkage of the bile salt pool is one of the main factors, if not the main factor in the production of lithogenic bile.

What causes the bile salt pool to shrink? This vital question has yet to be explored experimentally. However, by simple reasoning we can push the pathogenesis back one stage further and say that if, in the absence of gross bile salt malabsorption, the pool shrinks and stays small, then liver synthesis of bile salt must be pathologically suppressed. The normal homeostatic reaction to removing bile salts from the circulation is to increase synthesis of new bile salt. This is well shown by the effects of feeding cholestyramine, a bile salt-sequestrating resin. By feeding this resin, one can drain out of the body and into the faeces as much as 2 grams of bile salt in 24 hours (Grundy et al, 1971). Nevertheless, when normal subjects are kept on long term cholestyramine, they maintain a normal size bile salt pool (Garbutt & Kenney, 1972). Their livers have responded to the drain on the bile salt pool by greatly increasing the synthesis of new bile salt. In gallstone patients, the synthesis rate of bile salt is normal. This shows that, in them, the liver has failed to rise to the challenge of a depleted bile salt pool. Clearly, something must be constraining the liver, putting a check on its synthetic mechanism.

The origin of lithogenic bile seems therefore to involve two biochemical abnormalities: excessive secretion of cholesterol into the bile, and suppressed liver synthesis of bile salts.

Turning now to aetiology, to the environmental factors responsible for these biochemical disturbances, we must start by studying the epidemiology of the disease.

THE EPIDEMIOLOGY OF CHOLESTEROL RICH GALLSTONES

Epidemiology gives clues to aetiology in three ways; (1) Geographical variations in prevalence; (2) Historical changes in incidence; and (3) Clinical associations with other diseases, on the grounds that related diseases are likely to share a common cause.

Unfortunately, statistics giving the true prevalence of gallstones are very scanty. The figures that are available are from autopsy series, which are inevitably selected. Therefore, in comparing different countries, one is forced to look for crude differences in prevalence. In spite of these limitations, certain generalisations are possible (Heaton, 1973). Firstly, the disease is common in all Western countries, including Australasia, Israel and White South Africa. In these countries, between a quarter and a half of the population can expect to get gallstones in their lifetime, though in 70 to 80% they will be asymptomatic. Secondly, gallstones are a great rarity in rural Africans and probably in rural Asians (Burkitt, 1973). In urbanised Africans, for example in Johannesburg, gallstones are seen to a certain extent, while in US Negroes they are probably almost as common as in whites. Similarly, in Japan, cholesterol-rich stones are uncommon in rural areas and in the labouring classes, but are quite common in the professional classes and in the cities generally.

These geographical variations suggest that the frequency of gallstones in different societies is roughly proportional to the degree of economic development or 'Westernisation'. Affluence as such is not the key factor, as we can see from American experience. Admittedly, four out of the last six Presidents of the USA lost their gallbladders, but the American Indians, who are the poorest group in the country, have the highest incidence of gallstones of any community in the world.

The modern Western way of life is also implicated by historical changes in gallstone incidence. For example, in Japan, which has developed very rapidly in the last 30 years, the post-mortem prevalence of gallstones has doubled in 15 years. Similarly, in the Canadian Arctic, cholelithiasis has appeared as a virtually new disease in the Eskimo, that is to say in those who have abandoned their primitive nomadic way of life and sought their fortune in the mushrooming townships like Inuvik. Even in Europe, the number of patients requiring surgery for gallstones has increased markedly since World War II. In the Bristol area, the frequency of gallbladder operations rose by 230 percent between 1950 and 1970 (Holland & Heaton, 1972). A similar increase occurred in Sweden in the immediate post-war period. A disturbing trend, which has been noted in both England and Sweden, is that there appears to have been a disproportionate increase in young people. Thus, in 1933, 1940 and 1950 only four percent of Bristol gallbladder operations were in the under thirty age group. In 1960 the figure was 6.7% and in 1970 it was 9.3%. In Sweden since the nineteen fifties it has become quite common to diagnose gallstones in 12 to 15 year old children (Nilsson, 1966). There seems little doubt therefore that cholelithiasis is increasing not only in developing countries but also in Western society. Rising incidence and involvement of younger people imply that the environmental factors causing the disease have intensified in recent years.

Any hypothesis for the cause of a disease must take into account its clinical associations. The diseases associated with cholesterol-rich stones are: gallbladder cancer, pancreatitis, terminal ileopathy, obesity, diabetes, and probably coronary heart disease (Kaye & Kern, 1971; Heaton, 1973). However, the first three of these are not relevant to the present discussion. Gallbladder cancer and pancreatitis are generally regarded as caused by the gallstones, while resection or disease of the terminal ileum is known to cause bile salt malabsorption and deficiency, and hence lithogenic bile.

Obesity, diabetes and coronary heart disease (CHD) have much in common. Like cholesterol gallstones, they are rare in primitive communities but common in 'civilised' countries. All four have become commoner in this country since the last war. All four are commonly associated with disturbed glucose tolerance and with alterations of blood lipids. Furthermore each disease is significantly associated with each of the other three. Thus, gallstone patients tend to be obese and diabetic or pre-diabetic (Braunsteiner et al, 1966; Hikasa et al, 1969), and they probably get an excessive amount of CHD (Heaton, 1973). Obese subjects have an excess incidence of gallstones, diabetes and CHD. Diabetics tend to be obese and to get more gallstones and CHD. Patients with CHD tend to be obese and diabetic; whether they get more gallstones is not known.

The overlap between these four metabolic diseases is so great, the quartet is so inextricably linked (Figure 8), that one is forced to conclude

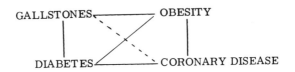

Figure 8. The network of associations. Each line represents a documented association

that all four share an important aetiological factor.

A NUTRITIONAL HYPOTHESIS

In his simple yet daringly original hypothesis, Cleave has postulated that many of the diseases of civilisation including gallstones, are caused by eating carbohydrate in refined form, especially as sugar (sucrose) and white flour (Cleave et al, 1969). Broadly speaking, he divides the effects of refining, that is of sugar refining and flour milling, into two distinct kinds — loss of fibrous residue or roughage from the diet, and production of concentrated, high energy food. The penalties of living on these foods are therefore altered gastrointestinal function, especially colonic stasis and its sequelae, and excessive energy intake or overconsumption. According to the Cleave hypothesis, the vast majority of 'civilised' people are obtaining too much energy and too little roughage from their diet, and it is merely individual differences in susceptibility which determine whether their excess energy intake leads to obesity, diabetes or coronary heart disease (or some combination of the three), and whether their lack of dietary fibre leads to constipation, diverticular disease or other colonic disorders. The 'fibre-deficiency' half of this concept has in the last few years received considerable support from the studies of Painter, Burkitt, Walker and Johnson, but Cleave himself stresses that fibre-depletion cannot be separated from over-consumption. Indeed he regards all these conditions, including gallstones, as manifestations of a single 'Saccharine Disease' (meaning sugar related, to indicate all dietary carbohydrate is absorbed as monosaccharides).

Does the Cleave hypothesis fit the facts as far as gallstones are concerned? Can it explain the epidemiology, clinical associations, and biochemical disturbances of the human disease, and is it consistent with the relevant animal experiments? Let us consider each point in turn.

First, epidemiology. Does the frequency of gallstones parallel the use of refined carbohydrate foods? The evidence is that it does. As Cleave and many others have shown, the changes in diet which occur with civilisation and economic development are chiefly in the carbohydrate fraction. Out go starchy staple foods, which are generally eaten whole or only partly refined, and in come sugar and white flour, which are both highly refined products,

and in most cases animal products increase too. However, in the case of
the Eskimo, consumption of animal products goes down as the incidence of
gallstones goes up. Remembering the post-war surge in gallstone cases, it
is important too to look at how diet has changed with post-war affluence. A
similar pattern emerges. Down go potatoes, which are unrefined, and bread,
that is the starchy staple foods, and up go the sugar-containing 'treats', the
confectionery, ice-creams, biscuits and cakes, as well as the convenience
foods (mostly containing sugar) and the fizzy drinks.

Secondly, does the refined carbohydrate hypothesis explain the clinical
associations of gallstones? The answer must be yes if refined carbohydrate
is involved in the genesis of obesity, diabetes and coronary disease. I am
not qualified to argue the case for and against diabetes and coronary disease,
but it seems self-evident that sugar if not white flour can cause obesity.
They are concentrated foods, high in calories but stripped of stomach-filling,
non-nutritive fibre. As cleave has shown, anyone satisfying his appetite on
such foods is bound to take in excess energy.

Thirdly, can the refined carbohydrate hypothesis explain the biochemical
disturbances which seem to underlie the secretion of lithogenic bile — oversecretion of cholesterol and undersynthesis of bile salts? The answer is yes.
Grundy et al (1972) measured the rate of cholesterol secretion in 23 American
Indian women and 13 Caucasian women. They also provided data on the

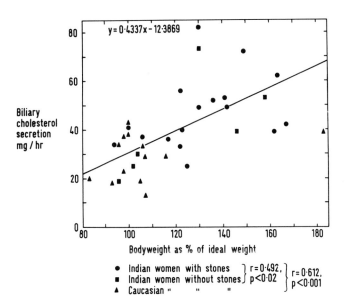

Figure 9. The relationship between bodyweight and biliary cholesterol secretion in
American women studied by Grundy et al, 1972

weight of these women in relation to their ideal weight. When cholesterol secretion is plotted against body weight a significant correlation emerges (Figure 9). As body fat goes up, so does bile cholesterol secretion. This important finding is new, but it might have been predicted. In 1971, Miettinen showed that, in a group of obese subjects, total body synthesis of cholesterol was increased to twice that of a non-obese control group. Since the liver is the chief site of cholesterol production, it is only to be expected that in obesity the secretion of the liver, that is the bile, will contain excess cholesterol. These facts provide at last a biochemical explanation for the long known association between obesity and gallstones. They also provide a clear link with refined carbohydrate, since a fundamental tenet of the Cleave hypothesis is that concentrated carbohydrate inevitably provides surplus calories. There is a crying need for experimental work to test this hypothesis, but what little has been done supports it. In Marseilles, Sarles et al (1970) found that 101 gallstone patients habitually consumed a higher calorie diet than 101 controls, and went on to show experimentally that raising the calorie intake causes a rise in the cholesterol concentration of bile.

Undersynthesis of bile salts is also explicable as an effect of refined carbohydrate. As long ago as 1958, Portman and Murphy showed that, when rats were taken off their normal (unrefined) chow diet and given a semi-synthetic diet rich in sucrose or refined starch, their bile salt pools shrank to half their normal size and their bile salt synthesis rates fell dramatically. Their livers, in fact, were grossly inhibited. These changes were partly reversed by adding cellulose to the diet. Other works have confirmed these findings but their relevance to human nutrition and disease has not previously been discussed. The mechanism whereby refined carbohydrate inhibits the liver is unknown, but a plausible link exists in the form of an aptly named substance, lithocholate. Western man produces about 100 mg lithocholate each day in his colon. It arises by the action of anaerobic bacteria on a major bile salt chenodeoxycholate. The vast majority of it is excreted but a small amount is absorbed and is found in the bile. Lithocholate is known to be toxic to liver microsomes in very small amounts and to inhibit at least one of the enzymes involved in bile salt synthesis (Nair et al, 1970). A low residue, Western-style diet favours the production of degraded bile acids such as lithocholate (Hill et al, 1971) and the associated colonic stasis would be expected to favour their absorption. It is possible therefore that on a refined, low-residue diet there is increased production and increased absorption of lithocholate, and that, on reaching the liver, lithocholate inhibits the synthesis of bile salt.

Fourthly and finally, is the refined carbohydrate hypothesis compatible with experimental work on the production of cholesterol gallstones in animals? Again, the answer is yes. To the best of this author's knowledge, all diets which have been successful in producing gallstones have contained a high proportion of purified sugar or refined starch. For example, in the much-used hamster model of Dam (1971), the diet contained 72% of glucose or sucrose. Similarly, Englert et al (1969) were able to force dogs to form gallstones by feeding a 50% sucrose diet.

SUMMARY

Cholesterol gallstones form because the liver secretes bile which is supersaturated with cholesterol (lithogenic bile). The biochemical explanation for this is twofold – oversecretion of cholesterol and undersecretion of bile salts, the latter being due to a reduced bile salt pool. The bile salt pool is small because liver synthesis of bile salt is inhibited. Epidemiologically, cholesterol gallstones are a disease of civilisation which is becoming commoner. Clinically, cholelithiasis is associated with obesity, diabetes and coronary thrombosis. Experimentally, diets which cause gallstones are rich in sugars or purified starch. All these facts are compatible with the hypothesis that cholelithiasis is caused by eating refined carbohydrate, and is part of the 'Saccharine Disease' of Cleave.

REFERENCES

Admirand, W. H. and Small, D. M. (1968) Journal of Clinical Investigation, 47, 1043

Bell, C. C., Vlahcevic, Z. R. and Swell, L. (1971) Surgery, Gynecology and Obstetrics, 132, 36

Braunsteiner, H., Dilauli, R., Sailer, S. and Sandhofer, F. (1966) Schweizerische Medizinische Wochenschrift, 96, 44

Burkitt, D. P. (1973) Personal communication

Cleave, T. L., Campbell, G. D. and Painter, N. S. (1969) Diabetes, Coronary Thrombosis and the Saccharine Disease. 2nd edition. Bristol, Wright

Dam, H. (1971) American Journal of Medicine, 51, 596

Englert, E., Harman, C. G. and Wales, E. E. (1969) Nature, London, 224, 280

Garbutt, J. T. and Kenney, T. J. (1972) Journal of Clinical Investigation, 51, 2781

Grundy, S. M., Ahrens, E. H. and Salen, G. (1971) Journal of Laboratory and Clinical Medicine, 78, 94

Grundy, S. M., Metzger, A. L. and Adler, R. D. (1972) Journal of Clinical Investigation, 51, 3026

Heaton, K. W. (1973) Clinics in Gastroenterology, 2, 67

Heaton, K. W. (1972) Bile Salts in Health and Disease. Edinburgh, Churchill Livingstone

Hikasa, Y., Matsuda, S., Nagase, M., Yoshinaga, M., Tobe, T., Maruyama, I., Shioda, R., Tanimura, H., Muraoka, R., Muroya, H. and Togo, M. (1969) Archiv Japanische Chirurgie, 38, 107

Hill, M. J., Crowther, J. S., Drasar, B. S., Hawksworth, G., Aries, V. and Williams, R. E. O. (1971) Lancet, i, 95

Holland, C. and Heaton, K. W. (1972) British Medical Journal, 3, 672

Isaksson, B. (1954) Acta Societatis Medicorum Upsaliensis, 59, 277

Kaye, M. D. and Kern, F. (1971) Lancet, i, 1228

Lancet (1968) i, 1416

Miettinen, T. (1971) Circulation, 44, 842

Nair, P. P., Garcia-Lilis, C. and Mendeloff, A. I. (1970) Journal of Nutrition, **100**, 698

Nakayama, F. and van der Linden, W. (1971) American Journal of Surgery, **122**, 8

Nilsson, S. (1966) Acta Chirurgica Scandinavica, **132**, 275

Pomare, E. W. and Heaton, K. W. (1972) Unpublished studies

Portman, O. W. and Murphy, P. (1958) Archives of Biochemistry and Biophysics, **76**, 367

Redinger, R. N. and Small, D. M. (1972) Archives of Internal Medicine, **130**, 618

Sarles, H., Hauton, J., Planche, N. E., Lafont, H. and Gérolami, A. (1970) American Journal of Digestive Diseases, **15**, 251

Shaffer, E. A., Braasch, J. W. and Small, D. M. (1972) New England Journal of Medicine, **287**, 1317

Small, D. M. (1970) Advances in Internal Medicine, **16**, 243

Small, D. M., Bourges, M. and Dervichian, D. G. (1966) Nature, London, **211**, 816

Sternby, N. H. (1968) Acta Pathologica et Microbiologica Scandinavica Supplement 194

Sutor, D. J. and Wooley, S. E. (1971) Gut, **12**, 55

Vlahcevic, Z. R., Bell, C. C., Buhac, I., Farrar, J. T. and Swell, L. (1970) Gastroenterology, **59**, 165

Vlahcevic, Z. R., Bell, C. C., Gregory, D. H., Buker, G., Juttijudata, P. and Swell, L. (1972) Gastroenterology, **62**, 73

The Dissolution of Gallstones

R HERMON DOWLING

INTRODUCTION

The tradition of 'cutting for stone' is not confined to the urinary tract and until recently, if treatment was indicated for gallstones, the only remedy was surgery. Within the past five to ten years, considerable advances have been made in our understanding of the physicochemical changes in bile which lead to the formation of gallstones, and it now seems that the application of these principles may be adapted to promote gallstone dissolution.

THE COMPOSITION OF GALLSTONES
AND THEIR SUITABILITY FOR DISSOLUTION THERAPY

(a) Classification of Gallstone Types

In any consideration of gallstone dissolution, the size, shape, crystal structure and matrix organisation of the stone are of fundamental importance. Although the size, shape and crystal composition of gallstones have been well studied in different communities, there is little information about the skeletal matrix and 'cement' substances of gallstones, or about how these substances may influence the rate of gallstone dissolution.

It has been known for more than 150 years that, in Westernised societies, the majority of gallstones consist predominantly of cholesterol, whether analysed chemically or by X-ray crystallographic techniques (Sutor & Wooley, 1971). At present, gallstone dissolution is confined to stones consisting predominantly of cholesterol, which may be arbitrarily defined as those containing more than 70% of cholesterol by weight on chemical assay. Pure cholesterol gallstones are comparatively rare and the majority of cholesterol stones are of the mixed variety. Many of these contain a black nucleus with brown staining of the interior due to bile pigment but on analysis the major component is still cholesterol. Only trace amounts of pigment are required to produce heavy staining of the stone. Mixed stones may also contain calcium salts, mucopolysaccharides and small quantities of bile acids and fatty

379

acids. In this country calcium carbonate is a common component of gallstones (Sutor & Wooley, 1971).

So-called 'pigment' stones are comparatively rare, except in association with haemolytic diseases and in hepatic cirrhosis, where there is an increased incidence of this type of stone (Nicholas et al, 1972). Although, clinically, pigment stones are easily identified as soft, black, crumbly stones, on crystallographic analysis, such stones are frequently shown to consist of the calcium salts of phosphate, carbonate and palmitate, together with calcium bilirubinate. At present there is no known method for dissolution of these stones.

Having considered gallstone composition, how can we predict the gallstone type in a given patient?

(b) Prediction of Gallstone Type

There is no certain way of predicting gallstone composition, but it is usually possible to make an accurate guess by considering:

    i)   Epidemiological data for the given population

    ii)   Radiological appearance of the stone

    iii) Examination of bile obtained by duodenal drainage —

                — lipid composition

                — presence of microcrystals

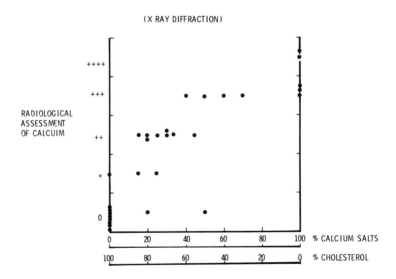

Figure 1. Relationship between the calcium (and cholesterol) content of gallstones, as measured by X-ray crystallographic techniques, and the radio-opacity of the stones graded arbitrarily from 0 (radiolucent) to ++++ (heavily radio-opaque), from cholecystography (Bell et al, 1972b)

Epidemiological studies (Comess et al, 1967; Sampliner et al, 1970; Friedman et al, 1966; Malhotra, 1968; Nakayama & Miyaka, 1970; Nakayama & van der Linden, 1971) and analysis of stones from different countries (Maki, 1966; Russell et al, 1968; Sutor & Wooley, 1971; Sutor & Gaston, 1972) show marked differences in the prevalence of gallstones and their chemical composition.

The X-ray appearance may also be helpful in predicting the composition of the stone. In general, cholesterol gallstones are radiolucent, while 'pigment' stones are usually radio-opaque, due to the presence of calcium salts. Figure 1 shows the relationship between the radiological appearance of gallstones and their subsequent composition as analysed by X-ray diffraction techniques (Sutor & Wooley, 1971). There is a roughly reciprocal relationship between the proportion of cholesterol and the proportion of calcium salts in any given stone and, as might be expected, the greater the proportion of calcium, the more radio-opaque the stone. Occasionally, however, predominantly calcium-containing 'pigment' stones may be radiolucent and indistinguishable on cholecystography from cholesterol gallstones.

The third method of predicting gallstone composition is by examining bile-rich fluid aspirated from the duodenum after intravenous cholecystokinin in the fasting subject. As discussed by Dr Heaton, the majority of patients with cholesterol gallstones have an abnormal bile composition. When the bile salt, phospholipid and cholesterol content of their bile is represented by a single point on the triangular coordinate diagram (Admirand & Small, 1968) most, but not all, patients have bile which is overloaded with cholesterol.

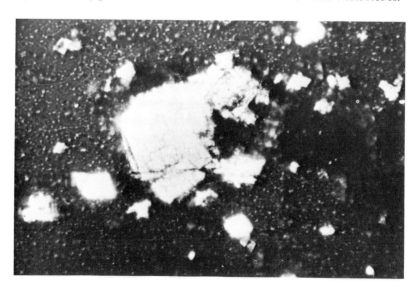

Figure 2. Microcrystals of cholesterol in a drop of bile from a patient with cholesterol gallstones, as seen by polarising microscopy.

Whole fresh bile analysed in this way may be abnormal either because it is supersaturated with cholesterol or because it contains a suspension of microcrystals, as illustrated in Figure 2. In our experience, approximately 50% of patients with cholesterol gallstones have microcrystals of cholesterol in their bile. However, cholesterol microcrystals may occasionally be found in bile from patients without gallstones. The presence of microcrystals is therefore not specific for patients with cholesterol gallstones (Juniper & Burson, 1957).

There is, therefore, no certain way of predicting gallstone composition, but in this country, radiolucent gallstones in a patient with an abnormal bile composition, particularly if accompanied by cholesterol microcrystals in bile, are most likely to be predominantly cholesterol and therefore suitable for dissolution therapy.

METABOLIC DEFECTS TO BE CORRECTED IN GALLSTONE DISSOLUTION THERAPY

Dr Heaton has already stressed the importance of a reduced bile acid pool and of an increased secretion of biliary cholesterol as the basic metabolic defects which lead to the formation of an abnormal or 'lithogenic' bile supersaturated with cholesterol.

(a) Increased Cholesterol Secretion

The increased cholesterol secretion has been shown by an intestinal perfusion technique (Grundy & Metzger, 1972) which has been used to study North American Indian women (Grundy et al, 1972) who have a very high incidence of cholesterol gallstones (Comess et al, 1967; Sampliner et al, 1970). A similar **pathological** secretion of excess biliary cholesterol has yet to be shown in Caucasian patients with gallstones. However, there is no known way of reducing the **proportion** of cholesterol in human bile. Therapeutic attention has therefore been directed towards expansion of the bile acid pool.

(b) Reduced Bile Acid Pool

The effect of a reduction in pool size has been studied in the Rhesus monkey (Dowling et al, 1971) and in the dog (Wheeler & King, 1972). With a reduced bile acid pool, and low bile acid secretion rates, there is a relatively greater proportion of cholesterol in bile. In other words, at low bile acid secretion rates, for every mole of bile acid produced (and for every mole of lecithin, since phospholipid secretion closely follows bile acid secretion — Swell et al, 1968) there is relatively more cholesterol, which results in the formation of a lithogenic bile. The results of recent perfusion studies in man (Northfield & Hofmann, 1972) support this hypothesis and suggest that there may be a diurnal variation in bile lipid composition: normal individuals occasionally

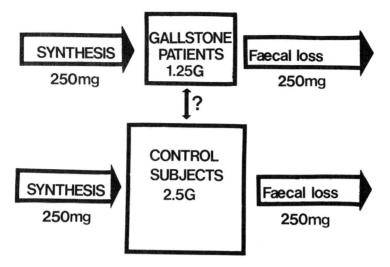

Figure 3. Regulation of bile acid pool size. In the steady state, bile acid synthesis matches faecal excretion. The reduced bile acid pool in patients with cholesterol gallstones is therefore independent of hepatic synthesis. (Values quoted are hypothetical but are based on published results from several centres)

secrete abnormal bile but patients with cholesterol gallstones have more hours of lithogenic bile each day.

(i) **Regulation of the bile acid pool size.** If reduction in bile acid pool size produces an abnormal bile, then expansion of the pool ought to reverse the abnormality, result in a bile less than fully saturated with cholesterol and ultimately promote gallstone dissolution.

The more basic question of what regulates the size of the bile acid pool remains unsolved. As is shown in Figure 3, in the steady state, bile acid synthesis matches faecal excretion and the pool size is independent of bile acid input and output. **Initially,** an acquired reduction in pool size must have been due either to reduced synthesis or increased loss, but the sensing or homeostatic mechanism which resets the pool at the new lower level is not known.

(ii) **Expansion of the bile acid pool.** Can the size of the bile acid pool be increased? Recent studies from our laboratory suggest that in experimental animals the pool may be increased in three different ways:

1) by increasing bile acid absorption from the intestine
2) by increasing bile acid synthesis in the liver
3) by bile acid feeding.

In the rat, active bile acid transport was increased from ileum made hyperplastic by jejunectomy (Perry et al, 1972) and as a result there was a

30% increase in the size of the bile acid pool (Mok et al, 1973). Similarly, when hepatic bile acid synthesis was increased by the microsomal enzyme inducing agent, phenobarbitone, there was a comparable increase in the size of the pool. In Rhesus monkeys with a virtually intact enterohepatic circulation (Dowling et al, 1968) both phenobarbitone (Redinger & Small, 1973) and bile acid feeding (Bell et al, 1972a) also increased the size of the bile acid pool. When the primary bile acid, chenodeoxycholic acid, was fed in a dose of 150mg/day, there was a significant increase in bile volume, bile acid secretion rate and pool size, but there was no change in bile acid concentration nor in the number of times the pool circulated per day (Figure 4).

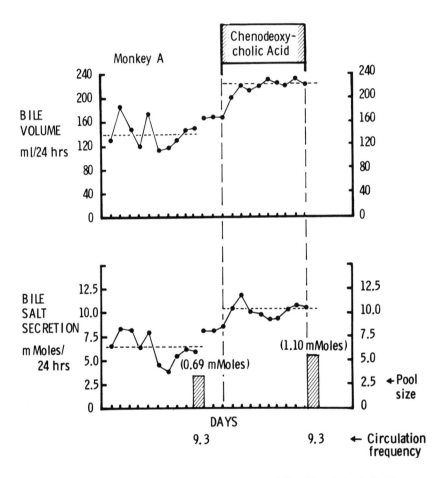

Figure 4. Example of how bile acid feeding can increase bile acid pool size in the Rhesus monkey with an 'intact' enterohepatic circulation. Chenodeoxycholic acid (150mg/day) increased bile volume and bile salt secretion. The bile salt pool size (hatched bars, lower panel) increased from 0.7 to 1.1 mmoles but the number of times the pool circulated/24 hr remained constant at 9.3 (Bell et al, 1972a)

In all three experimental situations, the bile acid pool size was **normal** before treatment and, apart from two of the three monkeys studied by Redinger and Small (1973) expansion of the pool did not improve cholesterol solubility in bile. However, repletion of a **diminished** pool should increase bile acid and phospholipid secretion rates and as a result enhance cholesterol solubility in bile (Wheeler & King, 1972). In the next section we will consider the experimental evidence supporting this thesis.

GALLSTONE DISSOLUTION IN VITRO

(a) Cholesterol Solubility

Cholesterol consists of a steroid ring and a side chain. With the exception of a solitary water-loving group (an hydroxyl group at the 3 beta position) the entire cholesterol molecule is hydrophobic and is, therefore, virtually insoluble in water. Bile salts can solubilise moderate amounts of cholesterol in vitro — differing bile salts having different capacities to dissolve cholesterol Deoxycholate, for example, whether free or conjugated with glycine or taurine, solubilises more cholesterol than cholate or chenodeoxycholate (Neiderhiser & Roth, 1968; Earnest & Admirand, 1971) but the difference between the different bile acids diminishes in the presence of phospholipids (Hegardt & Dam, 1971). Isaksson (1954) showed that cholesterol solubility in bile salt solutions was greatly enhanced by the addition of phospholipids and this observation has been confirmed repeatedly (Johnston & Nakayama, 1957; Nakayama & Johnston, 1960; Neiderhiser et al, 1966; Hegardt & Dam, 1970). The principal phospholipids in human bile are lecithins, which have a uniform effect on cholesterol solubility, irrespective of their variable fatty acid components (Saunders & Wells, 1969; Neiderhiser & Roth, 1972).

The solubility of cholesterol in mixtures of bile salt (sodium cholate) and phospholipid (lecithin) was more accurately defined by Bourgès et al (1967) who plotted their results on triangular coordinates to form a phase diagram (see previous section). In their studies, they defined a boundary zone which indicated the limits of cholesterol solubility both in vitro and in human bile (Admirand & Small, 1968). Recently, the exact position of the boundary line of cholesterol solubility has been challenged. In different studies, different limits for the micellar solubilisation of cholesterol have been defined (Dam & Hegardt, 1971; Mufson et al, 1972; Higuchi et al, 1972; Holtzbach et al, 1972). These apparent variations are largely due to differences in the physicochemical techniques used to define equilibrium conditions for cholesterol solubility (Mufson et al, 1972) and it now seems likely that the true boundary line is nearer the base of the triangle than that suggested by Admirand & Small (1968). However, since it takes 8-14 days to reach this true equilibrium (Mufson et al, 1972) the physicochemically defined boundary may have little relevance to cholesterol solubility in human bile, in which lipid composition may vary considerably throughout the day (Shaffer et al, 1972).

(b) Gallstone Solubility

As with crystalline cholesterol, Isaksson (1954) also showed that intact human cholesterol gallstones dissolved slowly in bile salt solutions but as the bathing detergent solution became saturated with cholesterol, there was a progressive reduction in the rate of dissolution. Gallstone dissolution by bile salt solutions has also been confirmed more recently (Earnest & Admirand, 1971) as has the enhancing effect of adding lecithin to the bile salt solutions (Small, 1970).

GALLSTONE DISSOLUTION IN EXPERIMENTAL ANIMALS

(a) Dissolution in the Gallbladder

It has been known since Naunyn's studies in 1892 that human gallstones, when placed in the gallbladder of the dog, dissolve rapidly, and at least 12 different publications have supported Naunyn's original observation (reviewed by Johnston & Nakayama, 1957). Human gallstones also dissolve rapidly in the gallbladders of other animal species, such as sheep, pigs and goats (Lutton & Large, 1957). In contrast, gallstones placed in the gallbladder of the Rhesus monkey dissolve much more slowly (Nakayama & Johnston, 1960).

These observations may be explained by considering bile lipid composition in the different animal species. Pig and dog bile, for example, contains very little cholesterol, and these undersaturated solutions, therefore, have a large cholesterol solubilising capacity (Small, 1972).

(b) Factors Influencing the Rate of Gallstone Dissolution

We have studied the rate of gallstone dissolution in the bile of Rhesus monkeys, the composition of which (Campbell et al, 1972) is fairly similar to that of humans (Admirand & Small, 1968).

The experimental model originally designed to study the effects of controlled interruption of the enterohepatic circulation (EHC) (Dowling et al, 1968) was modified to include a small glass chamber containing a human gallstone (Figure 5). In this way, the influence of stone composition, bile composition and stone surface area on the rate of gallstone dissolution could all be studied (Bell et al, 1972b).

Figure 6 illustrates the results of one study using this model when bile composition remained constant but when there were different amounts of cholesterol in 3 different stones. As a control, an almost pure cholesterol gallstone (95% cholesterol by weight on chemical assay) was placed in water and removed at regular intervals for weighing. Since cholesterol is virtually insoluble in water, there was no change in the weight of the control stone. In

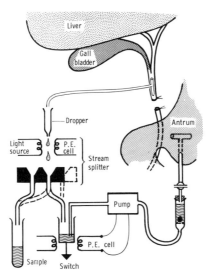

Figure 5. Schematic outline of experimental model used to study the rate of human gall-stone dissolution in Rhesus monkey bile. Bile from a chronic bile fistula was returned to the upper intestine through an electronic stream splitter which diverted every 20th drop of bile to a sampling tube and returned the remaining 95% to the upper intestine, thus maintaining a virtually intact enterohepatic circulation (Dowling et al,1968). The model is modified to include a small glass chamber with a perforated glass platform which supported a human gallstone (Bell et al, 1972b).

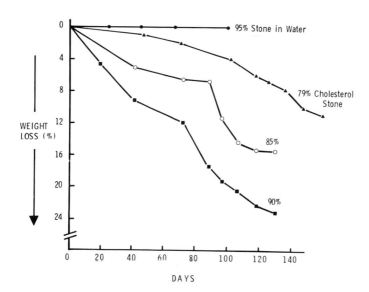

Figure 6. Human cholesterol gallstone dissolution in Rhesus monkey bile in vivo using the model illustration in Figure 5. The most rapid weight loss was seen with the 90% cholesterol gallstone (see text — Bell et al, 1972b).

387

contrast, the three stones exposed to monkey bile, containing 79, 85 and 90% cholesterol respectively, lost weight progressively, the most rapid dissolution being associated with the greatest amount of cholesterol in the stone.

When stone composition remained constant but the percentage saturation of bile changed by only 15%, there was a marked difference in gallstone dissolution rate, the most rapid weight loss being found with the less saturated bile.

Similarly, stone surface area influenced gallstone dissolution rates. When a large, single gallstone segment and 12 small cubic segments of identical chemical composition, and each weighing the same, but with markedly different surface areas, were exposed to bile from the same Rhesus monkey, the rate of dissolution was more rapid with the greater surface area of the 12 small segments, even when measured by crude planimetry. However, scanning electron microscopy shows that the surface architecture of gallstones is often far from smooth (Wolpers, 1972) and while dissolution may be related to the **apparent** surface area, it is impossible to calculate the **true** microsurface area with any degree of accuracy.

Is gallstone dissolution simply a surface phenomenon, or can the detergent action of bile salts penetrate the interstices between the crystalline structure of the stone to leach cholesterol from the interior? Figure 7 (a & b) shows the effect of exposing a human gallstone of mixed composition to the detergent action of dog bile. After exposure to this under-saturated solution, the surface became irregular and pitted with cracks and crevasses which suggest that dissolution is not simply a surface phenomenon but rather that it resembles the disintegration of a block of ice exposed to above zero temperature.

(c) Influence of Calcification on Gallstone Dissolution

In clinical practice, gallstones are frequently found to have a radio-opaque rim due to deposition of calcium salts on the surface of the stone. In vitro studies with dog bile suggest that while calcification markedly inhibits the rate of gallstone dissolution, it does not completely prevent very gradual reduction in gallstone weight.

From these studies of gallstone dissolution in animal bile in vivo and in vitro, it seems that gallstone dissolution is most rapid with small gallstones rich in cholesterol when the bile is less than saturated with cholesterol. The presence of a calcified rim slows, but may not completely prevent, gallstone dissolution.

However, in practical terms, the only variable which may be modified in human gallstone treatment is bile composition.

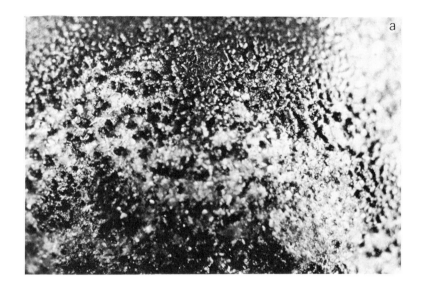

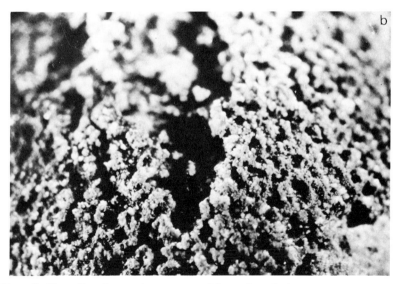

Figure 7. Dissecting microscopic appearance of the surface of a 'mixed' human gallstone (a) before, and (b) after exposure to dog gallbladder bile in vitro. Before dissolution the lighter patches consisted of cholesterol while the darker coarsely granular areas contain calcium salts. After exposure to the detergent action of bile, the cholesterol has been dissolved to give a pitted irregular surface (Bell et al, 1972b)

(a) Phospholipid Feeding

Several studies have suggested that the concentration of phospholipid is low in bile from patients with cholesterol gallstones (Tompkins et al, 1967; Anderson & Bouchier, 1969). It is not surprising, therefore, that feeding phospholipids has been advocated as a method for enhancing cholesterol solubility in bile. However, a brief consideration of phospholipid metabolism after oral feeding suggests that this form of treatment is unlikely to be of practical value in dissolving gallstones.

Lecithin, the principal phospholipid in bile, consists of a phosphoryl choline group with two fatty acid tails. When lecithin is given by mouth, it is hydrolysed in the small bowel lumen by pancreatic phospholipase which removes one fatty acid group from the lecithin molecule to yield the water-soluble lysolecithin. Although lysolecithin is mainly re-esterified within the intestinal epithelium and the newly formed lecithin then transported via lymph chylomicra to the systemic circulation, only a small percentage of this will find its way to the liver, and from thence be excreted in bile. In fact, Saunders (1970) has shown that there is no significant enterobiliary circulation of lecithin. In spite of this, there is some evidence that large doses of lecithin may increase both the phospholipid:cholesterol ratio and the cholesterol holding capacity of T-tube bile (Tompkins et al, 1970). When these authors fed twenty 500mg capsules of commercial 'lecithin' per day to patients recovering from cholecystectomy, they showed that the mean phospholipid: cholesterol ratio increased from 2.9 before treatment to 5.2 after 10 days' therapy. However, there are many problems in interpreting such data. The commercial phospholipid used contained only 32% phosphatidyl choline (lecithin). The studies were carried out on an abnormal population (patients with cholecystectomy for cholelithiasis) in the early stages after surgery when the enterohepatic circulation was at least partially interrupted by T-tube drainage of the common bile duct. There were no control studies during the same period when recovery from surgery spontaneously improves bile composition (Dowling et al, 1970; Small et al, 1972) and since bile salt concentrations were not measured simultaneously the true effect of lecithin feeding on cholesterol solubility cannot be assessed. Furthermore, in another study, feeding 20 G lecithin/day did not change the lecithin:cholesterol ratio in bile-rich duodenal-fluid after 14 days' treatment (Thistle & Schoenfield, 1968). Thus it seems that lecithin feeding will not be useful in gallstone treatment.

(b) Bile Acid Feeding

(i) **Clinical studies with chenodeoxycholic acid.** We have already seen from experimental animal studies that bile acid feeding can increase the size of the bile acid pool (Bell et al, 1972a) and if the pool size was depleted before treatment, this alone should improve cholesterol solubility in bile, irrespective of the type of bile acid fed. Recent evidence suggests that one particular bile acid, chenodeoxycholic acid, may promote gallstone dissolution by a second mechanism. Thistle and Schoenfield (1971a) fed a variety of bile acids to normal volunteers and showed that the only substance to increase the ratio of bile salts + phospholipid (the solubilisers) over cholesterol (the material to be dissolved) was chenodeoxycholic acid. Further studies from the Mayo Clinic (Thistle & Schoenfield, 1971b) showed that this bile acid, when fed to young North American Indian women of the Chippewa tribe who had a 'lithogenic' bile but no gallstones, changed bile from being a supersaturated solution to being a normal micellar solution. Moreover, oral chenodeoxycholic acid (0.75 - 4.5 G/day) given to patients with cholesterol gallstones, expanded their depleted bile acid pool (Danzinger, 1972) and promoted gallstone dissolution in 4 out of 7 patients (Danzinger et al, 1972).

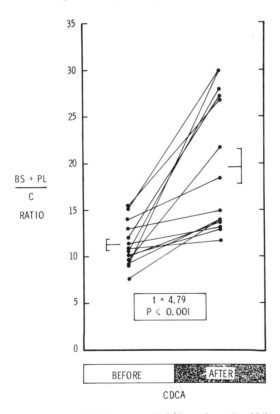

Figure 8. The 'cholesterol solubilising capacity' (the molar ratio of bile salts plus phospholipid over cholesterol) of bile-rich duodenal-fluid before and three months after treatment with chenodeoxycholic acid (0.75-1.25 G/day) in patients with presumed cholesterol gallstones (Bell et al,1972c; Dowling & Bell,1973)

Our own initial experience with chenodeoxycholic acid in the treatment of gallstones with smaller doses (0.5 - 1.25 G/day) than those previously used has recently been reported (Bell et al, 1972c; Dowling & Bell, 1973). After three months' treatment, the cholesterol solubilising capacity of bile (the ratio of bile salts + phospholipid:cholesterol) was increased in every

Table I. Effect of oral chenodeoxycholic acid (0.75 - 1.5 G/day for six months on gallstone size as measured by cholecystography in 15 patients with radiologically 'functioning' gallbladders (Bell et al, 1972c)

Radiolucent gallstones (12 patients)		
Initial gallstone size	Number of patients	Effect of treatment
Small	4	Stones disappeared
Medium	3	Stones significantly smaller
Large	5	No change in gallstone size
Radio-opaque gallstones (3 patients)		
Small	1	Stones disappeared
Medium/Large	2	No changes

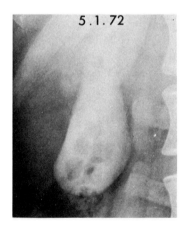 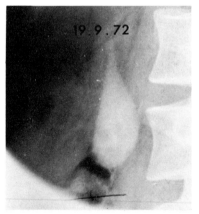

Figure 9. Example of reduction in gallstone size.
(a) Cholecystogram in January, 1972 showing 5 medium sized radiolucent gallstones. Treatment with chenodeoxycholic acid was started in March, 1972.
(b) Repeat cholecystogram (after fatty meal), in September, 1972 showing diminution in gallstone size. The vertebral bodies show that both X-ray films have comparable magnification

patient (Figure 8). The effect of treatment on gallstone size was assessed by cholecystography and the results are summarised in Table I. Of the 12 patients with radiolucent stones after 6 months' treatment, in 4 patients who had small gallstones the stones had disappeared; in 3 patients with medium sized stones there was a significant reduction in gallstone size (Figures 9 a & b) while in 5 patients with large stones there has, as yet, been no change in gallstone size. With the exception of one patient, who had small, faintly calcified gallstones and who had an attack of biliary colic which may well have heralded the disappearance of the gallstones, there has been no change in gallstone size in patients with calcified gallstones.

The results in man, therefore, confirm the general pattern of results seen in experimental animals. The most rapid dissolution occurred with small radiolucent gallstones, presumably rich in cholesterol, with a high surface area:weight ratio.

(ii) Dissolution or disappearance? The response to medical treatment for gallstones is judged on the basis of cholecystographic studies before and after therapy. Accepting the limitations of this technique to demonstrate residual gravel and small stones, does gallstone disappearance really mean that the stones have dissolved?

Spontaneous gallstone disappearance is well recognised and this subject has recently been reviewed (Wolpers, 1968). Some cases of gallstone disappearance are due to small stones passing down the biliary tree: occasionally the stones may disappear due to fistula formation between gallbladder or biliary tree and intestine but there remains a group of patients in whom the gallstones have spontaneously dissolved. However, spontaneous dissolution is comparatively rare and could not explain the results obtained with chenodeoxycholic acid (Bell et al, 1972c). In untreated patients, the spontaneous disappearance rate for single cholesterol stones is 0.8% and for multiple cholesterol stones is 6.7% in 230 patients followed for an average period of 7 years (Wolpers, 1972). In other words, the maximal disappearance rate was less than 1% per year. In our own study, 8 of 15 patients with a radiologically functioning gallbladder showed disappearance or reduction in gallstone size after only 6 months' treatment with chenodeoxycholic acid. However, the most convincing evidence that bile acid feeding causes gallstone dissolution comes from serial X-rays showing progressive reduction in gallstone size (Figure 9 and Danzinger et al, 1972).

(iii) An exclusive response to chenodeoxycholic acid? It is not yet known whether the beneficial action of bile acid feeding is confined to chenodeoxycholic acid or whether other bile acids will be equally effective. The response to treatment with other bile acids is now being tested in carefully controlled prospective double blind clinical trials at Hammersmith Hospital and elsewhere and preliminary studies suggest that chenodeoxycholic acid is indeed superior to the other primary bile acid, cholic acid (Thistle & Hofmann, 1972). Why should this be so? Two possible explanations have been advanced. First, Mosbach (1972) has suggested that while exogenous bile acid feeding ought to suppress endogenous bile acid synthesis from cholesterol, chenodeoxycholic acid does not appear to have this effect. In the rat, sodium taurocholate depressed hepatic cholesterol 7 alpha hydroxylase activity (the rate limiting enzyme in the conversion of cholesterol to bile acids) while sodium taurochenodeoxycholate did not. If these results may be extrapolated to man, it would seem that the benefits of exogenous chenodeoxycholate may be added to unsuppressed endogenous bile acid synthesis. Secondly, bile acids are known to influence both the synthesis and secretion of biliary phospholipids and, to a lesser extent, the secretion of biliary cholesterol. Again, preliminary studies suggest that chenodeoxycholic acid selectively increases phospholipid secretion without a parallel increase in cholesterol output, thus enhancing the cholesterol solubilising capacity of bile (Hoffman et al, 1972).

(iv) Complications of treatment. The complications of bile acid therapy may be considered under two headings: the side effects of chenodeoxycholic acid itself (Table II) and the complications due to gallstones.

Table II. Complications of medical gallstone treatment
(18 patients treated for 6 months)

Due to untreated stones	Due to chenodeoxycholic acid
Cholecystitis (1 patient ➤ surgery)	Gastric irritation (none)
Obstructive jaundice (1 patient ➤ surgery)	Loose stools (in approximately 50% of patients for first few weeks)
Biliary colic (3 patients — conservative treatment)	Hepatic dysfunction (slight rise in hepato-cellular enzymes: low BSP retention)
Dyspeptic symptoms (? improved)	Cholesterol accumulation (no change in serum cholesterol)

Fortunately the possible complications which were predicted for chenodeoxycholic acid treatment (Small, 1971) have not been prominent. Bile acids in the stomach have been implicated as a factor causing gastric ulcer (Rhodes et al, 1969) but none of our patients had gastric symptoms. Loose stools occurred in 50% of the patients during the initial weeks of treatment, but almost invariably settled spontaneously. Cholestasis could occur if lithocholate, the bacterial metabolite of chenodeoxycholic acid was formed (Palmer, 1969) but only trace amounts have been found in bile after treatment (Danzinger et al, 1972) and there has been no rise in serum 'biliary tree' enzymes. The levels of one hepatocellular enzyme (isocitric dehydrogenase) did rise in some patients but there has been no increase in BSP excretion. Hypercholesterolaemia was also predicted as a complication of exogenous bile acid feeding, but there was no change in fasting serum cholesterol levels measured monthly during chenodeoxycholic acid therapy.

Since treatment with chenodeoxycholic acid may take 12-18 months or more, during this time the patient is liable to the complications of any untreated gallstones. These include cholecystitis, which occurred in one patient with a 'non-functioning' gallbladder, and obstructive jaundice, which developed in a second patient who had common duct stones before therapy started. Both of these patients were referred for surgery. Biliary colic, which occurred in three patients, was managed conservatively.

(c) Retained Common Duct Stones

A frequent problem in clinical practice is the stone (or stones) which have been left in the biliary tree after cholecystectomy. Until now, expectant, conservative management and re-operation were the only alternatives available. However, recent studies suggest that dissolution may be possible in situ.

In patients who do not have T-tubes draining the common bile duct, bile acid feeding should again improve cholesterol solubility in bile, and if the mechanical problems of stones in the biliary tree can be avoided, such treatment should be effective in the management of choledocholithiasis. Trials with bile acid feeding in this group of patients are in progress but at present no results are available.

In patients with T-tubes in situ, a different principle has been used with apparent success. Way et al (1972) infused 100 mmolar sodium cholate through the horizontal limb of the T-tube at a rate of 30ml/hr. Here the aim was to provide a high detergent concentration locally rather than to change bile composition in toto. Such large quantities of bile acids passing through the ampulla of Vater cause considerable diarrhoea but feeding high doses of the bile acid binding resin cholestyramine (2 G/hr) minimised this complication.

During control periods when saline was infused through the T-tube there was no change in gallstone size, nor were the stones flushed through the sphincter of Oddi into the duodenum. However, when sodium cholate was infused, 6 out of 8 single stones and 5 out of 9 multiple stones disappeared in 3-14 days. These results are puzzling since the rate of gallstone dissolu-

lution, even for small pure cholesterol stones, is very much slower than that
observed during sodium cholate infusion. Furthermore, other investigators
have been unable to repeat this therapeutic success but if Way et al's (1972)
findings are confirmed, bile acid infusion through T-tubes will be invaluable
for this complication of cholecystectomy. The place of other detergents,
organic solvents and even heparin (Gardner, 1972) as alternatives to sodium
cholate for T-tube infusions has yet to be consolidated.

FUTURE PROBLEMS IN HUMAN GALLSTONE DISSOLUTION

Many problems remain to be answered: Which is the best bile acid to use?
What is the optimum dose? Are there other long term complications of bile
acid treatment? Will synthetic detergents be found to replace naturally
occurring bile acids? Once gallstones have dissolved, will maintenance
therapy be necessary, or will bile composition revert to its abnormal pre-
treatment state when bile acid feeding is stopped? Will gallstones re-form,
and if so, how soon? These questions provide clinical investigators with an
exciting challenge for the future. In the meantime 'cutting for stone' remains
the routine management for most patients when treatment is indicated for
gallstones.

SUMMARY

Human cholesterol gallstones dissolve in solutions of bile salts and particularly in mixtures of bile salts and phospholipids. Cholesterol gallstones also
dissolve in animal bile in vivo, the most rapid dissolution occurring in bile
of animals which has a large cholesterol solubilising capacity. In Rhesus
monkeys with an intact enterohepatic circulation, the most rapid rate of gallstone dissolution was found with small, radiolucent gallstones rich in cholesterol, in bile which was less than fully saturated with cholesterol.

In patients with cholesterol gallstones, there are two metabolic abnormalities: excess secretion of biliary cholesterol and a diminished bile acid pool
associated with an abnormal bile, which is supersaturated with cholesterol.
Since little is known about reducing excess biliary cholesterol secretion,
treatment has been directed towards expansion of the bile acid pool. Experimentally, the bile acid pool may be expanded by increasing intestinal bile
acid absorption, by stimulating hepatic bile acid synthesis and by bile acid
feeding. Bile acid feeding with chenodeoxycholic acid also repletes the bile
acid pool size in gallstone patients, improves cholesterol solubility in bile
and promotes gallstone dissolution. The complications of bile acid treatment
are discussed.

ACKNOWLEDGMENTS

Thanks are due to my former colleague, Dr Donald Small, who stimulated my interest in this exciting area. It is also a pleasure to acknowledge the help of my colleagues, Mrs J White, Drs H Y I Mok, P M Perry, B Whitney and particularly Dr G D Bell, whose work is quoted in this review. I also wish to thank Weddel Pharmaceuticals for their financial support in many of the studies cited in this chapter.

REFERENCES

Admirand, W. H. and Small, D. M. (1968) Journal of Clinical Investigation, **47**, 1043

Anderson, F. and Bouchier, I. A. D. (1969) Nature, **221**, 372

Bell, G. D., Nundy, S. and Dowling, R. H. (1972a) Proceedings of the 9th International Congress in Gastroenterology, Paris, July, 1972

Bell, G. D., Sutor, D. J., Whitney, B. and Dowling, R. H. (1972b) Gut, **13**, 836 (Abstract)

Bell, G. D., Whitney, B. and Dowling, R. H (1972c) Lancet, ii, 1213

Bourgès, M., Small, D. M. and Dervichian, D. G. (1967) Biochimica et biophysica acta, **144**, 189

Campbell, C. B., Burgess, P., Roberts, S. A. and Dowling, R. H. (1972) Australian and New Zealand Journal of Medicine, **1**, 49

Comess, L. J., Bennett, P. H. and Burch, T. A. (1967) New England Journal of Medicine, **277**, 894

Dam, H. and Hegardt, F. G. (1971) Zeitschrift für Ernährungswissenschaft, **10**, 239

Danzinger, R. G. (1972) in 'Bile acids in human diseases', (Ed) P. Back and W Gerok. F. K. Schattauer Verlag, Stuttgart, New York. Page 167

Danzinger, R. G., Hofmann, A. F., Thistle, J. L. and Schoenfield, L. J. (1972) New England Journal of Medicine, **281**, 1

Dowling, R. H., Mack, E., Picott, J., Berger, J. and Small, D. M. (1968) Journal of Laboratory and Clinical Medicine, **72**, 169

Dowling, R. H., Mack, E. and Small, D. M. (1970) Journal of Clinical Investigation, **49**, 232

Dowling, R. H., Mack, E. and Small, D. M. (1971) Journal of Clinical Investigation, **50**, 1917

Dowling, R. H. and Bell, G. D. (1973) Lancet, i, 267 (letter)

Earnest, D. E. and Admirand, W. H. (1971) Gastroenterology, **60**, 772 (Abstract)

Friedman, G. D., Kammel, W. B. and Dawber, T. R. (1966) Journal of Chronic Diseases, **19**, 273

Gardner, B. (1972) in Way et al, 1972 Annals of Surgery, **176**, 347

Grundy, S. M., Adler, A. L. and Metzger, A. L. (1972) Journal of Clinical Investigation, **51**, 3026

Grundy, S. M. and Metzger, A. L. (1972) Gastroenterology, **62**, 1200

Hegardt, F. G. and Dam, H. (1971) Zeitschrift für Ernährungswissenschaft, **10**, 223

Higuchi, W. I., Prakongpan, S., Surpuriya, V. and Young, F. (1972) Science, **178**, 633

Hoffman, N. E., Donald, D. E. and Hofmann, A. F. (1972) Proceedings of American Association for the Study of Liver Diseases, Chicago, October, 1972 (abstract)

Holtzbach, R. T., Marsh, M. and Olszewski, M. (1972) Gastroenterology, **62**, 850 (abstract)

Isaksson, B. (1954) Acta Societatis Medicarum Upsaliensis, **59**, 296

Johnston, C. G. and Nakayama, F. (1957) Archives of Surgery, **75**, 436

Juniper, K. Jr. and Burson, E. N. Jr. (1957) Gastroenterology, **32**, 175

Lutton, R. G. and Large, A. M. (1957) Surgery, **42**, 488

Maki, T. (1966) Annals of Surgery, **164**, 90

Malhotra, S. L. (1968) Gut, **9**, 290

Mok, H. Y. I., Perry, P. M. and Dowling, R. H. (1973) Clinical Science, **44** (in press)

Mosbach, E. H. (1972) in 'Bile acids in human diseases'. (Ed) P. Back and W. Gerok. F. K. Schattauer Verlag, Stuttgart, New York. Page 89

Mufson, D., Meksuwan, K., Zarembo, J. E. and Ravin, L. J. (1972) Science, **177**, 701

Nakayama, F. and Johnston, C. G. (1960) Proceedings of the Society for Experimental and Biological Medicine, **104**, 73

Nakayama, F. and Miyaka, H. (1970) American Journal of Surgery, **120**, 794

Nakayama, F. and van der Linden, W. (1971) American Journal of Surgery, **122**, 8

Naunyn, B. (1892) Klinik der Cholelithiasis Leipzig, F. C. W. Vogel

Neiderhiser, D. H., Roth, H. P. and Webster, L. T. Jr. (1966) Journal of Laboratory and Clinical Medicine, **68**, 90

Neiderhiser, D. H. and Roth, H. P. (1968) Proceedings of the Society for Experimental and Biological Medicine, **128**, 221

Neiderhiser, D. H. and Roth, H. P. (1972) Biochimica et biophysica acta, **270**, 407

Nicholas, P., Rinaudo, P. A. and Conn, H. O. (1972) Gastroenterology, **63**, 112

Northfield, T. C. and Hofmann, A. F. (1972) Proceedings of American Association for the Study of Liver Diseases, Chicago, October, 1972 (abstract)

Palmer, R. H. (1969) in 'Bile salt metabolism'. (Ed) E. Schiff, J. B. Carey Jr and J. M. Dietschy. Charles C Thomas, Springfield, Illinois. Page 184

Perry, P. M., White, J. and Dowling, R. H. (1972) Gut, **13**, 845 (abstract)

Redinger, R. N. and Small, D. M. (1973) Journal of Clinical Investigation, **52**, 161

Rhodes, J., Barnardo, D. E., Phillips, S. F., Raulstad, R. A. and Hofmann, A. F. (1969) Gastroenterology, **57**, 241

Russell, I. S., Wheeler, M. B. and Freake, R. (1968) British Journal of Surgery, **55**, 161

Sampliner, R. E., Bennett, P. H., Comess, L. J., Rose, F. A. and Burch, T. A. (1970) New England Journal of Medicine, **283**, 1358

Saunders, D. R. and Wells, M. A. (1969) Biochimica et biophysica acta, **176**, 828

Saunders, D. R. (1970) Gastroenterology, **59**, 848

Shaffer, E. A., Braasch, J. W. and Small, D. M. (1972) New England Journal of Medicine, **287**, 1317

Small, D. M. (1970) Advances in Internal Medicine, **16**, 243

Small, D. M. (1971) New England Journal of Medicine, **284**, 214

Small, D. M. (1972) Postgraduate Medicine, **51**, 187

Small, D. M., Dowling, R. H. and Redinger, R. N. (1972) Archives of Internal Medicine, **130**, 552

Sutor, D. J. and Wooley, S. E. (1971) Gut, **12**, 55

Sutor, D. J. and Gaston, P. J. (1972) Gut, **13**, 64

Swell, L., Bell, C. C. Jr. and Entenman, C. (1968) Biochimica et biophysica acta, **164**, 278

Thistle, J. L. and Schoenfield, L. J. (1968) Clinical Research, **16**, 450 (abstract)

Thistle, J. L. and Schoenfield, L. J. (1971a) Gastroenterology, **61**, 488

Thistle, J. L. and Schoenfield, L. J. (1971b) New England Journal of Medicine, **284**, 177

Thistle, J. L. and Hofmann, A. F. (1972) Proceedings of American Association for the Study of Liver Diseases, Chicago, October, 1972 (abstract)

Tompkins, R. K., Cornwell, D. G., Sprecher, D. W. and Zollinger, R. M. (1967) Surgical Forum, **18**, 411

Tompkins, R. K., Burke, L. G., Zollinger, R. M. and Cornwell, D. G.

(1970) Annals of Surgery, **172**, 936

Way, L. W., Admirand, W. H. and Dunphy, J. E. (1972) Annals of Surgery, **176**, 347

Wheeler, H. O. and King, K. K. (1972) Journal of Clinical Investigation, **51**, 1337

Wolpers, C. (1968) Deutsche Medizinische Wochenschrift, **93**, 2525

Wolpers, C. (1972) in 'Bile acids in human diseases'. (Ed) P. Back and W. Gerok. F. K. Schattauer Verlag, Stuttgart, New York. Page 171.

The Gut as an Endocrine Organ

A G E PEARSE

"The stomach, whatever sentimentalists may say to the
contrary, being the true seat of the emotions."

Norman Douglas: Old Calabria

I suppose that nobody would question the fact that the gastrointestinal tract
produces a number of polypeptides which have been established, by proper
physiological tests, as hormones. On this basis alone the gut could properly
be regarded as an endocrine organ but the accumulated weight of evidence
has so far been considered insufficient to warrant such status. Investigations and speculations on gut endocrine functions have, in the past, been
directed chiefly to the hormonal activities of one section of its length either
upon another section, or upon the exocrine or endocrine pancreas. More
distant effects, physiological or otherwise, have received much less
consideration.

POLYPEPTIDES OF GASTROINTESTINAL ORIGIN

Those polypeptide products of the gut which have achieved at least the res-
pectability of a certified number of amino acid residues are listed in Table I.
The presence of a bracket around any number indicates a certain degree of
doubt as to its veracity.

Table I. Gastrointestinal polypeptides

Group I	Group II		Group III	Group IV
Gastrin 17	Gut glucagon	(29)	Motilin 22	–
CCK 33	Secretin	27		
	VIP	28		
	GIP	43		

A lack of structural criteria thus excludes bulbogastrone, enterogastrone and
other gastrones, for instance, and also incretin and a variety of similarly
ill-characterised products. Gut insulin is omitted, because it is recorded
only in the rat, and likewise Substance P for the joint reason that it is usually

400

derived, or at least obtained, from the hypothalamus. It is probably a neurotransmitter rather than a hormone (there is not much difference between these two at times).

The three known hormones of the pancreatic islets are shown in Table II. It is impossible to consider the endocrine gut and the islets as separate entities, different as their products may be in chemical respects and as their cells may be in terms of cytochemistry and ultrastructure.

Table II. Pancreatic polypeptides

Group I	Group II	Group III	Group IV
Gastrin (17)	Glucagon 29	-	Insulin 21+30

The relationships between the various groups, which are expressed in the two tables, usually amount to shared amino acid sequences of significant length. These sequences may or may not, of course, confer similarity of biological effects. The relationship between cholecystokinin-pancreozymin (CCK) and gastrin is confined to the terminal pentapeptide GLY-TRP-MET-ASP-PHE-NH$_2$, as shown by the studies respectively of Mutt and Jorpes (1968) and of Gregory et al (1964). This C-terminal sequence they share with the decapeptide caerulein from **Hyla caerulea** (Anastasi et al, 1967). A morphologist's view of the structure of CCK is shown in the molecular model,

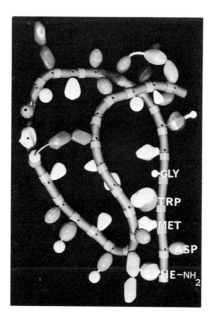

Figure 1. Molecular model of porcine CCK-PZ in which the amino acids of the C-terminal pentapeptide (glycine, tryptophan, methionine, aspartic acid, phenylalanine-amide) are labelled

constructed from Biobits (Smith & Smith, 1969), which is illustrated in
Figure 1. The C-terminal pentapeptide is labelled.

There are multiple similarities in the structures of glucagon and secretin
(Mutt et al, 1970) and between these two and gastric inhibitory polypeptide
(GIP – Brown & Dryburgh, 1971). Glucagon and secretin, but not GIP, share
their N-terminal histidyl-seryl sequence with another product of the gut, the
so-called vasoactive intestinal polypeptide (VIP – Said & Mutt, 1972). An
essentially dissimilar polypeptide is motilin, extracted from the first part of
the small intestine by Brown et al (1972), which resembles no known gastrointestinal hormone or polypeptide in terms of its chemical structure.

CELLULAR ORIGINS OF GASTROINTESTINAL POLYPEPTIDES

The cells which are responsible for the production of the polypeptide hormones of gut and pancreas belong to the so-called APUD series (Pearse,
1968 a & b, 1969; Pearse & Welsch, 1968). Historically they can now be
seen to be related to the cells (Helle Zellen) of the diffuse endocrine organ
of Feyrter (1938; 1954), but their recognition was independent of this concept,
being based on their common cytochemical and functional characteristics.
From the initial letters of the most constant of these cytochemical properties
the term APUD is derived (Amine content and/or Amine Precursor Uptake
and Decarboxylation).

Of the 20 members of the series no less than 11 are present in the gastrointestinal tract, and 3 in the pancreatic islets. The list, as it stands at
present, modified from the original list of the Wiesbaden agreement*, is
given in Table III.

Table III. Modified Wiesbaden classification

	Description(s)	Wiesbaden (amended)	Equivalent in Pancreas	Product
S	G, RO, V etc	G	none	Gastrin
T	A, II	A	A	Enteroglucagon
O	X, ND, III	D	D	-
M				
A	ECL, I variant	ECL	none	-
C				
H	EC, II	EC	EC	-
I	Large granule, II	L	A	Enteroglucagon
N	Small granule, IV	S	-	Secretin
T				
E	Intermediate, S variant	I	I	-
S				
T	D, X, V	D	D	-
I				
N	D_1	D_1	-	GIP
E	EC, I	EC	EC	-

* Proceedings of International Symposium Wiesbaden, 1969. F. K.
  Schattauer Verlag, Stuttgart.

The three APUD cells of the pancreatic islets are now usually called B (insulin), A (glucagon) and D (gastrin). There must be no confusion between this last cell and the gastrin-secreting G cell of the pyloric antrum. The two cells differ widely in their cytochemical and ultrastructural characteristics for reasons which are not well understood but which are considered to be due primarily to differences in the storage form of their respective gastrins.

DEMONSTRATION AND IDENTIFICATION OF ENDOCRINE CELLS IN THE GUT

The whole series of studies carried out by Feyrter on his diffuse endocrine (clear cell) system was based on two characteristics, or three if the clarity (emptiness) of the clear cell in conventionally stained preparations is counted. The other characteristics were argentaffinity (capacity to reduce silver solutions) and argyrophilia (capacity to take up and retain silver salts subsequently reduced by chemical methods). The second of these procedures remains popular as a means of demonstrating, in one preparation, the great majority of the granulated endocrine cells which are present at each level in

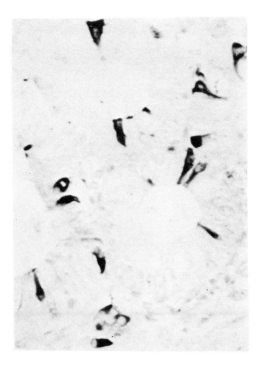

Figure 2. Preparation of human gastric fundus stained by the Grimelius technique. Shows a number of endocrine cells, only one or two of which are enterochromaffin cells. Note apical extensions, reaching the gland lumen in many instances. x 360

403

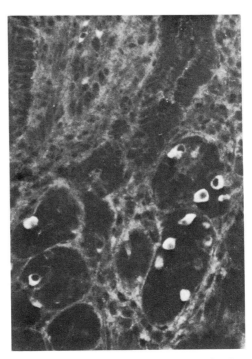

Figure 3. Indirect immunofluorescence shows the normal G cell population of
the mid-zone of the human pyloric glands.   x 320

the gut.   A silver-stained preparation of the mid-zone of the glands in the
human gastric fundus is shown in Figure 2. Other staining and cytochemical
techniques have been used for distinction of the various cell types from each
other but, today, virtually all such identification is carried out by immunofluorescence, for specific hormones or polypeptides, combined with ultrastructural studies.   The normal G (gastrin) cell population of the human
antrum is shown in Figure 3 while Figures 4 and 5 show, respectively, the
immunofluorescence of gut glucagon and, the ultrastructural appearance of,
a typical A cell of the fundus.   At the present time only five of the eleven
endocrine cells of the gut have been shown to be associated with a definite
polypeptide product.   These are the G cell (**gastrin** – McGuigan, 1968;
Bussolati & Pearse, 1970; Pearse & Bussolati, 1970), the S cell (**secretin** –
Bussolati et al, 1971; Polak et al, 1971a), The L cell (**enteroglucagon**) and the
A cell (**enteroglucagon** – Polak et al, 1971b; Polak et al, 1971d), and the D_1
cell (**gastric inhibitory polypeptide** — Polak et al, 1973a).

It is usually considered that the hormonal product of the enterochromaffin
cell is 5-hydroxytryptamine and it cannot be doubted that this is at least one
of its products. Since, however, the storage granule protein (polypeptide) is
also secreted, it remains possible that this has a physiological function.

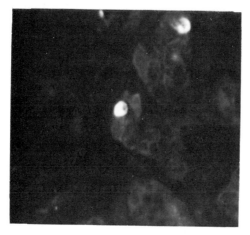

Figure 4. Indirect immunofluorescence shows, in the fundic glands of a young dog, two (enteroglucagon) cells reacting with anti-porcine pancreatic glucagon. x 400

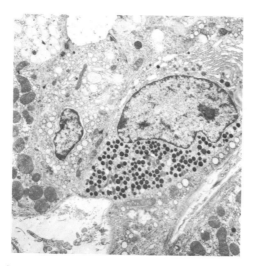

Figure 5. Electronmicrograph of a preparation from human fundus. Shows a typical A cell with round, electron-dense, granules which are situated predominately at the base of the cell.
x 9000

THE DISTRIBUTION OF ENDOCRINE CELLS IN THE GUT

Whatever may ultimately be shown to be the true function of each and every type of endocrine cell in the gastrointestinal mucosa it can be said with certainty that there is a spectrum of endocrine cells, extending from eosophagus to rectum, which are capable of responding not only to autonomic stimuli, but also to mechanical (pressure) and intraluminal (physical or chemical) stimuli, by discharge of their secretory granules directly into the bloodstream. The zones occupied by each cell type have no distinct boundaries. Several cell types are present together in any given territory, described in gross terms. In the histological sense, however in terms of levels within the gastrointestinal glands, the tenancy of a single cell type is often quite distinct. The situation is illustrated diagrammatically in Figure 6.

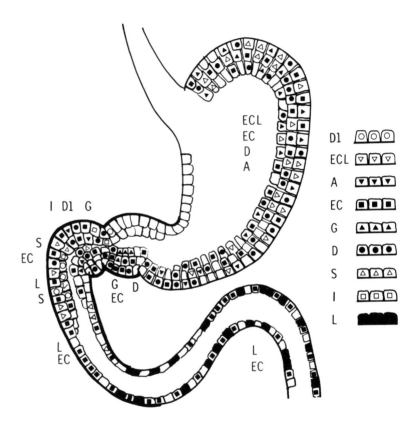

Figure 6. The Gastrointestinal Endocrine Cellular Spectrum

QUANTIFICATION OF THE NORMAL ENDOCRINE CELL

Using a Television Image Conversion Analyser it is possible to compute the relative area of the glands occupied by endocrine cells. For this purpose these can be demonstrated either in toto, as by the Grimelius (1968) technique illustrated in Figure 2, or by specific immunofluorescence. If the total volume occupied by the glands of any region can be ascertained, it is then

406

possible to estimate roughly the total endocrine cell mass of that region.
Calculations carried out in this way for the fundus of the human stomach
indicate that the volume of endocrine cells is at least equivalent to that of
the pituitary gland. If the antrum is added it must necessarily be even
greater. It is probable that the mass of any single endocrine cell in the gut
will prove greater than that of the parathyroid glands.

QUANTIFICATION OF ENDOCRINE HYPERPLASIAS

In this category, published work has been confined largely to the gastrin-
secreting G cells (Polak et al, 1971c; Polak et al, 1972). The degree of
antral G cell hyperplasia has been assessed in samples from cases of hyper-
parathyroidism, acromegaly, Type I Zollinger-Ellison Syndrome and
pernicious anaemia. In the first and second of these conditions the degree of
hyperplasia may rise to as high as 16x. In the third condition it may exceed
30x and in pernicious anaemia it is possibly even higher. Because in this
condition many of the antral G cells are empty, and their immunofluorescent
gastrin content thus imperceptible, an accurate estimate is difficult to obtain.

PHYSIOLOGICAL AND PATHOLOGICAL RESPONSES IN
GUT ENDOCRINE CELLS

In this field of investigation little effective work has yet been done. Forss-
mann and Orci (1969) demonstrated a secretory cycle in the gastrin-producing
(G) cells of the pyloric antrum in the cat, by alternate fasting and feeding,
and Fujita and Kobayashi (1971) described the release of granules from the
D-like cell of the canine pylorus after administration of hydrochloric acid.
Both these studies were carried out with the electron microscope.

Little is known of the response of the endocrine cells in pathological
disorders. Changes in the fundus in pernicious anaemia were described by
Polak et al (1971e) and in the antrum in this condition by Creutzfeldt et al
(1971) and by Polak et al (1973b). The field remains an exceedingly promising one for future investigations.

CONCLUSION

The internal secretions of the gut were formerly considered to act locally,
on neighbouring regions of the gastrointestinal tract or at most, on the
closely associated exocrine pancreas and gallbladder. The close relationship
between the gut and the endocrine pancreas was expressed by Unger and
Eisentraub (1969) in the so-called entero-insular axis. It is not sufficiently
appreciated that there is a close relationship between the gut APUD cells and
those situated elsewhere (Pearse & Polak, 1971), although Unger (1971)
suggested that 'the gut is a large endocrine gland that sends a signal to the
appropriate homeostatic regulator, depending on the character and magnitude
of an incoming solute', and Care et al (1971) have shown, for instance, that

gastrin (pentagastrin) stimulates the secretion of calcitonin. These relationships require much further study and elucidation.

It can be assumed that absolutely nothing can happen in the gut, by eating and drinking, or to the gut, by autonomic stimulation, without a secretory response from some of its endocrine cells. Under normal conditions the balance of these endocrine secretions, acting locally or on neighbouring or distant cells or organs, is finely maintained. In abnormal conditions, however, the polypeptides secreted by the gut endocrine cells (or their products) may stimulate their distant APUD relations to unphysiological activity. Total discharge of one or many of the endocrine cell types in the gut may occur through physiological, pathological, or even psychological stimuli. The resulting rise in circulating level of any hormone (or breakdown product thereof) may cause widespread systemic upset or even central vascular upsets like migraine.

"If I had control of their" (the Italians') "nutrition for a few centuries I would undertake to alter their whole outlook on life, to convert them from utilitarians into romantics – were such a change desirable." This is perhaps no place to debate this particular hypothesis which is derived, as is my dedicatory sentence, from Norman Douglas. It may be appropriate to suggest, however, that the somatic and psychological expression of the gut as an organ of nutrition may be effected not only by absorption of exogenous materials but also through its multiplicity of internal secretions.

REFERENCES

Anastasi, A., Erspamer, V. and Endean, R. (1967) Experientia, **23**, 699
Brown, J. C. and Dryburgh, J. R. (1971) Canadian Journal of Biochemistry and Physiology, **49**, 867
Brown, J. C., Cook, M. A. and Dryburgh, J. R. (1972) Gastroenterology, **62**, 401
Bussolati, G., Capella, C., Solcia, E., Vassallo, G. and Vezzadini, P. (1971) Histochemie, **26**, 218
Bussolati, G. and Pearse, A. G. E. (1970) Histochemie, **21**, 1
Care, A. D., Bates, R. F. L., Swaminathan, R. and Ganguli, P. C. (1971) Journal of Endocrinology, **51**, 735
Creutzfeldt, W., Arnold, R., Creutzfeldt, C., Feurle, G. and Ketterer, H. (1971) European Journal of Clinical Investigation, **1**, 461
Feyrter, F. (1938) 'Über diffuse endokrine epitheliale Organe'. J. A. Barth, Leipzig
Feyrter, F. (1954) 'Über die peripheren endokrinen (parakrinen) Drüsen des Menschen', W. Maudrich, Vienna
Forssmann, W. G. and Orci, L. (1969) Z. Zellforsch, **101**, 419
Fujita, T. and Kobayashi, S. (1971) Z. Zellforsch, **116**, 52
Gregory, R. A., Hardy, P. M., Jones, D. S., Kenner, G. W. and Sheppard, R. C. (1964) Nature (London), **204**, 931
Grimelius, L. (1968) Acta Societatis medicorum Upsaliensis, **273**, 243
McGuigan, J. E. (1968) Gastroenterology, **55**, 315
Mutt, V. and Jorpes, J. E. (1968) European Journal of Biochemistry, **6**, 156
Mutt, V., Jorpes, J. E. and Magnusson, S. (1970) European Journal of Biochemistry, **15**, 513
Pearse, A. G. E. (1968a) Proceedings of the Royal Society. Series B. Biological Sciences, **170**, 71

Pearse, A. G. E. (1968b) In 'The Physiology of Gastric Secretion', Universitetsforlaget, Oslo, page 92

Pearse, A. G. E. (1969) Journal of Histochemistry and Cytochemistry, 17, 303

Pearse, A. G. E. and Bussolati, G. (1970) Gut, 11, 646

Pearse, A. G. E. and Polak, J. M. (1971) Histochemie, 27, 96

Pearse, A. G. E. and Welsch, U. (1968) Z. Zellforsch, 92, 596

Polak, J. M., Bloom, S., Coulling, I. and Pearse, A. G. E. (1971a) Gut, 12, 605

Polak, J. M., Bloom, S., Coulling, I. and Pearse, A. G. E. (1971b) Gut, 12, 311

Polak, J. M., Bloom, S. R., Kuzio, M., Brown, J. C. and Pearse, A. G. E. (1973a) Gut (in press)

Polak, J. M., Bussolati, G. and Pearse, A. G. E. (1971c) Virchows Archiv Abteilung B. Zellpathologie, 9, 187

Polak, J. M., Coulling, I., Bloom, S. and Pearse, A. G. E. (1971d) Scandinavian Journal of Gastroenterology, 6, 739

Polak, J. M., Coulling, I., Doe, W. and Pearse, A. G. E. (1971e) Gut, 12, 319

Polak, J. M., Hoffbrand, A. V., Reed, P., Bloom, S. and Pearse, A. G. E. (1973b) Scandinavian Journal of Gastroenterology (in press)

Polak, J. M., Stagg, B. and Pearse, A. G. E. (1972) Gut, 13, 501

Said, S. I. and Mutt, V. (1972) European Journal of Biochemistry, 28, 199

Smith, I. and Smith, M. J. (1969) Education in Chemistry, 6, 2

Unger, R. H. (1971) New England Journal of Medicine, 285, 443

Unger, R. H. and Eisentraub, A. M. (1969) Archives of Internal Medicine, 123, 261

Radioimmunoassay of Gastrointestinal Hormones

S R BLOOM

The first hormone which was recognised 71 years ago, came from the gastro-intestinal tract and was called secretin (Bayliss & Starling, 1902). In spite of this early start the concept of gastrointestinal endocrinology has only recently become important. The actions of known hormones are still being ascertained and their overall effect is unknown. Professor Pearse in his paper has mentioned that the histology of the gut shows a very considerable mass of endocrine tissue and this implies a significant function in normal physiology. There are several human diseases of the gut where hormonal imbalance may be considered to be the underlying cause. Perhaps the most important example is duodenal ulceration but motility problems such as spastic colon and unexplained diarrhoea or constipation can also be included. As well as their role in normal gut physiology gastrointestinal hormones may well play an important part in general metabolism. The composition of ingested food is sampled first by mucosal endocrine cells which are there-fore in a good position to elicit a rapid metabolic response. A classical example of this is the much larger insulin release after oral glucose than after the same amount of glucose given intravenously (McIntyre et al, 1964). It is thus conceivable that metabolic disease may also be the result of gut endocrine pathology.

BIOASSAY

The main reason for the primitive state of gastrointestinal endocrinology was until recently the reliance on bioassays. These have three main drawbacks. Firstly they are very insensitive and thus cannot measure hormone levels in plasma. Secondly they are not specific and only give accurate results if a single completely purified hormone is used. Finally, such assays are very laborious and thus they are too expensive for use in routine patient care.

RADIOIMMUNOASSAY

The first radioimmunoassay was reported in 1959 by Berson and Yalow. This type of assay is not only highly specific and extremely sensitive, but its reagents are easy to handle. Indeed many firms are now profiting from the sale of radioimmunoassay kits through the post. A trained technician can handle at least two hundred plasma samples a day so that labour costs are not excessive. In spite of this, several different laboratories are in the process of automating the system. Thus once an acceptable radioimmunoassay has been developed exploitation should be rapid. The essential requirements are milligrams of the partially purified hormone, to raise an antiserum and micrograms of completely pure material for use as standards and for iodination.

It is important when interpreting immunoassay results to know where errors may occur. Firstly, there may be methodological errors in the assay, for example the use of bad standards that have become degraded with time, or radioactive tracer hormone that has been structurally damaged during iodination. Secondly, breakdown of hormone may occur in the blood withdrawn from the patient. This can be prevented by addition of an inhibitor and rapid centrifugation so that the plasma can quickly be deep frozen. Thirdly, the measurement of a hormone in plasma depends on estimating the percentage of that hormone bound by antibody. Any factor which impairs antibody binding therefore appears to be similar to the hormone and gives falsely high answers. Such factors include raised blood urea, abnormal plasma proteins and haemoglobin released by haemolysis during blood sampling. Finally, errors may occur due to the wrong specificity of the antibody used. This can either be too wide, in which case the assay will measure also other related hormones, or too narrow so that the assay is very good at measuring breakdown fragments without biological importance. Thus, there are at least four important ways of getting totally erroneous results. Radioimmunoassays are also relatively inaccurate. The same sample assayed in two assays rarely gives answers less than 10% apart. However, this is of little consequence as significant changes in hormone level are usually much in excess of 100%.

SOURCES OF PURE HORMONE

Before a hormone can be measured by radioimmunoassay it must be obtained pure. The gut hormones were not completely purified until recently and this is the main reason why their radioimmunoassays are only just being developed.

The peptide hormones of the gastrointestinal tract are all rapidly destroyed by proteolysis and yet have to be extracted from tissues extremely rich in proteolytic enzymes. The endocrine cells are not gathered in a single organ, as elsewhere in the body, but are scattered diffusely in the

411

mucosa. Thus, the very small quantities of labile hormone have to be snatched away from rapid destruction by enzymes. Many techniques have been tried but the one that has proved most commonly successful is to start by plunging the fresh tissues into boiling water which quickly destroys the proteolytic enzymes. Professors Jorpes and Mutt were the first to purify one of the gastrointestinal hormones when they obtained pure secretin in 1961. For 10mg of hormone they required the guts of 10,000 pigs. Since then they have purified cholecystokinin and pancreozymin (Jorpes et al, 1964) and shown these two hormonal activities to be inseparable, in other words, produced by a single substance. Secretin is unstable, losing all biological activity in aqueous solution in a few hours. Pancreozymin cholecystokinin is even more unstable, and it has proved very difficult to obtain significant quantities of the pure hormone.

Recently Professor Mutt has investigated the presence of other peptides in the final liquors and purified two substances that appear biologically active, gastric inhibitory peptide and vasoactive intestinal peptide. Gastric inhibitory peptide (Brown et al, 1970), which is obtained from the 10% pure cholecystokinin, can inhibit even histamine stimulated gastric secretion and therefore may be identical with enterogastrone. Vasoactive intestinal peptide (Said & Mutt, 1970) which comes from the final secretin purification fractions, causes vasodilation and also stimulates pancreatic bicarbonate flow. It seems likely that further biologically active peptides will be extracted and it is necessary to decide if such substances warrant the term hormone. This is most convincingly done by measuring the rise in plasma peptide level by radioimmunoassay after natural stimuli, such as food ingestion, and comparing it with the plasma level produced by the least amount of the purified substance necessary to produce a biological effect. This test has not been applied to any of the peptides mentioned so far. Gastrin, on the other hand, has proved to be a hormone by these criteria. It was first obtained pure in 1964 by Gregory and Tracy by similar methods to those used for secretin and later synthesised (Anderson et al, 1964) and thus made available in bulk. The main action of gastrin is to stimulate acid production from the stomach. The synthetic C terminal fragment does this every bit as effectively as the whole molecule and is now in routine clinical use as a gastric function test, replacing the histamine test.

PLASMA GASTRIN

Gastrin is released from the antrum of the stomach by several stimuli, including neutralisation of gastric acid, distension, protein ingestion and hypoglycaemia (Ganguli & Hunter, 1972; Stadil, 1972). Research is in progress to find a suitable maximal stimulus for gastrin release so that a measure of the functioning mass of gastrin cells can be obtained. Because of the pos-

Table I. Fasting plasma gastrin levels in pg per ml in controls and duodenal ulcer patients

		Controls	DU
A	Byrnes et al, 1970	400	1300
	Reeder et al, 1970	63	106
	Feurle et al, 1972*	100	240
B	Hansky and Cain, 1969	113	53
	Trudeau and McGuigan, 1971	85	78
	Stadil and Rehfeld, 1971	93	76
	Ganguli and Hunter, 1972	105	91
	Schrumpf and Sand, 1972	62	62

*Approximate values only

sibility that duodenal ulceration might be caused by high gastrin levels, several research groups have examined fasting blood from normal patients and patients with duodenal ulcers. The results are not in agreement (Table I).

The reason for the discrepancy between the group A and the group B results shown in the table is unknown. The majority of the workers in the field now favour the interpretation of group B which suggests that gastrin levels are slightly lower in duodenal ulcer patients passively reflecting the higher acid output, and that gastrin is not important in aetiology. Patients with gastric ulcer, hypochlorhydria, achlorhydria and pernicious anaemia have elevated plasma gastrins (Ganguli & Hunter, 1972), presumably because of lack of gastric acid to inhibit gastrin release.

In 1955, Zollinger & Ellison described a syndrome of excessive gastric acid secretion and severe peptic ulceration associated with an endocrine tumour of the pancreas. Gastrin was isolated from the tumour in 1967 by Gregory and colleagues and following the development of a radioimmunoassay very high plasma gastrin levels were found (McGuigan & Trudeau, 1968).

Until recently the diagnosis of the Zollinger-Ellison syndrome was made by gastric acid studies alone, but now help is obtained from the fasting gastrin level which is always above the range in normal subjects. Patients with pernicious anaemia also have elevated fasting gastrin levels, but are unlikely to have duodenal ulceration and so do not enter the differential diagnosis. In a recent series of patients with the Zollinger-Ellison syndrome (Lewin et al, 1972) under half had gastric acid secretory patterns suggestive of the disease, but all had diagnostic plasma gastrin elevation.

413

A single fasting blood sample is very much more convenient than a nasogastric tube and therefore plasma gastrin measurement is now the test of choice for screening duodenal ulcer patients.

SECRETIN

Radioimmunoassay of secretin has proved difficult because it has no tyrosine for coupling with radioactive iodine. The use of synthetic secretin with a tyrosine substituted for the N terminal histidine overcomes this problem (Bloom & Ogawa, 1973). Natural secretin is very unstable and care must be taken both in the collection of plasma specimens and during the assay to prevent proteolysis by the addition of the proteolytic enzyme inhibitor aprotinin (Trasylol).

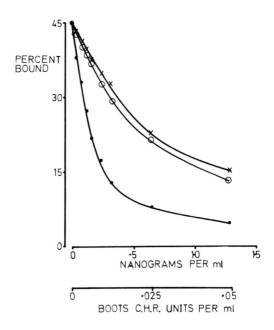

Figure 1. Standard curves obtained with Squibb synthetic secretin X and pure porcine secretin O, both in nanograms, and Boots secretin ●, measured in Crick Harper Raper units. From the curves one 100 unit vial of Boots secretin is equivalent to 10μg of pure porcine secretin

Using pure natural porcine secretin from the Karolinska Institute, Stockholm, or Squibb synthetic secretin as standards, Boots secretin appears to contain 10μg per standard vial (Figure 1). Bioassay (Grossman, 1969), however, would indicate it contained only a third of this quantity and this suggests the presence of a large amount of immunoreactive material whose biological action is impaired. The unknown effect of this degraded material and the fact that Boots secretin also contains enteroglucagon, vasoreactive intestinal peptide and, on occasions, insulin suggests that results previously obtained with this product ought to be checked with the pure material.

Fasting levels of secretin are below 100 pg/ml and are lowered by alkali and raised with acid ingestion (Figure 2). Secretin levels are not altered by oral glucose (Bloom & Ogawa, 1973). Preliminary studies (Bloom et al, 1973c) show that an amount of intraduodenal 0.1N HCl just sufficient to inhibit pentagastrin-stimulated gastric acid production causes a rise in plasma

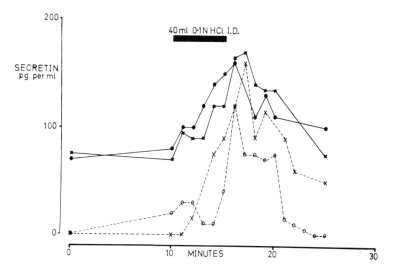

Figure 2. Peripheral plasma secretin levels following intraduodenal acid infusions in four volunteers. Two had a previous vagotomy and pyloroplasty, indicated by dotted lines

secretin of about 150 pg/ml. Infusion of pure secretin to produce similar inhibition of gastric acid results in plasma secretin levels that are several fold higher. This indicates that the release of secretin by acid is not the sole mechanism for gastric acid inhibition. No study has yet been undertaken to examine secretin levels in duodenal ulcer patients.

PANCREATIC GLUCAGON

Pancreatic glucagon is considered with the other gastrointestinal hormones because it bears a close structural resemblance to secretin, enteroglucagon and gastric inhibitory peptide and also because it has a wide range of gastrointestinal actions. These include stimulation of bile flow and intestinal secretion, inhibition of gastric acid and pancreatic juice flow, and inhibition of gut motility.

415

Basal levels are under 100 pg/ml and rise by about 50 pg/ml after eighteen hours starvation. Glucagon is released by elevated plasma amino acids and also by pancreozymin, itself released by intraduodenal amino acids. Pancreatic glucagon shows a moderate rise during hypoglycaemia and because of its classical action in releasing liver glycogen, glucagon has been thought of as a hormone of glucose lack.

Direct stimulation of the splanchnic nerves in the adrenalectomised calf produces a very large rise in peripheral plasma pancreatic glucagon - Figure 3 (Bloom et al, 1973b). The peak rise in response to fairly severe insulin hypoglycaemia is less than a tenth as great.

In conscious baboons, trained to sit quietly in a restraining chair, fear induced by a sudden very loud noise causes a large and rapid elevation in plasma glucagon - Figure 4 (Bloom et al, 1973a). This glucagon rise is simi-lar in pattern to the response to splanchnic nerve stimulation, and again many

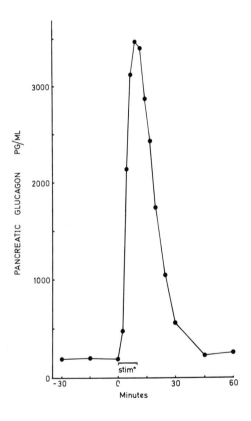

Figure 3. Mean peripheral plasma glucagon levels in two Jersey calves under Nembutal anaesthesia. The bar indicates a ten minute splanchnic nerve stimulation at 10 cps

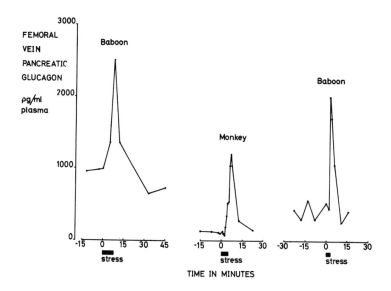

Figure 4. Effect of sudden loud noise in three chair-restrained baboons or monkeys on the peripheral plasma pancreatic glucagon concentration

fold larger than that seen with hypoglycaemia. Glucagon is therefore better regarded as a hormone of stress, causing elevation of blood glucose in preparation for an emergency. Its gastrointestinal actions, such as general inhibition of motility and acid secretion, now become more understandable as being appropriate to a stress situation.

ENTEROGLUCAGON

Enteroglucagon was discovered because of its interference in the radioimmunoassay for pancreatic glucagon. It has not so far been purified because it is very unstable in dilute solution. In the absence of any pure hormone it has to be assayed by utilising its cross reaction with certain pancreatic glucagon antibodies. Unlike secretin and pancreozymin, enteroglucagon is maximal in the lower small intestine and this could indicate a different type of function. A patient with an enteroglucagon tumour (Bloom, 1972) showed villous hypertrophy and jejunal stasis (Gleeson et al, 1971). These actions may indicate a role for enteroglucagon in preventing unabsorbed food passing too low in the small intestine and so being wasted.

Enteroglucagon is released by sugars and long chain triglycerides and in normal persons an enteroglucagon rise is easily detectable after a 50g oral glucose load. Levels are more than proprtionately larger after a 100g load, however, and much greater still after 200g. Presumably this is because relatively more of the glucose can reach the enteroglucagon cells in

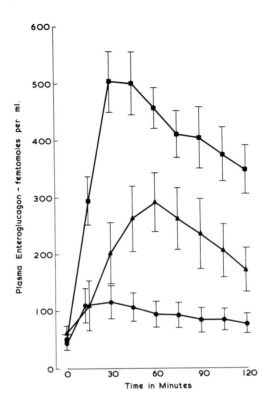

Figure 5. Mean values of plasma enteroglucagon after oral glucose. The zero point represents the average of the two fasting values. Preoperative patients are represented by ●———●, symptom free postoperative patients ▲———▲ , and post-operative patients with the dumping syndrome ■———■ . SEM indicated as vertical bars. Reproduced by kind permission of the editor of the Lancet

the jejunum and ileum by overwhelming the efficient absorption processes in the upper intestine.

After gastric operations, and particularly when dumping symptoms occur, glucose moves extremely rapidly down the small intestine and so releases very large amounts of enteroglucagon - Figure 5 (Bloom et al, 1972). Entero-glucagon release is therefore an indirect measure of small bowel motility and it is interesting to note that its release has also been found excessive in reactive hypoglycaemia (Rehfeld et al, 1973).

OTHER HORMONES

No satisfactory radioimmunoassay for cholecystokinin pancreozymin has yet been reported, although several attempts to assay it have been made. The main problems are poor antigenicity, difficulty in iodinating the sulphated tyrosine and instability in plasma. Professor Brown in Vancouver has set up an assay for gastric inhibitory peptide and reports a plasma rise after oral glucose (Brown, 1972) which is compatible with the inhibition of gastric acid previously noted under these circumstances. No plasma assays have been reported for either motilin or for vasoactive intestinal peptide as they have only become available very recently.

CONCLUSIONS

Gastrointestinal endocrinology is still in a very rudimentary state. Its possible importance is difficult to assess at this stage, but histologically there appears to be a complex and numerous endocrine cell system. The initial step in unravelling the situation is to purify and characterise all extractable peptides with biological action. A great deal has, in fact, been achieved in this direction in the last two decades by Professors Jorpes and Mutt in Stockholm. Then it is necessary to set up radioimmunoassays to measure the plasma levels of these peptides, both to demonstrate that they are present in the plasma, and to establish the normal physiological fluctuations. Finally when this is done it is possible to examine pathological states for clues to aetiology and treatment. At present only in the Zollinger-Ellison syndrome is the goal realised. In this situation gastrin measurement by radioimmunoassay has become the investigation of choice and is so simple to perform that routine screening of all duodenal ulcer patients has been suggested. It is easy to predict that this is only the beginning and that within a few years every hospital will require access to a multiple gastrointestinal hormone radioimmunoassay service.

REFERENCES

Anderson, J. C., Barton, M. A., Gregory, R. A., Hardy, P. M., Kenner, G. W., MacLeod, J. K., Preston, T., Sheppard, R. C. and Morley, J.S. (1964) Nature, **204**, 933
Bayliss, W. M. and Starling, E. H.(1902) Proceedings of the Royal Society of London, **69**, 352
Berson, S. A. and Yalow, R. S .(1959) Journal of the New York Academy of Science, **82**, 338
Bloom, S. R. (1972) Gut, **13**, 520
Bloom, S. R., Daniel, P. M., Johnston, D. I., Ogawa, O. and Pratt, O. E. (1973a) Quarterly Journal of Experimental Physiology, **58**, 99
Bloom, S. R. and Ogawa, O. (1973) Journal of Endocrinology (in press)
Bloom, S. R., Royston, C. M. S. and Thompson, J. P. S. (1972) Lancet, **11**, 789
Bloom, S. R., Vaughan, N. J. A. and Edwards, A. V. (1973b) Diabelogia (in press)
Bloom, S. R., Ward, A. S . and Ogawa, O. (1973c) unpublished observations
Brown, J. C. (1972) personal communication
Brown, J. C., Mutt, V. and Pederson, R. A. (1970) Journal of Physiology, **209**, 57
Byrnes, D. J., Young, J. D., Chisholm, D. J. and Lazarus, L. (1970) British Medical Journal, **2**, 626
Feurle, G., Ketterer, H., Becker, H. D. and Creutzfeldt, W. (1972) Scandinavian Journal of Gastroenterology, **7**, 177
Ganguli, P. C. and Hunter, W. M. (1972) Journal of Physiology, **220**, 499

Gleeson, M. H., Bloom, S. R., Polak, J. M., Henry, K. and Dowling, R. H. (1971) Gut, **12**, 773

Gregory, R. A., Grossman, M. I., Tracy, H. J. and Bentley, P. H. (1967) Lancet, **ii**, 543

Gregory, R. A. and Tracy, H. J. (1964) Gut, **5**, 103

Grossman, M. I. (1969) Gastroenterology, **57**, 767

Hansky, J. and Cain, M. D. (1969) Lancet, **ii**, 1388

Jorpes, J. E. and Mutt, V. (1961) Acta chemica Scandinavica, **15**, 1790

Jorpes, J. E., Mutt, V. and Toczko, K. (1964) Acta chemica Scandinavica, **18**, 2408

Lewin, M. R., Stagg, B. H. and Clark, C. G. (1972) Gut, **13**, 849

McGuigan, J. E. and Trudeau, W. L. (1968) New England Journal of Medicine, **278**, 1308

McIntyre, N., Holdsworth, C. D. and Turner, D. S. (1964) Lancet, **ii**, 20

Reeder, D. D., Jackson, B. M., Ban, J. L., Davidson, W. D. and Thompson, J. C. (1970) Surgical Forum, **21**, 290

Rehfeld, J. F., Heding, L. G. and Holst, J. J. (1973) Lancet, **i**, 116

Said, S. I. and Mutt, V. (1970) Science, **169**, 1217

Schrumpf, E. and Sand, T. (1972) Scandinavian Journal of Gastroenterology, **7**, 683

Stadil, F. (1972) Scandinavian Journal of Gastroenterology, **7**, 225

Stadil, F. and Rehfeld, J. F. (1971) Scandinavian Journal of Gastroenterology, Suppl. 9, 61

Trudeau, W. L. and McGuigan, J. E. (1971) New England Journal of Medicine, **284**, 408

Zollinger, R. M. and Ellison, E. H. (1955) Annals of Surgery, **142**, 709

Hormone Secreting Tumours and the Gut

C C BOOTH

The relationship between tumours of the endocrine glands and recognisable clinical syndromes has been established since the nineteenth century. The association between acromegaly and tumours of the pituitary, for example, was described by Brigidi in 1877 and by Pierre Marie in 1886. It is, however, perhaps paradoxical that although the first hormone to be discovered, secretin, was an alimentary hormone, no tumour involving excess secretin secretion has hitherto been described in man and other endocrine tumours of the gut have been reported only within recent years. The purpose of this paper is first to describe the best recognised syndrome in which there is excessive secretion of an alimentary hormone, the Zollinger Ellison syndrome, and then to outline the features of two other recently described endocrine tumours involving the gut.

THE ZOLLINGER ELLISON SYNDROME

In 1955, Zollinger and Ellison described the association between gastric hyper-secretion, severe and recurrent peptic ulceration and non-beta islet cell tumours of the pancreas. A potent gastric secretogogue was extracted from the tumour obtained from a patient with the Zollinger Ellison syndrome in 1960 (Gregory et al, 1960), and the identity of this material with gastrin was subsequently established (Gregory et al, 1964; Gregory & Tracy, 1964; Gregory et al, 1967). More recent work has demonstrated that the pancreatic tumour in the Zollinger Ellison syndrome may secrete gastrins of unusually high molecular weight — 'big gastrin' (Gregory & Tracy, 1972).

CLINICAL SYNDROMES RESEMBLING ZOLLINGER ELLISON SYNDROME

Although gastric hypersecretion and intractable peptic ulceration have most frequently been described in association with a gastrinoma of the pancreas, it is now clear that there are a number of other situations in which a similar clinical syndrome may occur. It has been recognised for some years that

421

surgical exploration of the pancreas in a patient with Zollinger Ellison syndrome may reveal no evidence of tumour and in such patients hyperplasia only of the D cells of the pancreas, which secrete gastrin, has sometimes been demonstrated (Polak et al, 1972). In other cases, hyperplasia of the antral G cells has been shown without evidence of tumour in the pancreas and quantitative studies have suggested that in such patients the degree of hyperplasia may reach as much as 20-30 times the normal situation. The suggestion has also been made that a gastrin producing tumour may arise from the antral G cells and a single interesting patient has been described in whom there was an infiltrating tumour of the stomach, the cells of the tumour apparently containing gastrin as demonstrated by immunofluorescence (Royston et al, 1972).

There are therefore four distinct situations which may lead to gastric hypersecretion and peptic ulceration as a result of excessive gastrin production. These are:

1. Pancreatic D-cell hyperplasia
2. Pancreatic gastrinoma
3. Antral G-cell hyperplasia
4. G-cell tumour of the stomach

Clinical Features

The clinical features of the Zollinger Ellison syndrome have been well established by detailed studies on nearly a thousand cases described since 1955. Peptic ulceration is intractable and recurrent. Ulceration may occur in the jejunum as a result of the highly acid pH found in the upper intestine. Ulcers may be multiple, and may recur after operations such as partial gastrectomy or vagotomy and drainage procedures. Diarrhoea frequently occurs and may be the presenting symptom. The cause of the diarrhoea appears to be inactivation of pancreatic lipase (Summerskill, 1959), precipitation of the conjugated bile salts and, in some cases, there may actually be damage to the jejunal mucosa. Excessive secretion of other hormones causing diarrhoea, however, has not been excluded in such patients.

The association of the Zollinger Ellison syndrome with tumours of other endocrine glands, particularly the pituitary, parathyroid or adrenal, has been recognised for many years and is usually referred to as the 'pluriglandular syndrome'.

The diagnosis can be suspected by the demonstration of formidable gastric hypersecretion, 24-hour secretion rates reaching as high a figure as 12 litres in individual cases (Donaldson et al, 1957). The establishment of the diagnosis now rests, however, on measurement of the serum gastrin level by radioimmunoassay, levels being increased by ten to a hundred fold in the Zollinger Ellison syndrome.

Treatment clearly depends on the type of Zollinger Ellison syndrome

encountered. If there is a pancreatic gastrinoma, however, it is preferable
to advise total gastrectomy rather than simple removal of the pancreatic
tumour alone. This is because gastrinomas may be multiple and they may
also metastasize. Since over-secretion of gastrin may therefore continue
following removal of a single tumour and since death in the Zollinger Ellison
syndrome is usually due to the complications of the severe and intractable
peptic ulceration, many surgeons recommend total gastrectomy as an essential part of treatment.

VERNER-MORRISON SYNDROME

There is another syndrome in which a non-beta islet cell tumour of the pancreas is associated with severe watery diarrhoea, but, in contrast to the
Zollinger Ellison syndrome, there is usually gastric hyposecretion or achlorhydria (Murray et al, 1961). This syndrome was first described by Verner
and Morrison in 1958. Peptic ulceration does not occur but the watery diarrhoea, which is so severe in some cases as to deserve the name 'pancreatic
cholera' (Matsumoto et al, 1966), may lead to marked hypokalaemia which is
difficult to correct without intravenous potassium infusions. The term WDHA
syndrome' was coined by Marks et al in 1967 to denote the main features of
watery diarrhoea, hypokalaemia and achlorhydria. The condition is much
more rare than the Zollinger Ellison syndrome and the total number of cases
reported is only 40. There has been considerable speculation as to the nature
of the hormone secreted in the Verner Morrison syndrome. Zollinger's
group have suggested that secretin might be responsible and Barbezat and
Grossman (1971) have speculated that combined production of gastrin and
glucagon may be involved.

A patient with this syndrome was referred to the Hammersmith Hospital
in 1972 by Dr C Foster-Cooper. The characteristic features of watery diarrhoea, severe hypokalaemia and hypochlorhydria were present. At laparo-
tomy (Professor R B Welbourn) a pancreatic tumour measuring 1. 5cm in
circumference was removed and multiple hepatic metastases were found in
the liver. Despite treatment with 5-fluorouracil and oral corticosteroids, the
patient died four months post-operatively. Studies of the hepatic metastases
showed the characteristic histological features of a non-beta islet cell tumour.
which on immunofluorescence showed negative results for gastrin, caerulein,
secretin, glucagon, calcitonin, ACTH, insulin and motilin. There was, however, markedly positive fluorescence when an anti-serum against highly
purified porcine gastric inhibitory polypeptide (GIP) was used (Elias et al,
1972).

The findings in this patient therefore suggest that the Verner-Morrison
syndrome is due to a pancreatic tumour producing GIP. Further work is
necessary, however, to extract pure GIP from the tumour and in order to

423

determine whether there are any other gastrointestinal hormones secreted by the tumour.

ENTEROGLUCAGON SECRETING TUMOUR

A remarkable patient in whom an endocrine tumour involving the kidney was found to secrete enteroglucagon, was described by Gleeson et al in 1971. The patient was a 44-year old woman who was referred to the Hammersmith Hospital complaining of polyuria, intractable constipation and oedema. Clinical examination revealed severe generalised pitting oedema and there was evidence of chronic constipation. Investigations revealed hypoalbuminaemia (serum albumin levels ranging from 1.8 to 2.0g/100ml) and steatorrhoea (faecal fat excretion 20g/24 hours), but there was no evidence of protein losing enteropathy. A Schilling test demonstrated subnormal vitamin B12 absorption. Barium examination of the gastrointestinal tract showed evidence of marked intestinal dilatation and there was remarkably slow intestinal transit. Biopsy of the small intestinal mucosa surprisingly showed striking elongation of the villi due to apparent hypertrophy. Following a urinary tract infection, an intravenous pyelogram was performed and this revealed the tumour of the kidney, which was subsequently removed surgically by Mr G Chisholm. On light microscopy histological examination strongly suggested an endocrine tumour and on electron microscopy the characteristic secretory granules of such a tumour were seen. Immunofluorescent studies then demonstrated negative fluorescence when anti-sera against gastrin, calcitonin, growth hormone and ACTH were used, but there was a very strongly positive reaction with anti-glucagon serum. Subsequent analysis of the glucagon derived from the tumour indicated that it was enteroglucagon (Bloom, 1972).

The findings in this patient are unique and have not been described before or since. They strongly suggest that enteroglucagon can so delay intestinal transit as to cause severe constipation and steatorrhoea. The reason for the intestinal hypertrophy is uncertain, but it may be related to the secretion by the tumour of another hormone with trophic effects on the small intestinal epithelium.

CONCLUSIONS

The hormone secreting tumours described in this paper are all 'Apudomas'. They are tumours of the endocrine cells of the gastrointestinal tract, the cells described by Professor A G E Pearse as APUD cells. Why such a cell should be producing a tumour of the kidney in the patient with the enteroglucagonoma must remain uncertain. It appears, however, that such tumours may secrete a wide variety of different hormones and it seems likely that further syndromes involving hypersecretion of the gastrointestinal hormones remain to be described. The results in the Verner-Morrison syndrome, where oversecretion of GIP appears to be responsible for the diarrhoea, and in the patient with the enteroglucagon secreting tumour which caused severe constipation, are particularly interesting since they stimulate the suggestion that patients with chronic unexplained diarrhoea or constipation may be suffering from hyperplasia of the cells responsible for secreting either GIP or enteroglucagon. The endocrinology of the gastrointestinal tract represents one of the most fascinating interfaces in medicine and a great deal more remains to be discovered than has hitherto been established.

REFERENCES

Barbezat, G. O. and Grossman, M. J. (1971) Lancet, i, 1025

Bloom, S. R. (1972) Gut, 13, 520

Donaldson, R. M., von Eigen, P. R. and Dwight, R. W. (1957) New England Journal of Medicine, 257, 965

Elias, E., Polak, J. M., Bloom, S. R., Pearse, A. G. E., Welbourn, R. B., Booth, C. C., Kuzio, M. and Brown, J. C. (1972) Lancet, ii, 791

Gleeson, M. H., Bloom, S. R., Polak, J. M., Henry, K. and Dowling, R. H. (1971) Gut, 12, 773

Gregory, H., Hardy, P. M., Jones, D. S., Kenner, G. W. and Shepherd, R. C. (1964) Nature (Lond.), 204, 931

Gregory, R. A., Grossman, M. I., Tracy, H. J. and Bentley, P. H. (1967) Lancet, ii, 543

Gregory, R. A. and Tracy, H. J. (1964) Gut, 5, 115

Gregory, R. A. and Tracy, H. J. (1972) Lancet, ii, 797

Gregory, R. A., Tracy, H. J., French, J. M. and Sircus, W. (1960) Lancet, i, 1045

Marks, I. N., Bank, S. and Louw, J. H. (1967) Gastroenterology, 52, 695

Matsumoto, K. K., Peter, J. B., Schultze, R. G., Hakim, A. A. and Franck, P. T. (1966) Gastroenterology, 50, 231

Murray, J. S., Paton, R. P. and Pope, C. E. (1961) New England Journal of Medicine, 264, 436

Polak, J. M., Stagg, B. H. and Pearse, A. G. E. (1972) Gut, 13, 501

Royston, C. M. S., Brew, D. St.J., Garnham, J. R., Stagg, B. H. and Polak, J. (1972) Gut, 13, 638

Summerskill, W. H. J. (1959) Lancet, i, 120

Zollinger, R. M. and Ellison, E. H. (1955) Annals of Surgery, 142, 709

The Lilly Lecture

The Enigma of Cystic Fibrosis: A Tangle of Biochemical and Cellular Clues

ALEXANDER G BEARN

When it is considered that cystic fibrosis is one of the commonest inherited diseases of man its delineation as a distinct entity has emerged surprisingly slowly. For decades, patients with cystic fibrosis have died with the confident clinical label of coeliac disease, infantile bronchopneumonia, or steatorrhoea of unknown aetiology (di Sant' Agnese & Talamo, 1967; Lobeck, 1972). It was not until Dorothy Anderson in 1938 defined a group of patients in whom steatorrhoea was associated with cystic and fibrotic changes in the pancreas at autopsy that cystic fibrosis as a specific disease was first recognised (Figures 1 and 2). These studies accented and made historic the case report published by Fanconi two years earlier (Fanconi, 1936). Although the disease was originally described as an acquired primary pancreatic disorder, it is

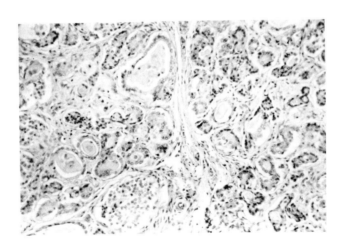

Figure 1. The pancreatic acini are distended by inspissated, laminated eosinophilic concretions. Many of the acini are distorted and have flattened epithelium. Some interstitial fibrosis is present

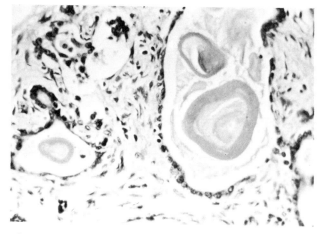

Figure 2. The laminated appearance of the inspissated pancreatic secretions is characteristic. Acinar atrophy and interstitial fibrosis are evident

now appreciated that cystic fibrosis is a recessively inherited multisystem disease with the brunt of damage falling on the exocrine system.

During the last thirty-five years, but particularly during the last twenty, the world literature on cystic fibrosis has grown exponentially; the descriptive biology of cystic fibrosis in clinical and pathological terms has become well recognised and the natural history of the disease fully documented. In sharp contrast to the wealth of information on the clinical and pathological aspects of the disease the primary inherited defect remains quite unknown, despite the fact there has been no shortage of talented investigators who have devoted their energies towards elucidating the underlying molecular cause for the disease. Much of the aetiological mystery which surrounds the disease centres on the unusual plethora of biochemical and cellular abnormalities which have been uncovered, none of which appears to represent the primary defect. Before embarking on a discussion of the possible significance of some of the investigations carried out in our laboratory and in those of others who are also studying the disease from a molecular viewpoint, a number of the cardinal clinical features of the disease will be recalled.

CLINICAL

Before the dawn of the antibiotic era, diarrhoea and infection in the early months of life were responsible for a large fraction of the infantile mortality even in those countries where general hygiene was good. Although it has been said that 10-20% of patients with cystic fibrosis may present with meconium ileus at birth, most patients with the disease will present with a failure to thrive, chronic diarrhoea or recurrent respiratory infections. In 1968, 597 patients with cystic fibrosis died in the US of whom 126 (21%) died

427

under one year of age and 372 (64%) under the age of 10 (Vital Statistics of the United States, 1968). In this country Edwards (1971) has calculated that in round numbers there are about 500 children with cystic fibrosis born each year. Although the introduction of antibiotics and specialised medical and nursing care has significantly decreased the mortality in the early years, the disease is a constant threat to life and it is exceptionally rare to be able to delay a fatal outcome beyond the 25th year of life.

GASTROINTESTINAL SYMPTOMATOLOGY

The most dramatic gastrointestinal manifestation of cystic fibrosis is small intestinal obstruction at birth, or shortly thereafter, and is due to blockage of the terminal ileum with inspissated meconium. Although this manifestation of cystic fibrosis occurs in only some 15-20% of patients it is pathognomonic of the disease (Figure 3). Meconium ileus is all too often lethal and may

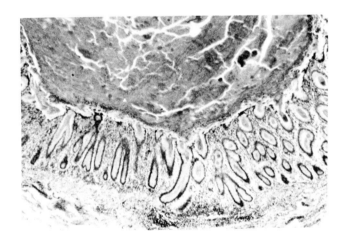

Figure 3. Densely viscid secretions are present within the intestinal glands of the appendix. The material filling the lumen is coarsely clumped and eosinophilic

affect more than one member of a family. More usually the child with cystic fibrosis is normal at birth but his enfeebled first year of life is characterised by a failure of thrive, poor weight gain and the passage of frequent foul smelling stools. The profound steatorrhoea that results from pancreatic insufficiency may, if vitamin supplements are omitted, lead to symptoms and signs of a deficiency of Vitamin A. This deficiency of Vitamin A led some early investigators to suggest that the entire syndrome of cystic fibrosis could be accounted for by a lack of this vitamin. The medical misfortunes of the infant with cystic fibrosis of the pancreas in the first year of life are not confined to the alimentary system. Although the very earliest descriptions of

428

cystic fibrosis did not emphasise pulmonary involvement, it quite quickly
became apparent that a variable degree of bronchial and pulmonary disease
was usually present. The pulmonary symptoms are due to the secretion by
the bronchial glands of a viscid mucus which by leading to bronchial obstruction predisposes the infant to recurrent pulmonary infections, progressive

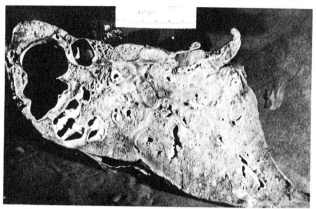

Figure 4. The upper apical one-third of the lung of this 26-year old patient with cystic
fibrosis is replaced by inter-communicating smooth-walled cysts, the residue of
severe bronchiectasis. The lower two-thirds of the lung are consolidated by terminal
staphylococcal pneumonia

Pulmonary Function Tests

R.Z.	Age (Yrs.)	VC (Liters)	FEV(1) (Liters)	PaO$_2$ (mm Hg)
Nov. 1965	17	4.5	4.1	-
Sept. 1968	20	4.1	3.3	79.6
Dec. 1969	21	4.3	3.5	-
Jan. 1973	25	3.5	2.5	65
Predicted value		4.7	4.0	90

VC   Vital Capacity.

FEV(1)   Forced Expiratory Volume in 1 second.

PaO$_2$ Partial pressure of oxygen in arterial blood.

Figure 5. Sequential pulmonary function tests on male patient with cystic fibrosis. The
sharp decrease in FEV$_1$ is particularly noteworthy

fibrosis, bronchiectasis, emphysema and in some instances cor pulmonale (Figure 4). The age at which respiratory symptoms become prominent and the rate of progression of the pulmonary disease determine, in large part, the prognosis (Figure 5).

GENETICAL CONSIDERATIONS: A REASON FOR OPTIMISM

One of the most imaginative and fruitful biological hypotheses of this century was advanced by Sir Archibald Garrod in his Croonian Lectures in 1908 in which he developed the theme that genes control the synthesis of proteins, many of which have an enzymatic function. Garrod was led to this biological generality by studying certain hereditary diseases, that he called inborn errors of metabolism, in which he postulated that the normal wild-type gene responsible for the synthesis of a particular enzyme had been replaced by a mutant gene. If the mutant gene was present in a homozygous state no enzyme was synthesised and resulted in an inborn error of metabolism. The implication for physicians of the one gene-one enzyme hypothesis was clearly seen by Garrod but only in the last 25 years has the clinical harvest begun to be reaped. If a disease is shown to be inherited in a simple recessive fashion it follows that the primary inherited abnormality must be a deficient or deformed protein which will frequently play a crucial enzymatic function in the biological economy of man. However complex the clinical picture, however many organ systems are involved, and however many biochemical or cellular abnormalities can be defined there is one, and only one, primary inherited abnormality and this single abnormality determines, in the last analysis, all the signs and symptoms of the disease. The concept of a pedigree of causes was enunciated by Grüneberg (1947) to emphasise that tracing the relationship between the primary inherited abnormality and the clinical and pathological features of the disease may be complex and indirect.

INCIDENCE OF THE DISEASE

Cystic fibrosis is the commonest inherited disease of the white population. In the last twenty years an attempt has been made to obtain information on the frequency of the disease in different populations. As a result of these studies it appears now well-established that the frequency of the disease in most white populations is approximately 1/2,000-1/3,000 (Danks et al,1965; Bearn,1972). The variation in frequency is remarkably small. The highest figure recorded is from a small canton in Switzerland; the lowest from Sweden (Table I). A careful and extensive recent population study from Victoria, Australia gives a frequency for the disease of 1/2,500 (Danks et al,1965). The disease is rare in the American Negro, even more rare in the black African, and almost unknown in Oriental populations (Bearn,1973). The frequency of the disease coupled with its lethality raises the question of

Table I. The incidence of cystic fibrosis in different populations
(Adapted from Bearn, 1973)

UK	1:2,900
USA	
Hawaii	1:3,800
Ohio	1:3,700
New England	1:2,400
FRANCE	1:3,200
WEST GERMANY	1:3,300
SWEDEN	1:7,200
CZECHOSLOVAKIA	1:3,000
AUSTRALIA	
Victoria	1:2,500

whether there are under certain environmental circumstances, powerful selective forces operating which would favour the heterozygote. Indeed it has been suggested that the striking racial variation may have its root cause in the operation of selective factors which act unfavourably in hot climates. Although no convincing evidence for such presumed heterozygous advantage has been advanced, it can be calculated that a mere 2% advantage of the heterozygote is sufficient to achieve genetic equilibrium; the likelihood of being able to identify such a small advantage is remote. While heterozygous advantage remains a theoretically attractive explanation for the frequency of the cystic fibrosis gene it must be admitted that random genetic drift could also account for the high frequency.

FORMAL GENETICS

The autosomal recessive nature of cystic fibrosis is beyond serious cavil. The disease occurs equally in both sexes, is common in sibs and does not show parent-child transmission. A series of detailed and well executed family studies indicate the expected maximum likelihood estimate of the segregation ratio in sibs to be approximately 0.25 (Danks et al, 1965).

Although the frequency of the disease in first cousins is that which would be expected if cystic fibrosis were determined by a single gene, the possibility of genetic heterogeneity (Bearn, 1972) is raised by certain investigations that will be discussed later. Although the recognition that cystic fibrosis was clearly inherited in a recessive fashion became evident in the forties it is worth nothing that Garrod had already labelled the disease an inborn error of metabolism in 1912 (Garrod & Hurtley, 1912). In the Quarterly Journal of Medicine in 1912 Garrod and Hurtley reported a family with 'Congenital Family Steatorrhoea'. In this historic but rather neglected paper Garrod

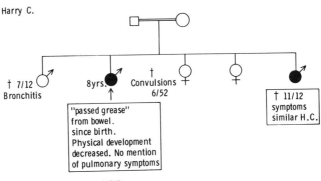

Figure 6. Pedigree of Sir Archibald Garrod's patient with 'congenital family steatorrhoea'

reported a 12-year old boy who 'passed grease from the bowel'. He noted that the parents of the patient were first cousins and that a younger sib had an identical disease (Figure 6). With his customary clairvoyance, he wrote "It seems probable that our patient is the subject of an inborn error, hitherto undescribed, and on a par with such anomalies as alkaptonuria and cystinuria".

From a biological viewpoint the disease can be considered a conditional lethal. Not only do patients with the disease usually die before reproductive age but males are almost uniformly sterile. Recent evidence suggests that reproductive failure may be associated with a failure of the normal vas deferens to develop. Aspermia and abnormal sperm are commonly seen. Females with cystic fibrosis may be fertile (Kaplan et al, 1968; Taussig et al, 1972).

HETEROZYGOTES

It has been periodically and plausibly suggested by a number of investigators that heterozygous carriers for the cystic fibrosis gene may be more susceptible to respiratory disease. Since heterozygotes for cystic fibrosis account for 4% of the white population they could indeed comprise a significant fraction of patients with chronic respiratory disease. With this in mind, Hallett and co-workers (1965) compared 132 heterozygous carriers for cystic fibrosis and 118 normal controls, but were unable to establish any difference in pulmonary disease between the heterozygous and the control group. This finding was not altogether unexpected since on theoretical grounds it could again be argued that so far from the heterozygotes being at increased risk for respiratory or other diseases they might, under certain environmental circumstances, be at a distinct biological advantage.

BIOCHEMICAL ABNORMALITIES

Those who were persuaded by the predominance of symptoms related to pancreatic insufficiency that the disease was a primary disorder of pancreatic function, as well as those who ascribed the disease to an excessive viscosity of mucous secretions, had to abandon their respective positions when, in 1953 di Sant' Agnese and his colleagues published their classic paper in which they showed that patients with cystic fibrosis secrete sweat with an increased sodium and chloride content. This important biochemical finding had its origin in the astute clinical observations of Kessler and Andersen (1951) that 5 of 10 children admitted to the hospital with dehydration and collapse during a heat wave in August 1948 were cystic fibrotics. The observation that patients with cystic fibrosis have an increased sweat sodium and chloride gave hope to those who were beginning to agree with Garrod's forgotten suggestion of forty years earlier that an inborn error of metabolism was the primary abnormality in cystic fibrosis.

SWEAT ELECTROLYTES

The intervening twenty years since sweat electrolytes were found to be abnormal in cystic fibrosis have fully confirmed the validity of the early observations. Yet despite the regularity of the electrolyte disturbance the relationship to the primary abnormality has remained enigmatic.

It seems clear that the electrolyte perturbation which affects sodium, chloride, and to a lesser extent potassium transport is present at birth and continues throughout life. In normal individuals there is a tendency for the sweat electrolytes to increase in concentration with age and thus there is a greater need for caution in interpreting sweat electrolytes in the adolescent or adult patient suspected of having cystic fibrosis (di Sant' Agnese & Talamo, 1967). It is curious that even twenty years after the original observation the precise physiological nature of the sweat defect remains elusive. Patients with cystic fibrosis have an active sodium transport in the kidneys, the sodium pump in the red cells appears to function normally (Lobeck, 1966); and although the salivary glands are frequently enlarged in cystic

433

fibrosis they are morphologically normal. The most likely explanation for the increased sweat and salivary electrolytes in cystic fibrosis is a defective reabsorption of electrolytes across the tubules. A promising lead to explain the inhibition of sodium reabsorption in this disease has come from the observations of Mangos and his colleagues (Mangos & McSherry, 1967a, b). Suspicious that the sweat gland might be producing a substance that inhibited the reabsorption of electrolytes they devised a micro-puncture system in rats that enabled them to perfuse the duct system of the salivary glands in a retrograde fashion. Using this retrograde perfusion technique they introduced different substances into the duct and observed their effects on sodium reabsorption. Ouabain was found to inhibit sodium reabsorption and cyanide, in appropriate concentrations, abolished sodium reabsorption completely. More importantly, these investigators showed that retrograde perfusion of the duct system with sweat obtained from patients with cystic fibrosis inhibited sodium transport while sweat obtained from age-matched controls had no effect. When heparin was mixed with saliva before retrograde injection the inhibitory effect was abolished (Mangos & McSherry, 1968).

Fractionation of the factor by column chromatography has disclosed three peaks of activity (Mangos & McSherry, 1967a, b). The greatest activity was found in the fraction of high molecular weight. Later this fraction was shown to have a dyskinetic effect on rabbit tracheal cilia. When rats are given isoproterenol the salivary glands enlarge, the excretion of sodium and chloride in the sweat increases sharply and a factor with dyskinetic effect on tracheal cilia can be detected in serum (Mangos et al, 1969).

SPOCK FACTOR

In 1967 Spock and his colleagues at Duke University reported the remarkable observation that the serum from patients with cystic fibrosis disorganized the synchronous beating of cilia of rabbit tracheal explants, incubated for 4-6 days in culture. This asynchrony and premature cessation of all ciliary movement was seen in all 75 patients studied and was not present in 75 controls (Spock et al, 1967). Asynchrony and inhibition was also found in 18 heterozygous parents but only when the euglobulin fraction of serum was used, suggesting the possibility that although the factor responsible was present in the heterozygote it existed at a lower concentration. Chemically, the substance in serum that was responsible for this phenomenon was heat labile and non-dialysable. It was found in the euglobulin fraction and behaved on sephadex G-200 chromatography as a 19S macroglobulin.

These imaginative observations of Spock evoked great interest and soon a number of laboratories began to look more closely for substances in cystic fibrosis serum which had this unpredictable and somewhat bizarre biological effect.

In 1969, Besley, Patrick and Norman at Great Ormond Street investigated

434

the effect of cystic fibrosis serum on cilia derived from the fresh water mussel Dreissensia, a mollusc found in abundance in the lakes and waterways of England (Besley et al, 1969). Confirming the results of Spock they observed inhibition of ciliary motility when cystic fibrosis serum was added to the mussel preparation. A similar inhibitory effect was also observed with serum from the heterozygous parents of those affected with cystic fibrosis. A troublesome idiosyncratic feature of the biological system emerged when it was observed that the ability of serum to inhibit the cilia was dependent, at least in part, on seasonal variations. Between April and June the ability of molluscan cilia to discriminate between normal serum and cystic fibrosis serum was of a high order of magnitude. Between September and April this magical talent waned since even control serum would inhibit ciliary activity of molluscs during the winter months. Although the reason for this seasonal difference in responsivess is not entirely explicable it may be related to excessive production of mucus by the mussel in winter months.

OYSTER CILIA TEST

NL
SERUM

CF
SERUM

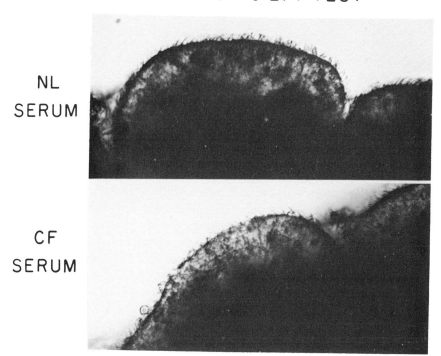

Figure 7. Comparative effect of normal and cystic fibrosis serum on oyster cilia. The upper frame show normally beating oyster cilia; the lower frame oyster cilia show morphological disruption and cessation of movement (after 30 min)

Crawfurd in 1969, using the same ciliary preparation, and observing the same seasonal variations, tested 13 patients all of whom were positive and 163 obligate heterozygotes of whom all but 13 were positive. Among the control group 12 of 163 serum samples tested gave positive reactions.

In 1969, Bowman and her colleagues at the University of Galveston, conveniently located in the molluscan paradise of the Gulf of Mexico, took astute advantage of the gastronomically prized Gulf oyster Crassotrea virginica, and selected this celebrated mollusc as a ready source of cilia. In their initial paper the serum from all 47 patients and 19 heterozygotes with cystic fibrosis caused ciliary inhibition, whereas only 2 of 64 individuals without cystic fibrosis caused ciliary inhibition in an equivalent period of time (Figure 7). In 1970, Bowman and her colleagues reported on the nature of the inhibitor in more chemical detail. The inhibitor was cationic, eluted with the immunoglobulin G fraction and appeared on gel filtration to have a molecular weight of 125,000 to 150,000. The data could not distinguish between two possibilities. Was the factor responsible for the inhibition IgG or was it due to a small molecular weight substance bound to gamma globulin? As will be discussed later these two possibilities are not yet fully resolved.

SALIVARY TRYPSIN-LIKE ACTIVITY

Human saliva contains trypsin which hydrolyses a variety of substrates and which can be inhibited by soybean inhibitor. Rao and Nadler (1972) supposed that the presence of the Mangos factor, a cationic protein in the saliva and sweat, might be due to the lack of an enzyme which normally hydrolyses the factor. To test this hypothesis they compared the trypsin-like activity of the saliva in normal and control subjects and found a considerable decrease in the patients with cystic fibrosis. The authors further supposed that the trypsin-like activity might be due to a deficiency of kallikrein. Direct testing of kallikrein activity, and kallikrein activity inhibited by soybean inhibitor were significantly reduced in the plasma of patients with the disease and, to a variable extent, in obligate heterozygotes (Rao et al, 1972). This interesting observation has recently been investigated in our laboratory (Harpel et al, 1973) and the deficiency of kallikrein claimed by these authors could not be confirmed. Further investigations to clarify these observations are urgently needed.

STUDIES OF CYSTIC FIBROSIS IN FIBROBLASTS

Once cystic fibrosis was determined to be a disease inherited in a recessive fashion it followed that there must be two abnormal genes in every cell in the body, and by the same orthodox genetical reasoning the parents of those affected who were obligate heterozygotes must have one abnormal gene in every cell. With these facts in mind we decided, in the summer of 1967, to investigate the morphological, histological and biochemical characteristics of cultured fibroblasts derived from the skin of patients with cystic fibrosis.

For many years the assumption had been somewhat cavalierly made that the fibroblast, because of its simple nature, would be able to exhibit only a limited number of biochemical characteristics and be able to synthesise only a restricted number of enzymes and proteins — indeed merely those necessary for its survival. However, earlier findings in our laboratory, in which a cellular abnormality had been detected in the fibroblasts derived from patients with the mucopolysaccharidoses, encouraged us to believe that cellular abnormalities might be detected in cystic fibrosis. Although on simple inspection the fibroblasts appeared morphologically normal they stained metachromatically when exposed to the cationic dye Toluidine Blue 0 (Danes & Bearn, 1968). Toluidine Blue not only stains mucopolysaccharides metachromatically but it also reacts with a number of negatively charged cellular substances including lipids and nucleic acids. The non-specificity of the metachromatic reaction was investigated further by exposing the cells to another dye, Alcian blue (Danes et al, 1970). Alcian blue will bind and precipitate mucopolysaccharides even at high electrolyte concentrations; increasing the concentration of inorganic electrolytes will cause the non-specific staining of anions to disappear. Cystic fibrosis fibroblasts did not show alcianophilia at high electrolyte concentrations ($0.3m$ $MgCl_2$) and thus it could be concluded on histochemical grounds that the metachromatic staining with Toluidine Blue 0 was unlikely to be due to mucopolysaccharides. Direct analysis of the fibroblast for increased mucopolysaccharides, however, has given rather equivocal results (Matalon & Dorfman, 1968; Danes & Bearn, 1969). The results recently obtained in our laboratory have not disclosed any consistent increase in mucopolysaccharides although in some instances an increased quantity was observed (Danes & Bearn, 1969). The situation can probably be summarized by saying that while the fibroblasts of certain patients with cystic fibrosis may have an increased mucopolysaccharide content this is not a usual finding and should probably no longer be emphasized.

Increasing application of metachromatic staining of fibroblasts from patients with cystic fibrosis and their families has led (Danes & Bearn, 1969; Bearn & Danes, 1969) to a refinement of the cellular abnormalities. Without doubt, however, the most interesting and reproducible of these refinements was the qualitative observation that there were a small proportion of patients with unequivocal cystic fibrosis whose fibroblasts showed no cellular metachromasia when stained with Toluidine Blue 0. Closer inspection of the metachromatic classes suggested the possibility of additional heterogeneity.

The metachromasia observed in the cells of certain patients with cystic fibrosis took on an added significance when it was shown that obligate heterozygotes, the parents of those affected with the disease, also showed metachromasia (Danes & Bearn, 1969; Bearn & Danes, 1969). The metachromasia observed in heterozygotes, however, could not be distinguished from the metachromasia seen in affected individuals. Family studies revealed that where it was possible to examine the fibroblasts from both grandparents, 2 of the 4 grandparents showed metachromasia. Metachromasia was also seen in some of the sibs of those affected. Most interestingly, the parents of those patients in whom metachromasia could not be demonstrated did not show metachromasia, none of the four grandparents showed metachromasia and metachromasia was not seen in the cells of unaffected sibs.

The finding of metachromatic and non-metachromatic sibships among patients with cystic fibrosis raises the possibility that the disease may be genetically heterogeneous. The fraction of patients with cystic fibrosis with ametachromatic fibroblasts is small. In one American population reported, the percentage of ametachromatic cystic fibrosis was approximately 13.0% (Danes & Flensborg, 1971); in a Danish population the fraction was approximately 25.0% (Danes, 1972). For a number of reasons the results obtained on the Danish population, however, cannot be considered as reliable as those of the American population and further studies are needed before the high figure of the Danish population are taken at face value. It will be recalled that the population studies carried out by Danks and his colleagues (1965), as well as the calculations of Crow (1965), in which the frequency of the disease in cousins was calculated, did not suggest genetic heterogeneity. The sensitivity of the method would probably not permit the detection of genetic heterogeneity if the less frequent gene accounted for only 10-20% of the patients studied. If the fraction of ametachromatic patients represented 40-45% of the patients studied genetic heterogeneity should be detected using the methodology of population genetics. In view of the necessary uncertainty of metachromasia it would seem prudent to classify a patient as belonging to the metachromatic or ametachromatic class only when at least one of the two parents show concordance. When this caveat is heeded approximately 20% of the white population appeared to belong to the ametachromatic class (Table II). It has not yet proved possible to examine the parents of the patients from Denmark. A critical purchase on the problem of genetic heterogeneity would be gained if it could be shown that the double heterozygote was normal. In practice one would hope to find a mating of a metachromatic and ametachromatic carrier. If a patient with the disease had one metachromatic parent and one ametachromatic parent who could be proved to be heterozygous for cystic fibrosis the case for multiple genetic loci would be virtually

Table II

Population	Number of patients	Metachromatic	Ametachromatic
New York City	20	16	4
Minneapolis	25	20	5
Total	45	36 (80%)	9 (20%)

In 41 of 45 patients both parents available and stained concordantly
In 4 of 45 patients one parent available and stained concordantly

excluded. The difficulty of defining an ametachromatic individual as a cystic fibrosis carrier is self-evident. If the linkage relationships of cystic fibrosis can be established then the finding of some patients in whom linkage cannot be demonstrated would support the concept of genetic heterogeneity very strongly. If all cases of cystic fibrosis, even those in whom ametachromasia was present, still exhibited the same degree of linkage genetic heterogeneity would be highly unlikely.

An ingenious experimental method to investigate genetic heterogeneity at the cellular level was devised by Neufeld and her colleagues and has been employed most successfully to investigate the genetic heterogeneity among the mucopolysaccharidoses (Fratantoni et al, 1968; Danes & Bearn, 1970). This method uses the principles of 'in vitro correction'. Cells of two types are mixed in vitro. If the two cells have an identical mutation the possibility of mutual correction of a cellular or biochemical anomaly is excluded. If, however, the two cells carry mutations at two different loci the correction of the cellular or metabolic error is possible. When cells derived from patients with metachromatic and ametachromatic classes were mixed no correction was observed.

It has been of some interest to study the extent to which metachromasia has been found in other cell types in cystic fibrosis. Fibroblast cultures established from organs as varied as adrenal, liver, pancreas, testis, thymus, and lung all showed metachromasia. An opportunity to investigate metachromasia in the organs of patients whose fibroblasts were ametachromatic has not presented itself.

The cultivation of skin fibroblasts takes time, and since metachromasia had been demonstrated previously in white cells derived from patients with the mucopolysaccharidoses, the possibility that white blood cultures derived from patients with cystic fibrosis might also show metachromasia was explored (Danes et al, 1969). The data obtained on a number of kindreds with cystic fibrosis indicated that, provided the technical precaution of adding heparin to the cultured cells is taken, it is possible to classify patients with cystic fibrosis into metachromatic and ametachromatic classes. The 'technical precaution' of adding heparin is of considerable interest. Heparin is, of course, a negatively charged substance, which in sufficient concentration will stain metachromatically. However, in the amounts used, metachromasia in normal white cells could not be induced in white cells derived from normal individuals. Further studies using labelled heparin might be instructive.

Although cellular metachromasia has been useful in extending our knowledge of the cellular manifestations of cystic fibrosis some puzzling and presently unexplained facts emerge. The cause for the metachromasia remains obscure. It is presently assumed that if a metachromatic carrier were to marry an ametachromatic carrier the children would be unaffected. This does not fit with the preliminary in vitro experience in which correction of the cellular phenotype cannot be achieved by mixing cells of the two phenotypes.

The inability to distinguish heterozygotes from homozygotes coupled with the non-specificity of cellular metachromasia limits sharply the potential use of this genetic marker in intrauterine diagnosis. The possibility of amniocentesis and genetic counselling could only be entertained if the cells from the first-born affected child and both parents yielded metachromatic fibroblasts. Secure postzygotic intrauterine distinction between homozygotes and heterozygotes would be of great value to those families who had already given birth to a child with cystic fibrosis; further work to achieve this goal is required.

ADDITIONAL CELLULAR AND IMMUNOLOGICAL ABNORMALITIES

LYSOSOMAL ABNORMALITIES

In addition to metachromasia a number of additional cellular abnormalities have been observed in fibroblast culture. In some hands cultures derived from patients with cystic fibrosis do not grow as rapidly and have markedly depressed collagen synthesis (Houck & Sharma, 1970). An increased glycogen content of the cells has been reported (Pallavicini et al, 1970). Bartman et al (1970) have found an increase in number and size of the lysosomes. Antonowicz, Sippell and Schwachman (1972) have reported a marked increase in the lysosomal enzyme α-glucosidase in cultured lymphoid cells derived from patients and heterozygotes. Other lysosomal enzymes including β-glucosidase, β-galactosidase, β-glucosomidase, N-acetyl-β-glucosominidase, arylsulfatase and acid phosphatase were the same in patients with cystic fibrosis as in control subjects. These observations have led the authors to suggest that cystic fibrosis may be a lysosomal disease.

RNA METHYLATION

Rennert and his colleagues have reported the finding of undermethylated RNA in fibroblasts and short-term lymphocyte cultures obtained from patients with cystic fibrosis and in heterozygous carriers (Rennert et al, 1972a, b). This puzzling finding had as its origin the observation that methionine deficient dogs exhibit pathologic changes in the lung and the pancreas and that differentiation of pancreatic rudiments require methionine. Weisiger (1971) had also suggested that an abnormality of free radical metabolism may occur in cystic fibrosis. Although it is too early to interpret these results, and they have yet to be confirmed, it is worth recalling that under-methylation occurs in the methionine-requiring mutant in Escherichia coli described by Fleissner and Borek in 1962.

OPSONIC ABNORMALITIES

Good and his colleagues (Biggar et al, 1971) reported that sera of patients with cystic fibrosis did not promote normal phagocytosis of Pseudomonas aeruginosa by rabbit alveolar macrophages. This observation represents another new and puzzling addition to the host of biochemical and cellular abnormalities reported. The authors suggest that the defect may reside in a quantitative or functional defect of IgA antibodies. The results await confirmation.

RELATIONSHIP OF CELLULAR METACHROMASIA TO CILIARY INHIBITION

The multitude of cellular and biochemical irregularities which characterise the patient with cystic fibrosis is an affront to the principle of parsimony. In an effort to coalesce the cellular metachromasia and ciliary inhibition into biological harmony an investigation was carried out to determine whether material could be identified in fibroblast cultures derived from patients with

Table III. Effect of normal and cystic fibrosis serum on inhibition of oyster cilia

Subjects	Metachromatic staining	Genotype	No.	Elapsed time (min) to inhibit cilia	
				Serum	Medium
Cystic fibrosis	Metachromatic	Homozygotes	24	10-25	5-25
		Heterozygotes	24	10-40	5-25
	Ametachromatic	Homozygotes	12	60-120+	60-120+
		Heterozygotes	12	60-120+	60-120+
Normal	Ametachromatic		36	60-120+	60-120+

cystic fibrosis which would inhibit oyster cilia (Danes, 1972; Danes & Bearn, 1972; Bowman et al, 1973).

Sera obtained from patients and heterozygous carriers whose fibroblasts stained metachromatically in tissue culture appeared to inhibit oyster cilia rapidly whereas those whose fibroblasts were ametachromatic could not be readily distinguished from normal individuals. Moreover the medium in which metachromatic staining fibroblasts were grown tended to inhibit oyster cilia rapidly whereas the media derived from ametachromatic cultures usually did not (Table III). Media from cultures in which metachromatic fibroblasts had been grown but which were derived from patients with Hurler's Syndrome were seldom inhibitory to oyster cilia. Although the foregoing results must be taken as preliminary until the biological test system behaves in a more predictable fashion, it appears as though the factor in serum which inhibits oyster cilia in cystic fibrosis is only present when fibroblasts derived from patients are metachromatic. If fibroblasts derived from the patients are ametachromatic the serum will not inhibit the oyster cilia to the same degree. The data also appear to indicate that the medium in which metachromatic cystic fibrosis fibroblasts have been allowed to grow will inhibit oyster cilia while used medium derived from ametachromatic cystic fibrosis cultures will not. The possibility that a substance is synthesised or released from the metachromatic cells should be entertained but it is also possible that the cystic fibrosis fibroblasts fail to elaborate a substance that is present in normal fibroblasts and breaks down the ciliary inhibitory factor. The possibility that the factor is a gamma globulin is rendered far less likely since fibroblasts have not yet been shown to synthesise gamma globulin.

To investigate the nature of the factor further, collaborative studies have been undertaken with Bowman and her colleagues in Texas (Bowman et al, 1973). In 15 of 18 cystic fibrosis patients and in 8 of 10 heterozygotes an inhibitor was isolated. Fractionation of the fibroblast media revealed an inhibitor peak which did not react with antisera against gamma globulin, again suggesting that the ciliary inhibitor was not a gamma globulin. The observation that radioactive leucine added to the growing culture was also present in the peak that contained the inhibitory activity indicates that the inhibitor may be synthesised by the fibroblast. Although most of the experiments were conducted in the presence of foetal calf serum similar results were obtained when a purely synthetic medium containing no serum protein was employed.

The nature and physiological functions of the serum and tissue culture inhibitor remain elusive. Preliminary evidence suggests that the inhibitor is a small dialysable molecule which under certain circumstances can bind rather specifically to gamma G globulin. The apparent restriction of this inhibitor to the serum and tissue culture medium of those homozygous and heterozygous patients with cystic fibrosis in whom metachromasia can be demonstrated in their fibroblasts is puzzling.

SUMMARY

In this lecture I have not attempted to review all the biochemical abnormalities in the serum in cystic fibrosis, and with a few exceptions, I have confined my remarks to those abnormalities which currently seem most promising. Despite the difficulties that surround the interpretation of the many biochemical and cellular clues in cystic fibrosis, we hope that our studies, as well as those being performed in other laboratories throughout the world, will prove relevant to our eventual understanding of the primary metabolic defect as well as the pathogenesis and treatment of the disease.

Three hundred years ago the Earl of Rochester in a somewhat different context expressed my present position regarding cystic fibrosis. "Before I got married", said that profligate and famous Earl in 1670, "I had six theories about bringing up children; now I have six children and no theories." Yet, the enigma of the inborn error of metabolism cystic fibrosis will, I feel sure, yield to the scientific approach to medicine. The abnormal protein, probably an enzyme, whose deficiency causes cystic fibrosis, remains to be discovered. I suspect that day will dawn before the end of this decade. Goethe the poet philosopher with the mind of a scientist once said, "Even in science we can never really know, we must always do." What we must do is to return to the laboratory and to the bedside.

ACKNOWLEDGMENTS

The research carried out in my laboratory and reported in this lecture was made possible by a grant from The National Foundation-March of Dimes.

I am very greatly indebted to my colleague, Dr B Shannon Danes, without whose collaboration this research could not have been carried out. In addition, I am most pleased to record my indebtedness to Dr Danes as well as to Dr Barbara H Bowman and Dr Hartwig Cleve for their stimulating and critical discussions. Dr John Ellis and Dr Renate Dische gave invaluable help in the selection of the illustrative pathological material.

REFERENCES

Andersen, D. H. (1938) American Journal of Diseases of Children, **56**, 344
Antonowicz, I., Sippell, W. G. and Schwachman, H. (1972) Pediatric Research, **6**, 803
Bartman, J., Wiesmann, U. and Blanc, W. A. (1970) Journal of Pediatrics, **76**, 430
Bearn, A. G. and Danes, B. S. (1969) Transactions of the Association of American Physicians, **82**, 248
Bearn, A. G. (1972) New England Journal of Medicine, **286**, 764

Bearn, A. G. (1973) 'Clinics in Gastroenterology'. (Ed) R. B. McConnell.
W. B. Saunders, Philadelphia (in press)
Besley, G. T. N., Patrick, A. D. and Norman, A. P. (1969) Journal of
Medical Genetics, **6**, 278
Biggar, W. D., Holmes, B. and Good, R. A. (1971) Proceedings of the
National Academy of Sciences, **68**, 1716
Bowman, B. H., Lockhart, L. H. and McCombs, M. L. (1969) Science,
164, 325
Bowman, B. H., McCombs, M. L. and Lockhart, L. H. (1970) Science,
167, 871
Bowman, B. H., Barnett, D. R., Matalon, R., Danes, B. S. and Bearn,
A. G. (1973) Proceedings of the National Academy of Sciences (in press)
Crawfurd, M. d'A. (1969) Proceedings of the 5th International Cystic
Fibrosis Conference. (Ed) D. Lawson. Cystic Fibrosis Research Trust,
London. Page 42
Crow, J. F. (1965) 'Genetics and the Epidemiology of Chronic Diseases'.
US Department of Health, Education and Welfare, Washington, DC.
Page 23
Danes, B. S. and Bearn, A. G. (1968) Lancet, **1**, 1061
Danes, B. S. and Bearn, A. G. (1969) Biochemical and Biophysical Research
Communications, **36**, 919
Danes, B. S. and Bearn, A. G. (1969) The Journal of Experimental Medicine,
129, 775
Danes, B. S., Foley, K. M., Dillon, S. D. and Bearn, A. G. (1969)
Nature, **222**, 5194
Danes, B. S. and Bearn, A. G. (1970) Proceedings of the National Academy
of Sciences, **67**, 357
Danes, B. S., Scott, J. E. and Bearn, A. G. (1970) Journal of Experimental
Medicine, **132**, 765
Danes, B. S. and Flensborg, E. W. (1971) The American Journal of Human
Genetics, **23**, 297
Danes, B. S. (1972) Birth Defects: Original Article Series, The National
Foundation, **8**, 2
Danes, B. S. and Bearn, A. G. (1972) The Journal of Experimental Medicine,
136, 1313
Danks, D. M., Allan, J. and Anderson, C. M. (1965) Annals of Human
Genetics, **28**, 323
di Sant' Agnese, P. A., Darling, R. C., Perera, G. A. and Shea, E. (1953)
Pediatrics, **12**, 549
di Sant' Agnese, P. A. and Talamo, R. C. (1967) New England Journal of
Medicine, **277**, 1287, 1343, 1399
Edwards, J. H. (1971) 'Seventh Symposium on Advanced Medicine'.
(Ed) I. A. D. Bouchier. Pitman Medical, London. Page 55
Fanconi, G. (1936) Wiener medizinische Wochenschrift, **86**, 753
Fleissner, E. and Borek, E. (1962) Proceedings of the National Academy of
Sciences, **48**, 1199
Fratantoni, J. C., Hall, C. W. and Neufeld, E. F. (1968) Proceedings of
the National Academy of Sciences, **60**, 699
Garrod, A. E. (1908) Lancet, ii, 1, 73, 142, 214
Garrod, A. E. and Hurtley, W. H. (1912) Quarterly Journal of Medicine,
6, 242
Grüneberg, H. (1947) 'Animal Genetics and Medicine'. Paul R. Hoeber,
New York
Hallett, W. Y., Knudson, A. G. and Massey, F. J. (1965) American
Review of Respiratory Disease, **92**, 714
Harpel, P., Danes, B. S. and Bearn, A. G. (1973) unpublished observations
Houck, J. C. and Sharma, V. K. (1970) Proceedings of the Society for
Experimental Biology and Medicine, **135**, 369
Kaplan, E., Shwachman, H., Perlmutter, A. D., Rule, A., Khaw, K-T.
and Holsclaw, D. S. (1968) New England Journal of Medicine, **279**, 65
Kessler, W. R. and Andersen, D. H. (1951) Pediatrics, **8**, 648
Lobeck, C. C. (1966) Third International Conference on Research on

Pathogenesis of Cystic Fibrosis of the Pancreas (Mucoviscidosis). (Ed) P. A. di Sant' Agnese. Wickersham Printing Co., Lancaster, Pennsylvania. Page 107

Lobeck, C. C. (1972) in 'The Metabolic Basis of Inherited Disease'. (Ed) J. B. Stanbury, J. B. Wyngaarden and D. S. Fredrickson. McGraw-Hill, New York. Page 1605

Mangos, J. A. and McSherry, N. R. (1967a) Pediatric Research, **1**, 436

Mangos, J. A. and McSherry, N. R. (1967b) Science, **158**, 135

Mangos, J. A. and McSherry, N. R. (1968) Pediatric Research, **2**, 378

Mangos, J. A., McSherry, N. R., Benke, P. J. and Spock, A. (1969) Proceedings of the 5th International Cystic Fibrosis Conference. (Ed) D. Lawson. Cystic Fibrosis Research Trust, London. Page 25

Matalon, R. and Dorfman, A. (1968) Biochemical and Biophysical Research Communications, **33**, 954

Pallavicini, J. C., Wiesmann, U., Uhlendorf, W. B. and di Sant' Agnese, P. A. (1970) Journal of Pediatrics, **77**, 280

Rao, G. J. S. and Nadler, H. L. (1972) Journal of Pediatrics, **80**, 573

Rao, G. J. S., Posner, L. A. and Nadler, H. L. (1972) Science, **177**, 610

Rennert, O. M., Frias, J. L., Julius, R. L. and LaPointe, D. (1972a) Clinical Pediatrics, **2**, 351

Rennert, O. M., Julius, R. L. and LaPointe, D. (1972b) Pediatrics, **50**, 485

Spock, A., Heick, H. M. C., Cress, H. and Logan, W. S. (1967) Pediatric Research, **1**, 173

Taussig, L. M., Lobeck, C. C., di Sant' Agnese, P. A., Ackerman, D. R. and Kattwinkel, J. (1972) New England Journal of Medicine, **287**, 586

Vital Statistics of the United States (1968) Section 1, Tables 1-22, 1-25; Section 2, Tables 2-5, 2-13, 2-14. US Department of Health, Education, and Welfare, Washington, DC.

Weisiger, J. (1971) Comments, GAP Conference of the National Cystic Fibrosis Foundation, West Palm Beach, Florida

Cumulative Index (Volumes 1-8) Sub-headings according to specialties

Author Index
(Volumes 1-8)